NUTRITION AND DIET RESEARCH PROGRESS

BEYOND DIET AND DEPRESSION

BASIC KNOWLEDGE, CLINICAL SYMPTOMS AND TREATMENT OF DEPRESSION

VOLUME 1

NUTRITION AND DIET RESEARCH PROGRESS

Additional books in this series can be found on Nova's website
under the Series tab.

Additional e-books in this series can be found on Nova's website
under the e-book tab.

NUTRITION AND DIET RESEARCH PROGRESS

BEYOND DIET AND DEPRESSION

BASIC KNOWLEDGE, CLINICAL SYMPTOMS AND TREATMENT OF DEPRESSION

VOLUME 1

SUSHIL SHARMA, PH.D.

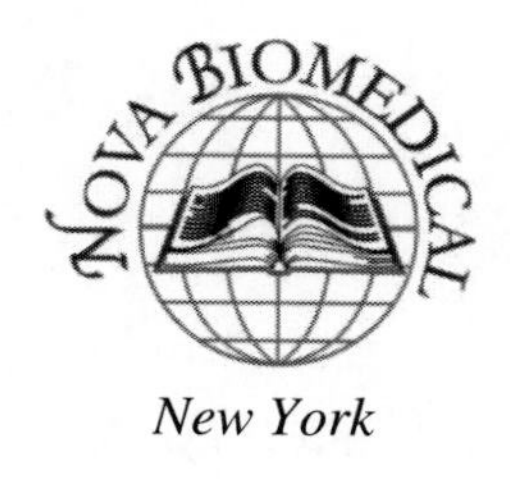

New York

Library of Congress Cataloging-in-Publication Data

ISBN: 978-1-63463-274-4

ISSN: 2375-3307

Published by Nova Science Publishers, Inc. † New York

Contents

Preface

Depression is characterized by sadness, purposelessness, irritability, and impaired body functions. Depression can be serious and often requires professional help or medication. Depression remains a significant health and economic challenge globally irrespective of increased investment in its recognition and treatment. According to World Health Organization (WHO), unipolar depression is expected to become one of the most leading causes of disease burden by 2030. Hence, the discovery of antidepressive foods is fascinating and could have significant impact globally. Indeed noncommunicable diseases are one of the most significant challenges health decision makers currently facing in Eastern Mediterranean countries where the transition is increasing morbidity of depression and mental diseases, cardiovascular diseases, diabetes, cancer, and respiratory diseases with a significant impact on the least disadvantaged populations.

Current treatment strategies focus primarily on biological and psychological pathways, ignoring the key contribution of lifestyle and dietary patterns. Metabolic syndrome (MetS) and depression are becoming most prevalent diseases globally, whose interaction needs further investigation. Dietary treatment for weight loss in patients with MetS may improve depressive symptoms, however, the precise pathways remain unknown.

There is emerging evidence to suggest that diet and nutrition play an important role in the risk, and the genesis of depression. However, there are limited studies regarding the therapeutic impact of dietary interventions on existing mental illness. Studies of single nutrients on depression have generated inconsistent results, and have failed to consider the complex interactions between nutrients. Several studies are now investigating the association of various dietary patterns and depression.

This book aims to accomplish the primary goal of health promotion by preventing depression among young adolescent women with pre and post-menstrual syndrome, pregnancy, hypothyroidism, diabetes, obesity, coelic diseases, drug addiction, and elderly patients with progressive neurodegenerative disorders, cardiovascular disorders, post-traumatic stress disorders, chronic pain, rheumatoid arthritis, fibromyalgia, cancer, and several other chronic illnesses. Diet, which targets multiple disease etiologies, can prevent the development of depressive and neurodegenerative disorders and the cognitive deficits. Increased prevalence of depressive and neurodegenerative diseases combined with the lack of effective pharmaceutical treatments and their deleterious side effects, has created a dire need for the development of effective therapies. As these disorders are multifactorial in origin; treatments directed to interfere at different mechanistic levels may be more effective than the traditional single-targeted pharmacological approach. A diet composed of zinc, melatonin, curcumin, piperine, eicosapentaenoic acid (EPA, 20:5, n-3), docosahexaenoic acid (DHA, 22:6, n-3), uridine, and choline has shown ameliorating effects on olfactory bulbectomized animals; a well-established experimental model of depression (Borre et al., 2013).

This book motivates to learn beyond diet and depression as diet alone may not be sufficient to completely cure a particular victim of severe depression. The chapters described in this book are based on the author's own research experience of over 30 years and from other internationally-recognized scientists. There are numerous risk factors associated with depression, which have been described in detail. The book provides an up to date knowledge about the therapeutic potential of dietary interventions, including Tryptophan-rich diet, Vitamin-B6, Melatonin, Coenzyme Q10, Antioxidants, Zinc, Iron, Folate, Vitamin B1, Vitamin B12, Vitamin D, Antioxidants, Moderate Exercise, and Natural Light to accomplish synergistic effect during the treatment of depression.

The primary objective of dietary interventions is to minimize the requirement of expansive pharmaceutical agents such as specific serotonin-reuptake inhibitors (SSRIs), Fluoxetine and other antidepressants with serious adverse effects including anorexia, weight loss, osteoporosis, and suicidal ideations.

There is now sufficient evidence to suggest that dietary manipulation can alleviate various symptoms of depression alone or in combination with well-established antidepressants. Each chapter brings new knowledge and recent references to the reader. This book is being introduced at an appropriate time and will be extremely useful for the prevention/treatment of depression by simple non-pharmacological dietary interventions with minimum or no adverse effects alone and/or in combination with well-established antioxidants and antidepressants currently available in the market as well as in our daily diet. It is envisaged that specific dietary interventions may either eliminate or reduce the requirement of antidepressant drugs with numerous deleterious adverse effects and cost in chronic diseases associated with severe depression.

This book will be a valuable source of information for the early management of depression in several clinical conditions including chronic psychiatric diseases, neurodegenerative diseases of aging, cancer, diabetes, cardiovascular diseases, neuropsychoendorcinological diseases, post-traumatic stress disorders, stroke, diabetes, eating disorders, chronic drug addiction, obesity, celiac disease, hypothyroidism, rheumatoid arthritis, fibromyalgia, chronic multi-drug-resistant malignancies, infections, and several other diseases where depression plays a significant impact on the health, wellbeing, and productivity of a victim.

In general, physicians try a battery of antidepressants for the clinical management of patients with MDD with limited success as the conventional antidepressant treatment may not be completely successful in every patient. On several occasions these patients may suffer from the adverse effects of the antidepressants including, anorexia, weight loss, and osteoporosis as mentioned earlier. Hence considerable attention is being focused on simple non-pharmacological dietary approaches for the clinical management of depression. A brief description of these dietary interventions is provided below as a general background information.

Tryptophan. Although several neurotransmitters including serotonin (5-HT), dopamine (DA), norepinephrine (NE) and γ-amino butyric acid (GABA) and their receptors may participate in the pathogenesis of depression; serotonergic mechanism proved highly significant in the clinical management of depression. Serotonin is synthesized in the CNS by its precursor, Tryptophan. Tryptophan can easily cross the blood brain barrier and converted to serotonin by enzymes, tryptophan hydroxylase and 5-HTP decarboxylase in the presence of pyridoxal phosphate, derived from vitamin B_6. As tryptophan is naturally less abundant in various protein-rich diets, it is important to select foods specifically rich in essential amino acid, tryptophan. Craving for fat and carbohydrate-rich diet particularly among obese persons is to enhance insulin secretion which augments tryptophan bioavailability in the CNS in order to augment 5-HT synthesis and hence alleviates symptoms of depression. Brain regional serotonin in the dorsal raphe and periaqueductal grey regions is significantly reduced in patients with depression. Recently we and other investigators reported that decreased level of brain region-specific 5-hydroxytryptamine (5-HT) is a major pathogenic factor in depression and its symptoms can be alleviated by consuming tryptophan-rich diet (Wurtman and Wurtman., 1995; Wurtman, 1995; Shabbir et al., 2013). Hence tryptophan–rich diet can be prescribed to patients with depression. As a matter of fact various healthy foods are rich in tryptophan. As such serotonin does not cross the blood brain barrier and has shorter half-life hence cannot be directly used for the treatment of depression. This concept arose from the observation that drugs augmenting extracellular levels of 5-HT have antidepressant action. Whether such drugs rectify a primary deficit of depression, remains unknown. A number of impairments in biomarkers of central 5-HT function have been reported in depressive patients, indicating that 5-HT deficiency could be present in depression, particularly in severely ill Parkinson's disease (PD) patients. The literature on putative 5-HT biomarker abnormalities and depression has been corroborated by demonstrating that such impairments occur as a consequence of reduced 5-HT(Ext) in a mouse model of 5-HT deficiency, the tryptophan hydroxylase 2 His(439) knockin (Tph2KI) mouse. These studies have provided further evidence for 5-HT deficiency in depression and the role of polymorphisms in the Tph2 gene as a factor in 5-HT deficiency (Jacobsen et al., 2012). (A detailed description of Tryptophan-rich food in alleviating depression is provided in one of the chapter in this book)

Kema et al., (1995) developed a high performance liquid chromatographic method with quaternary gradient elution and fluorometric detection for estimating tryptophan (TRP), 5-hydroxytryptophan, serotonin (5-HT) and 5-hydroxyindole-3-acetic acid (5-HIAA) in urine, platelet-rich plasma and (tumor) tissue of patients with carcinoid tumors. Prior to injection, urine samples are diluted and filtered. Platelet-rich plasma and tissue homogenates are pre-purified by C18 solid phase extraction. Detection limits are ~2 pmol. Results of urinary 5-HT and 5-HIAA compared with those of single component analyses. No consistent diurnal variations were found for TRP, 5-HT and 5-HIAA in 12-h urine samples from 15 healthy adults. Abstinence of 5-HT-rich foods reduced urinary levels of 5-HT and 5-HIAA. C18 extraction of indoles from protein-containing matrices was studied in platelet-rich plasma. This approach offers distinct advantages over single component analyses in the study of TRP metabolism in patients with carcinoid tumors and depression.

We have reported that depression is characterized by sadness, purposelessness, irritability, and impaired body functions. Depression causes severe symptoms for several weeks, and dysthymia, which may cause chronic, low-grade symptoms. Treatment of depression involves psychotherapy, medications, or phototherapy (Shabbir et al., 2013). Clinical and experimental evidence indicates that a healthy diet can reduce symptoms of depression. The neurotransmitter, serotonin (5-HT), synthesized in the brain, plays an important role in mood alleviation, satiety, and sleep regulation. Although certain fruits and vegetables are rich in 5-HT, it is not easily accessible to the CNS due to blood brain barrier. However the serotonin precursor, tryptophan, can readily pass through the blood brain barrier. Tryptophan is converted to 5-HT by tryptophan hydroxylase and 5-HTP decarboxylase, respectively, in the presence of pyridoxal phosphate, derived from vitamin B_6. Hence diets poor in tryptophan may induce depression as this essential amino acid is not naturally abundant even in protein-rich foods. Tryptophan-rich diet is important in patients susceptible to depression such as certain females during pre and postmenstrual phase, post-traumatic stress disorder, chronic pain, cancer, epilepsy, Parkinson's disease (PD), Alzheimer's disease (AD), schizophrenia, and drug addiction. Carbohydrate-rich diet triggers insulin response to enhance the bioavailability of tryptophan in the CNS which is responsible for increased craving of carbohydrate diets. Although serotonin reuptake inhibitors (SSRIs) are prescribed to obese patients with depressive symptoms, these are incapable of precisely regulating the CNS serotonin and may cause life-threatening adverse effects in the presence of monoamine oxidase inhibitors (MAOIs). However, CNS serotonin synthesis can be controlled by proper intake of tryptophan-rich diet. We highlighted the clinical significance of tryptophan-rich diet and vitamin B_6 to boost serotonergic neurotransmission in depression observed in various neurodegenerative diseases. However pharmacological interventions to modulate serotonergic neurotransmission in depression, remains clinically significant. Depression may also involve several other molecular mechanisms as yet remain to be further explored.

There is increasing evidence demonstrating that sleep has an influence on dietary choices. Both cross-sectional and epidemiologic studies have shown that those who sleep less are more likely to consume energy-rich foods (such as fats or refined carbohydrates), fewer portions of vegetables, and have more irregular meal patterns. The purpose of this book is to discuss the evidence linking diet and sleep and to determine whether what we eat and nutrients we obtain from the food before bed time matters. In addition, scientific evidence behind traditional sleep-promoting foods such as milk and some herbal products has been described. These are reviewed using data from clinical trials, mostly in healthy subjects. In addition, the author has discussed the possible mechanisms and summarized their findings that confirm a link between diet and sleep. Overall, foods impacting the availability of tryptophan, as well as the synthesis of serotonin and melatonin, may be helpful in promoting sleep. Although there are physiological connections, the clinical relevance needs to be studied further (Peuhkuri et al., 2012). Brain serotonin function promotes sleep regulation and cognitive processes, whereas sleep abnormalities and behavioral decline are attributed to deficient brain serotoninergic neurotransmission particularly in the aging subjects. Brain uptake of the serotonin precursor, tryptophan is dependent on nutrients that influence the availability of tryptophan via a change in the ratio of plasma tryptophan to the sum of the other large neutral amino acids (Trp: LNAA). It was tested whether evening consumption of α-lactalbumin protein with an enriched tryptophan content of 4.8 g/100 g increases plasma Trp: LNAA and improves alertness and performance on the morning after sleep, particularly in individuals with sleep abnormalities. Healthy subjects with or without mild sleep complaints participated in a double-blind, placebo-controlled study. The subjects slept for 2 separate nights so that morning performance could be evaluated after an evening diet containing either tryptophan-rich α-lactalbumin or tryptophan-low placebo protein. Evening dietary changes in plasma Trp: LNAA were measured. Behavioral measures of attention were recorded during a continuous performance task. Evening α-lactalbumin intake caused a 130% increase in Trp: LNAA before bed time and reduced sleepiness and improved sustained attention the following morning. Only in poor sleepers was accompanied by improved behavioral performance. Evening dietary increases in plasma tryptophan availability for uptake into the brain enhance alertness early in the morning after an overnight sleep, because of improved sleep (Markus et al., 2005). It is now known that sleep depends on the quantity and quality of the diet. Food deprivation results in a reduction in sleep duration. It has also been demonstrated that in the newborn, the supply of certain essential amino acids improves sleep through their action on the synthesis of specific neurotransmitters. A study was performed to test if the quantity and/or quality of dietary protein could improve the recovery of sleep during re-feeding after caloric deprivation. Sleep parameters were compared in rats fed ad libitum, food restricted during 4 days, or reefed isocalorically after food restriction with three dietary regimens varying in the amount (14% versus 30%) or quality (milk protein or α-lactalbumin) of protein. Sleep recovery, in particular slow-wave sleep, was improved in rats re-fed with α-lactalbumin, confirming the close relationship between feeding and sleep and that α-lactabumin could be used to improve sleep quality with nutritional disturbances such as food restriction, shift work, and Ramadan etc (Minet-Ringuet et al., 2004).

Vitamin B_6. We reported that vitamin B_6 is also equally important as an antidepressant as it is involved in the synthesis of several neurotransmitters including serotonin, dopamine, and GABA required for the normal CNS function. Vitamin B_6 (pyridoxine) from different dietary sources is converted to pyridoxal by pyridoxine oxidase, and pyridoxal is converted to pyridoxal phosphate by pyridoxal kinase. Pyridoxal phosphate (PLP) serves as a coenzyme for the metabolic activation of various decarboxylases including 5-HTP decarboxylase for the synthesis of serotonin. More specifically the neuroprotective role of pyridoxine is its involvement in the brain-regional synthesis of serotonin, dopamine, taurine, and GABA by acting as a coenzyme in the decarboxylation step (Dakshinamurti et al., (1990). Treatment of normal adult rats with pyridoxine or B-vitamin mixture resembling Neurobion (*E-Merck, Germany*) increased the synthesis of brain regional serotonin (Dakshinamurti et al., 2003). The author has several publications in this direction. (A detailed description of Vitamin B_6-rich food in alleviating depression is provided in this book)

Melatonin. Melatonin is synthesized by pineal gland and regulates the circadian rhythm and sleep-wakeful cycle. Recently its role as an antioxidant has also been reported. Serotonin is the precursor for the synthesis of melatonin which is derived from N-acetyl serotonin. Hence tryptophan in the diet and its metabolism remains of central importance for alleviating depression. Melatonin can also serve as anti-inflammatory, anti-apoptotic, and antidepressant agent and is being further explored for its clinical usefulness in depression in addition to its well-established role as a regulator of sleep-wake cycle. In fact subjects with sleep disorders also suffer from depression. Recent studies have demonstrated that Melatonin prevents methamphetamine-induced autophagy in cultured glioma cell lines (Nopparat et al; 2010; Jumnongprakhon et al., 2013). Hence Melatonin may be used as an antidepressant with no or minimum adverse effects. (A detailed description of tryptophan-rich food and melatonin in alleviating various symptoms of depression is provided in this book)

***Mitochondrial Bioenergetics in Depression*:** The author discovered Charnoly body (CB) which is formed as a result of mitochondrial degeneration due to nutritional and/or neurotoxic insult. Charnoly bodies are electron-dense, multi-lamellar, pleomorphic structures and are involved in apoptosis and neurodegeneration. Charnoly body formation occurs in the CNS (particularly hippocampus and hypothalamus) in depression. We have recently reported that CB formation can be inhibited by MTs as these metalloproteins serve as free radical scavengers in the CNS and cultured human dopaminergic (SK-N-SH and SHY-5Y) neurons (Sharma et al., 2013a; Sharma et al., 2013b). Free radicals are formed due to oxidative and nitrative stress in the mitochondria as a result of oxidative phsophorylation. (A detailed description of foods supplemented with Zn^{2+} in alleviating depression through MTs induction is provided in this Book)

Coenzyme Q_{10}. Coenzyme Q_{10} serves as a rejuvenator of the mitochondrial bioenergetics as it is required for the synthesis of rate limiting enzyme, ubiquinone-NADH oxidoreductase (complex-1). This enzyme complex is rate limiting and is involved in the mitochondrial oxidative phosphorylation for the synthesis of ATP. We discovered that CoQ_{10} can serve as an antioxidant and anti-inflammatory agent as it inhibits TNFα and NFκβ expression in homozygous weaver (wv/wv) mice exhibiting progressive neurodegeneration (Ebadi et al., 2004). CoQ_{10} stabilizes mitochondria in PD associated with severe depression (Ebadi et al., 2007). Furthermore, vitamin E and CoQ_{10} are localized primarily in the inner mitochondrial membrane to scavenge free radicals and reactive oxygen species (ROS) formed during oxidative phosphorylation and during oxidative stress. CoQ_{10} rejuvenates vitamin E during oxidative stress, hence both CoQ_{10} and Vitamin E act synergistically to provide neuroprotection. Hence additional supplementation of vitamin E and CoQ_{10} could be beneficial in depression. That induction of pro-inflammatory cytokines, NFκβ is suppressed by CoQ_{10} and MTs enhance CoQ_{10} synthesis, established the free radical theory of neurodegeneration and the therapeutic potential of CoQ_{10} and vitamin E (Ebadi and Sharma, 2006). Since MTs provide neuroprotection by boosting mitochondrial bioenergetics and monoaminergic neurotransmission, therapeutic interventions augmenting brain regional MTs may provide neuroprotection in depression (Sharma and Ebadi., 2008; Sharma and Ebadi., 2011a ; Sharma et al., 2013). We have recently reported that MTs provide neuroprotection by acting as a free radical scavenger to prevent CB formation implicated in apoptosis and progressive neurodegeneration. In addition to MTs and CoQ_{10}, several other potent antioxidants, anti-inflammatory, and antiapoptotic agents exist in our healthy diets about which very limited information is as yet available. Intensive studies are going on in this direction which will provide better therapeutic interventions for the clinical management of depression. The author has recently written a detailed chapter on “Antioxidants and Potential Therapeutics in Neurodegeneration” (Sharma and Ebadi, 2014). (A detailed description regarding CB formation and its involvement in major depressive disorders is provided in volume-2 of this book)

Antioxidants and Depression. Recently we and others have written an extensive reviews on the therapeutic potential of various antioxidants in progressive neurodegenerative disorders including PD, AD, HD, ALS, MS, and depression (Sharma and Ebadi 2014; Wurtman, 2013; Lang and Borgwardt, 2013). (A detailed description of various antioxidants-rich food in alleviating depression is also provided in this book)

Zinc. The bioavailability of Zn^{2+} is 50% among old subject >60 years of age due to improper mastication and irregular intestinal absorption. Physiological concentrations of Zn^{2+} provide advantage by augmenting MTs with anti-inflammatory, anti-apoptotic, and antioxidant properties. A detailed description of Zn^{2+} and MTs is provided in our recent publications (Ebadi et al., 2001; Sharma and Ebadi 2003; Ebadi and Sharma 2003; Sharma et al., 2004; Klongpanichapak et al., 2006; Sharma and Ebadi. 2013). Hence physiological supplementation of Zn^{2+} in the diet may alleviate depression. (A detailed description of Zn^{2+}-

supplemented diet in alleviating depression particularly among aging subjects is provided in this book)

Phototherapy. Photo-therapy can be effectively used for augmenting brain regional serotonin synthesis and hence alleviate depression in seasonal affective disorders (SAD). Natural sun light augments the synthesis of CNS serotonin, hence has significant impact on mood alleviation (Conti. 2008). Therefore, subjects suffering from SAD during winter can be effectively treated with a combination of tryptophan-rich diet and phototherapy without prescribing expansive antidepressants with serious adverse effects. Although phototherapy lamps are available to alleviate symptoms of depression in people suffering from seasonal affective disorders, a better option will be to visit tropical countries and/or Caribbean islands with lot of sunshine during winter for couple of weeks as a tourist. It is important to point out that the duration of the direct light and its intensity must be adjusted in a delicate way so that it does not cause impairment in vision. Particularly psoriasis patients should be very careful about direct exposure of their skin to sunlight. Using sun glasses and proper hydration are recommended during visit to the tropical countries or Caribbean islands even during winter (A detailed description of the therapeutic potential of phototherapy as a booster of serotonergic neurotransmission in depression is provided in one of our publications)

The last chapters are devoted to differential diagnosis and the significant beneficial effects of combined therapies with dietary interventions, natural light, and pharmacological agents in order to accomplish synergistic benefits for the clinical management of depression. A brief mention of electroconvulsive therapy (ECT) is also provided, where dietary interventions may have synergistic effect on the clinical outcome of patients with MDDs. There are several unknown neuroprotective agents and antioxidants in our diet which remain unknown and as yet undiscovered although we consume them routinely through our diet without even knowing their exact clinical significance. Hence a detailed future study on diet and its therapeutic potential in depression will go a long way in the clinical management of several patients of depression in future. Recently curcumin has emerged as a potent antidepressant; however its bioavalability in the CNS is a major challenge which is being resolved by employing modern nanotechnological approaches.

It is envisaged that the book will be a valuable source of recent knowledge about depression, emerging disease-specific biomarkers of depression and its alleviation by nonpharmacological dietary interventions with minimum and/or no adverse effects. Indeed dietary intervention is an economical therapeutic approach with allmost full compliance unlike conventional antidepressants associated with noncompliance, significant cost, and severe adverse effects. However one should not be carried away with an elusive idea that diet is the only solution to combat this complex disorder. In fact antidepressants have their own clinical significance in MDDs. Several potential synergistic or antagonistic interactions with diet may occur when antidepressant drugs are taken alone or in combination with specific diets. A limited information is as yet available in this direction. Although there are various types of balanced diets, Mediterranean diet has shown significant promise and universal acceptance as the healthiest diet to alleviate depression.

It is envisaged that this book will be a valuable source of recent knowledge about depression, emerging disease-specific biomarkers of depression and its alleviation by nonpharmacological dietary interventions with minimum and/or no adverse effects. Indeed dietary intervention is an economical and unique therapeutic approach with all most full compliance unlike conventional antidepressants associated with noncompliance, significant cost, and severe adverse effects. Hence it will gain more acceptance and popularity in the management of depression.

Experimental Models of Depression

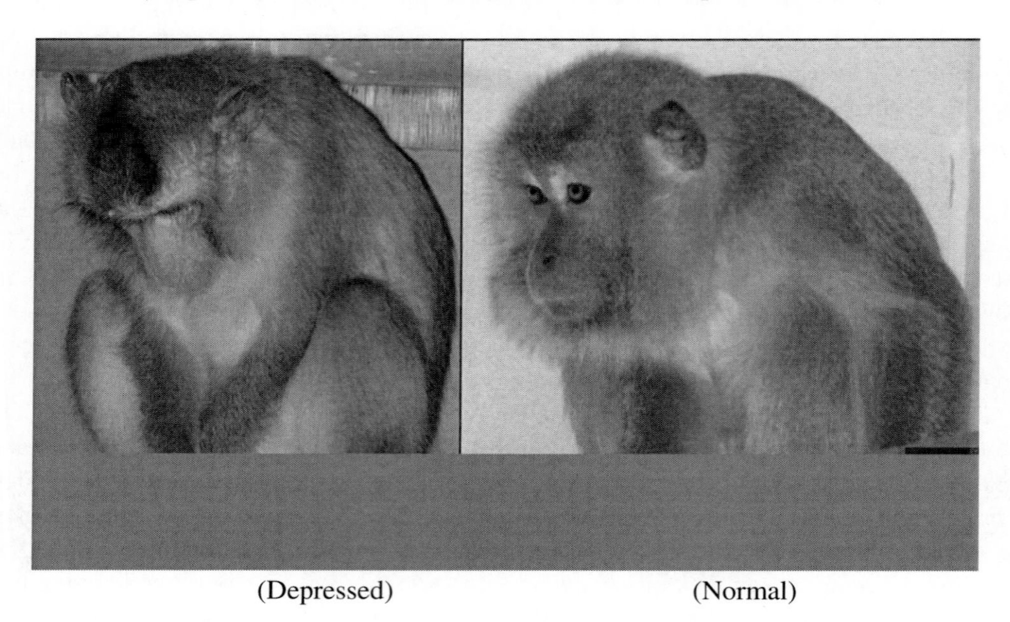

(Depressed) (Normal)

Acknowledgement: The author acknowledges with sincere thanks NIDA scientists, who developed this monkey model of depression to discover novel antidepressant for human mental illnesses. This picture was retrieved from the *Google* Search on animal model of depression.

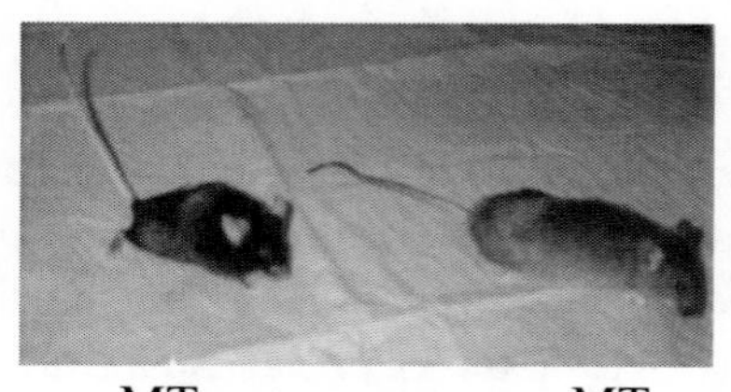

MT_{trans} MT_{dko}

The above picture represents the in-vivo model of mitochondrial complex-1 inhibitor, 1-methyl, 4-phenyl, 1,2,3,6-tetrahydropyridine (MPTP)- (10mg/kg, i.p)-induced neurotoxicity in metallothioneins transgenic (MT_{trans}) and metallothioneins double gene knock out ($_{MTtrans}$) Mouse after 7 days of treatment. MT_{dko} mouse was moderately obese, lethargic, and completely immbolized; whereas MT_{trans} mouse could still walk with its stiff legs and erect tail, confirming that MTs provide mitochondrial neuroprotection by inhibiting Charnoly body (CB) formation and by serving as free radical scavengers associated with numerous progressive neurodegenerative disorders including major depressive dorders (MDDs). (*Original contribution: Sharma & Ebadi; 2014*)

References

Borre, Y.E; Panagaki, T; Koelink, P.J; Morgan, M.E; Hendriksen, H; Garssen, J; Kraneveld, A.D; Olivier, B, (2014) Oosting RSNeuroprotective and cognitive enhancing effects of a multi-targeted food intervention in an animal model of neurodegeneration and depression. *Neuropharmacology*. 79, 738-749.

Conti, L. (2008) How Light Deprivation causes Depression. Scientific American. Aug 8.

Dakshinamurti, K; Sharma, S.K.; and Gieger J.D. (2003) Neuroprotective Actions of Pyridoxine. *Biochem. Biophys. Acta.* 1647: 225-229.

Dakshinamurti, K; Sharma, S. K; and Bonke, D. (1990) Influence of B-vitamins on binding properties of serotonin receptors in the CNS of rats. *Klin Wochenschr*. 68,142-145.

Ebadi, M; Sharma, S; Wanpen, S; Amornpan, A. (2004) Coenzyme Q_{10} Inhibits Mitochondrial Complex-1 downregulation and Nuclear Factor-kappa B Activation. *J. Cellular & Molecular Medicine*. 8, 213-222.

Ebadi, M;, and Sharma, S. (2003) Peroxynitrite and Mitochondrial Dysfunction in the Pathogenesis of Parkinson's disease. *Antioxidants & Redox Signaling* 5, 319-335.

Ebadi, M; and Sharma, S. (2006) Vitamin E and Coenzyme Q10 in Parkinson's disease. CAB International Encyclopedia of Vitamin E. Ed. V.R. Preedy and R.R. Watson), p 439-449.

Ebadi, M; Govitrapong, P;, Sharma. S; Muralikrishnan, D;, Shavali. S;, Pellet, L; Schaffer. R; Albano, C; and Ekens J. (2001) Ubiquinone (Coenzyme Q10) and Mitochondria in Oxidative Stress of Parkinson's disease. Biological Signals and Receptors. 10, 224-253.

Ebadi, M; Wanpen, S; Shavali, S; Sharma, S; El-Refae, H. (2007) Coenzyme Q_{10} stabilizes Mitochondria in Parkinson's disease. In Molecular Interventions in Life-Style-Related Diseases. Eds: M. Hiramatsu, T. Yoshikawa, L. Packer. P 127-153.

Greenberg, P.E; Kessler, R.C; Birnbaum, H.G; Leong, S.A; Lowe, S.W; Berglund, P.A; Corey-Lisle, P.K. (2003) The Economic Burden of Depression in the United States: How Did It Change Between 1990 and 2000? *Journal of Clinical Psychiatry*. 64, 1466-1475.

Jacobsen, J.P; Medvedev, I.O; Caron, M.G. (2012) The 5-HT deficiency theory of depression: perspectives from a naturalistic 5-HT deficiency model, the tryptophan hydroxylase 2Arg439His knockin mouse. *Philos Trans R Soc Lond B Biol Sci.* 367, 2444-2459.

Jumnongprakhon, P; Govitrapong, P; Tocharus, C; Tungkum, W; Tocharus, J. (2013) Protective Effect of Melatonin on Methamphetamine-Induced Apoptosis in Glioma Cell Line. *Neurotox Res*. Aug 23.

Kema, I.P; de Vries, E.G; Muskiet, F.A. (1995) Measurement of 5-HIAA in urine. Ann Clin Biochem. 32, 102-104.

Klongpanichapak, S; Govitropong, P; Sharma, S; and Ebadi, M. (2006) Attenuation of Cocaine and Methamphetamine neurotoxicity by Coenzyme Q_{10}. *Neurochem. Res.* 31, 303-311.

Lang, U.E; Borgwardt, S. (2013) Molecular mechanisms of depression: perspectives on new treatment strategies. *Cell Physiol Biochem.* 31, 761-777.

Markus, C.R; Jonkman, L.M; Lammers, J.H; Deutz, N.E; Messer, M.H; Rigtering, N. (2005) Evening intake of alpha-lactalbumin increases plasma tryptophan availability and improves morning alertness and brain measures of attention. *Am J Clin Nutr*. 81, 1026-1033.

Minet-Ringuet, J; Le Ruyet, P.M; Tomé, D; Even, P.C. (2004) A tryptophan-rich protein diet efficiently restores sleep after food deprivation in the rat., *Behav Brain Res.* 152, 335-340.

Nopparat, C; Porter, J.E; Ebadi, M; Govitrapong, P. (2010) The mechanism for the neuroprotective effect of melatonin against methamphetamine-induced autophagy., *J Pineal Res.* 49, 382-389.

Peuhkuri, K; Sihvola, N; Korpela, R. (2012) Diet promotes sleep duration and quality., *Nutr Res.* 32, 309-319.

Sharma, S; and Ebadi, M. (2014) Antioxidants as Potential Therapeutics in Neurodegeneration. Ed. I. Laher, Springer Verlag. Heidelberg, Germany. Chapter 91, p 2191-2273.

Sharma, S; Moon, C.S; Khogali, A; Haidous, A; Chabenne, A; Ojo, C. Jelebinkov, M; Kurdi, Y; Ebadi, M. (2013) Biomarkers of Parkinson's Disease (Recent Update)., *Neurochemistry International.* 63, 201-229.

Sharma, S; Rais, A; Sandhu, R; Nel, W; Ebadi, M. (2013a) Clinical significance of metallothioneins in cell herapy and nanomedicine., *International Journal of Nanomedicine.* 8, 1477–1488.

Sharma, S; and Ebadi, M. (2011a) Metallothioneins As Early & Sensitive Biomarkers of Redox Signaling in Neurodegenerative Disorders., *Journal of Institute of Integrative Omics & Applied Biotechnonogy (IIOAB Journal)* 2, 98-106.

Sharma, S; and Ebadi, M. (2011b) Therapeutic Potential of Metallothioneins as Anti-inflammatory Agents in Polysubstance Abuse., *Journal of Institute of Integrative Omics & Applied Biotechnonogy IIOAB Journal* 2, 50-61. Sharma, S; and Ebadi, M. (2008) Therapeutic Potential of Metallothioneins in Parkinson's Disease. Chapter 1, In New Research on Parkinson's Disease. Nova Science Publishers. Eds: T.F. Hahn and J. Werner. P 1-41.

Sharma, S; Refaey, H. El; and Ebadi, M. (2006) Complex-1 activity and ^{18}F-DOPA uptake in genetically engineered mouse model of Parkinson's disease and the neuroprotective role of coenzyme Q_{10}., *Brain Res. Bull.* 70, 22-32.

Sharma, S; Kheradpezhou, M; Shavali, S; EI Refaey, H; Eken, J; Hagen, C; and Ebadi, M. (2004) Neuroprotective Actions of Coenzyme Q_{10} in Parkinson's Disease., *Methods in Enzymology.* 382, 488-509.

Sharma, S.K; and Ebadi, M. (2003) Metallothionein Attenuates 3-Morpoholinosydnonimone (SIN-1)-Induced Oxidative and Nitrative Stress in Dopaminergic Neurons., *Antioxidants and Redox Signaling.* 5, 251-264.

Wurtman, R.J; Wurtman, J.J. (1995a) Brain serotonin, carbohydrate-craving, obesity and depression., *Obes Res. Suppl* 4, 477S-480S.

Wurtman, R.J. (1995b) Genes, stress, and depression., *Metabolism.* 54, (5 Suppl 1), 16-19.

Wurtman, R.J. (2013) Personalized medicine strategies for managing patients with parkinsonism and cognitive deficits., *Metabolism.* 62, S27-S29.

Acknowledgment

This book is dedicated to the memory of author's late mother whose nick name was "*Charnoly*." She motivated him to discover *Charnoly Body* (CB) as a universal biomarker of cell injury in the developing undernourished rat Purkinje neurons in India and later in the hippocampal CA-3 and dentate gyrus neurons in response to environmental neurotoxins and rigid structural analogs of glutamate; "*Kainic acid and domoic acid*" in Canada. Now it is known that almost all chronotoxins induce hippocampal CB formation to cause major depressive disorders and several progressive neurodegenerative diseases.

To make this book interesting and informative, the author has quoted the excellent work of several researchers, dieticians, scientists, and clinicians around the world. The author acknowledges with thanks their contribution in understanding this complex disorder with currently limited knowledge at the basic molecular level and effective treatment through dietary interventions.

The author is thankful to his family, friends, and colleagues who encouraged him to write "*Beyond Diet & Depression*".

Motivation and encouragement by Nadya Columbus, President, Nova Science Publishers, New York, U.S.A and the publication team is gratefully acknowledged.

Moral support by Dr. Kallol Guha, President, Saint James School of Medicine, Bonaire (The Netherlands) is also gratefully acknowledged.

About the Author

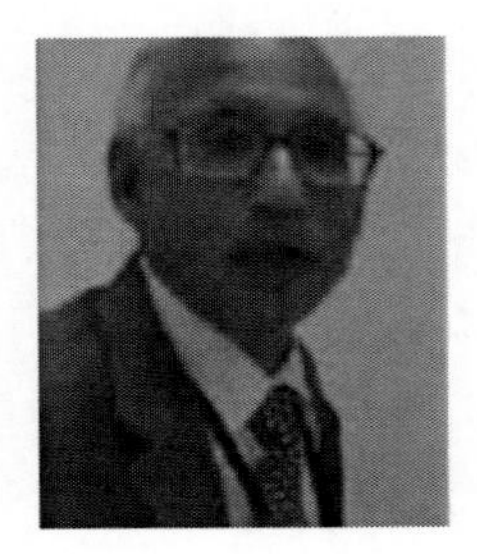

Sushil Sharma, Ph.D.; D.M.R.I.T
Professor of Pharmacology &
Course Director
Saint James School of Medicine
Plaza Juliana 4, Kralendijk
Bonaire, Dutch Caribbean
The Netherlands

Biography: Dr Sushil Sharma, is Professor and Course Director of Pharmacology at the Saint James School of Medicine, Bonaire. He received Ph.D. in Neuropharmacology from A.I.IM.S, New Delhi; Radiopharmaceutical Training from BARC, Bombay, GE, Siemens, Agilent Technologies, & Cardinal Health in USA; Served as Research Officer in AIIMS:1979-88); awarded Royal Society Fellowship (UK:1988-89); MHRC Post-doctoral Fellowship (Canada: 1989-91); Research Officer (University of Montreal:1993-94); Research Associate (McGill University:1994-95); Senior Scientific Officer (Clinical Research Institute of Montreal:1995-97); awarded Scientist E Rank in the Defence Research and Development Organization (DRDO) New Delhi (1997); Research Scientist (University of Manitoba:1997-99); Assistant Professor 2000-04; Associate Professor & Director (Research) UND School of Medicine, Grand Forks:2004-08); Associate Professor & Director (Methodist Hospital) & Research Scientist (University Texas Medical Center:2008-11). Organized and Chaired several World Conferences; was awarded 5 Gold Medals; Certificate of Honor IT Nano-2014 Conference, Boston. (Original Discoveries: Electromicroinjector; Charnoly Body in Purkinje Neurons, IL-10 Receptors on Cortical Neurons, & MTs-Gene-Manipulated Mice)

About This Book

Depression is a complex global health challenge with considerable economical and psychological burden. Women, adolescents, and aging subjects are highly vulnerable to suffer from depression. Depression is linked to numerous modifiable and non-modifiable risk factors. Its effective treatment involves both psychotherapy and/or chemotherapy. Currently available pharmacotherapeutical agents used for the treatment of depression have low margin of safety and reduced therapeutic index with deleterious adverse effects including osteoporosis, obesity, hypertension, diabetes, cardiovascular diseases, infertility and even fatalities if abused. It is now realized that healthy life style and consuming diets rich in Mediterranean component can ameliorate minor to moderate symptoms of depression. In this regard, tryptophan-rich diets, diets rich in omega-3 fatty acids such as fish, olive oil, and Flax seed oil, whole grains, soy bean, vitamin B_1, vitamin B_6, folate, and vitamin B_{12} along with iron and vitamin D3 are highly significant for alleviating various symptoms of depression. This book is divided in two volumes. Volume-1 provides basic knowledge of depression and the therapeutic potential of various healthy dietary interventions including tryptophan-rich diet and the diet rich in omega-3 polyunsaturated fatty acids. Furthermore, it provides basic knowledge for the clinical diagnosis and treatment of depression. In particular, this book describes various dietary interventions alone or in combination with pharmacological, and electroconvulsive therapy for the treatment of major depressive disorders. Although there is no firm evidence that healthy diets rich in tryptophan can act synergistically with the currently available psychopharmacotherapy of depression, evidence along these lines is gradually accumulating. Volume-2 is devoted to important diets and their impact on depression. It covers various aspects of disease-specific depression and its alleviation. This volume is focused on disease-specific depression and its prevention and/or treatment with specific dietary interventions. Furthermore, it highlights recently developed disease-specific biomarkers which can be used for the early clinical diagnosis and personalized treatment of depression. This volume is written with a primary objective to convey the important message that dietary interventions early in the course of depression might be beneficial to provide neuroprotection by inhibiting hippocampal and hypothalamic Charnoly body formation involved in depression and progressive neurodegeneration as a consequence of free radicals-induced compromised mitochondrial bioenergetics. There are numerous anti-inflammatory, antiapoptotic, and growth promoting antioxidants in our diet including flavonoids and polyphenols which can enter CNS without any allergic reaction about which very limited knowledge is yet available. This volume provides further insight along these directions and emphasizes the importance of antidepressant dietary regimens for healthy living at any age. There is no doubt that aging, obese subjects, drug addicts, and female patients with hypothyroidism, eating disorders, post-traumatic stress disorder, chronic diseases and pain experience severe depression. Hence it may be a better option to initiate safer and risk-free nonpharmacological approaches by selective dietary interventions, moderate exercise, and by refraining from substance abuse including coffee, cigarette smoking, and alcohol to remain healthy and productive throughout life. The last chapter is written particularly to provide emerging knowledge of novel biomarkers and therapeutic strategies (with theranostic potential) for the differential diagnosis and personalized treatment of depression.

The timely introduction of this book is intended for the benefit of general public and entire medical community interested in the effective clinical management of minor and major depressive disorders of diversified etiology with dietary interventions alone or in combination with psychopharmacotherapeutic approaches including electroconvulsive therapy and healthy lifestyle choices.

Words of Wisdom

There are primarily three types of diets; Rajas, Tamas, and Satvik. The behavior is modified depending on the type of diet consumed. Primary ingredients of Rajas diet are saturated fats and simple carbohydrates with high glycemic index; Tamas diet is rich in spices and substances of abuse; Satvik diet is composed of fruits, vegetables, and milk products containing healthy nutrients. Hence Satvik diet is the best for better health and wellbeing. A nutritious food may or may not be delicious and vice versa [Bhagvat Geeta; Indian Religious Book by Rishi Ved Vias]

Doctors are performing uncontrolled experiments on their patients, hoping that in some scattershot way they might hit on a solution. But of course drugs have dangerous interactions and most physicians are shooting in the dark with all the dangers that attend such bad marksmanship. [Dr. L.J Leonard]

Exercise is at least as good as antidepressants for helping people who are depressed. Physical exercise changes the brain regional levels of serotonin and increases endorphin levels. Exercise can increase the number of cells in the hippocampus [Dr. Gordon]

Abbreviations

Acetyl Choline: ACh
Alzheimer's disease: AD
Amyotrophic lateral sclerosis: ALS
Attention deficit hyperactivity disorder: ADHD
Blood Pressure: B.P
Body mass Index: BMI
Cerebrospinal fluid: CSF
Charnoly Body: CB
Compiterized Tomography: CT
C-Reactive Protein: CRP
D – Depressions; E – energy levels; A – anhedonia; D – death – thoughts about death and self harm – i.e. Risk! ; S – sleep pattern; W – worthlessness, guilt, A – appetite, M – mentation – decreased ability to think and concentrate, P – Psychomotor agitation and retardation: DEAD-SWAMP
Dihydroxy phenyl acetaldehyde (DOPAL)
Dihydroxy phenylacetic acid: DOPAC
Dopamine: DA
Electoencephalography: EEG
Electroconvulsive therapy: ECT
Gamma amino butyric acid: GABA
High density lipoprotein: HDL
Homeostatic assessment of insulin resistance: HOMA
Homovalinic acid: HVA
Human Immunodeficiency Virus/Acquired Immunodeficiency Disease: HIV/AIDs
Huntington's disease: HD
5-Hydrotryptophan: 5-HTP
5-Hydroxy indole acetic acid: 5-HIAA
Liver Function Test: LFTs
Low density lipoprotein: LDL
Macrophage inflammatory protein 1-β (MIP-1 β)
Magnetic Resonance Imaging: MRI
Major Depression: MD
Major Depressive Disorder: MDD

Metallothioneins-1 and 2: MT1/MT2
Monocyte chemotactic protein-1; MCP-1
Multiple Sclerosis: MS
Norepinephrine: NE
Parkinson's disease: PD
Positron Emission Tomography: PET
Rapid eyemovement sleep: REM sleep
Renal function tests: RFTs
Serotonin: 5-HT
Thyroid function tests: TFTs
Tumor necrosis factor alpha: TNF-α

Chapter 1

History of Depression

Abstract

In this chapter, a brief description of the history of depression is provided for the general knowledge of public and professionals. The chapter highlights original contributions of famous psychologists and doctors who understood, defined, and described this complex disorder. Various clinical symptoms of depression are also discussed for the information of physicians and patients. Based on these symptoms, the diagnosis of depression may be confirmed. (*For further details please refer to Encyclopedia of Depression*).

Keywords: Melancholy, Anhedonia, Antidepressants

What was once known as melancholia (now known as *depression, clinical depression*, or *major depression)* and presently referred to as major depressive disorder (MDD), has very interesting history. The glimpses of this history have been derived from the *Wikipedia, the free encyclopedia*. According to Greek health care system, there are primarily four tempraments: (i) sanguine; (ii) phlegmatic; (iii) melancholic; and (iv) choleric. The disease occurred due to an imbalance in any of these four body fluids, or humors. Hence personalities can be determined by the dominant humor in an individual. Hippocrates, *Aphorisms*, Section 6.23 describes the word "melas "black" and khole "bile. He described melancholia as a disease with mental and physical symptoms with fears and despondenciesm if remain untreated (Radden, 2003). Aretaeus observed dull or stern, dejected or torpid, without any cause in some of his patients. Although humoral theory remained unpopular in the beginning, Galen revived it. Melancholia was considered a broader concept than depression. Emphasis was directed to accumulation of the symptoms of sadness, dejection, and despondency, with fear, anger, delusions and obsessions (Jacquart, 1996). A Persian physicians developed the concept of melancholia. *Ishaq ibn Imran* and combined melancholia and phrenitis_(Haque 2004), whereas, Avicenna explained melancholia as a mood disorder where a person may become suspicious and develops phobias (Safavi-Abbasi 2007). He published the book "*The Canon of Medicine*"_, which became famous along with Hippocrates and Galen's wisdom (Daly, 2007).

Moral and spiritual theories also existed in those days, and in the medieval Europe, a malaise called acedia (*absence of caring*) was introduced, involving low spirits and lethargy with isolation (Burton, 2004). During 17th century, Burton wrote "*The Anatomy of Melancholy*" consisting of several theories and his own experiences. He suggested that melancholy could be overcome by a healthy diet, proper sleep, music, "*meaningful work*", and discussing the problem with a friend which is practiced even today (Jackson 1986). During the 18th century, the humoral theory of melancholia was challenged (*Etymology Dictionary, 2008*). Heinroth emphasized that melancholia was a disturbance of the soul due to moral conflict within the patient. Up to 30 different subtypes of melancholia and other terms were suggested. *Melancholia* and *Melancholy* were used until the 19th century, as a pathological condition and temperament respectively (Jacquart, 1996). The term *depression* was derived from the Latin verb *deprimere*, "to press down" in spirits (Wolpert 2008). It was used in 1665 by Richard Baker's *Chronicle* to refer to someone having "*a depression of spirit*", and by Johnson in 1753 (Berrios 1998) for the first time. An early usage referring to a psychiatric symptom was by Delasiauve in 1856, and by the 1860s it was referred to a *physiological and metaphorical lowering of emotional function* (Davison, 2008).

Since melancholia had been associated with learning and intelligence, a hazard of contemplation and creativity, the newer concept abandoned these associations and, in the 19th century was linked with women (Jacquart 1996). Although *melancholia* remained the diagnostic term, *depression* gained importance and became famous by the end of the century. Kraepelin was the first to use this term, referring to different kinds of melancholia as *depressive states* (Lewis 1934). Maudsley proposed *affective disorder*, whereas Kraepelin integrated all types of mood disorders into *manic–depressive insanity* (Schneider 1920). He described the underlying brain pathology and distinction between endogenous (*internal*) and exogenous (*external*) causes of depression (Schneider 1920). In 1920, Schneider coined the terms *endogenous depression* and *reactive depression* (Mapother 1926), which was challenged in 1926 by Mapother who found no difference between the two (Parker 1996). The Unitarian hypothesis became popular in the UK, while the binary view remained popular in the US, influenced by the work of Meyer and Freud (Carhart-Harris 2008). Meyer proposed a mixed social and biological framework emphasizing *reactions* in an individual's life, and proposed that the term *depression* should be used instead of *melancholia* (Schneider 1920). Freud stated that depression, or melancholia, results from loss and is more severe than mourning. He linked the state of melancholia to mourning in his 1917 paper "*Mourning and Melancholia" and* proposed that loss of a relationship through death or a romantic break-up, results in subjective loss; the depressed individual identifies with the object of affection through the *libidinal* cathexis of the ego. Such loss results in melancholic symptoms more prominantly than mourning. Not only is the outside world viewed negatively, but also the ego is compromised (Freud 1984). The patient's decline of self-perception is revealed in his belief of his own blame, inferiority, and worthlessness (*American Psychiatric Association 1968*). Freud also emphasized early life experiences as a predisposing factor in depression (Jacquart 1996).

The DSM-I (1952) contained *depressive reaction* and the DSM-II (1968) *depressive neurosis*, defined as reaction to internal conflict or an event, and included a depressive type of manic-depressive psychosis within major affective disorders (Freeman, Epstein & Simon 1987). In the mid-20th century, other theories were proposed. In addition, Existential and humanistic theories represented affirmation of individualism (Frankl 2000). Frankl linked depression to feelings of futility and meaninglessness_(Seidner and Stanley 2009). His logotherapy explained the filling of an "*existential vacuum*" associated with such feelings, useful for depressed adolescents (Blair 2004; Geppert 2006). Furthermore, May hypothesized that "*depression is the inability to construct a future*" and proposed that it occurs in the dimension of time than in space, and the depressed individual is ubable to look ahead in time adequately. Thus the "focusing upon some time *outside* the depression, gives the patient a perspective which may break the chains of the depression (Boeree 1998). Some psychologists emphasized that depression resulted from an incongruity between society and the individual's innate drive to self-actualize, or to realize one's full potential (Maslow 1971; Parker 2000). Maslow proposed that depression occurs when the world precludes a sense of "*richness" or "totality*" for the self-actualizer (Parker 2000). About half century ago, depression was either endogenous (melancholic), considered a biological condition, or reactive (neurotic), a reaction to stressful events (Akiskal and McKinney, 1975). Debate persisted during 20th century over whether a unitary or binary model of depression is a true reflection of the syndrome (Akiskal and McKinney 1975); in the former, there is a continuum of depression represented by severity and the result of a "*psychobiological final common pathway*" (Schildkraut 1965), whereas the latter conceptualizes a distinction between biological and reactive depressive syndromes (Mapother, 1926). Following the DSM-III publication, the Unitarian hypothesis of depression gained universal acceptance (Akiskal and McKinney, 1975).

In the mid-20th century, researchers proposed that depression was caused by a chemical imbalance in neurotransmitters in the brain; based on observations made in the 1950s of the effects of reserpine and isoniazid in altering monoaminergic neurotransmission and affecting depressive symptoms (Spitzer 1975). (Isoniazid *was the first compound named as antidepressant).* During the 1960s and 70s, manic-depression was referred to as a type of mood disorder (*commonly known as bipolar disorder*) which was delineated from (unipolar) depression. The terms unipolar and bipolar were introduced by Kleist (Lewis 1934), whereas the term *major depressive disorder* was introduced in the mid-1970s for diagnosis based on symptoms (Research Diagnostic Criteria, *building on earlier* Feighner Criteria), (Philipp 1991) and was incorporated into the DSM-III in 1980 (Gruenberg et al., 2005). The ICD-10 used the same criteria, with minor modifications, but using the DSM diagnostic threshold to distinguish a *mild depressive episode*, adding increased threshold for moderate and severe episodes (Gruenberg et al., 2005; *American Psychiatric Association 2000*). The ancient "*melancholia*" still exists as a melancholic subtype. The new definitions of depression were universally accepted, with some conflicting views, and the nomenclature continues in DSM-IV-TR, the latest version, published in 2000 (Bolwig et al., 2007). There have been some arguments for the return to the diagnosis of melancholia and some criticism of the diagnosis, related to the development and promotion of antidepressants and the biological model (David 1999; Fink et al., 2007). Recently Spanemberg et al., (2014) performed a study on 33 depressed patients and 54 healthy controls. Depressive patients exhibited higher IL-4, IL-6, and protein carbonyl content (PCC) than healthy controls. Thirteen of the depressed patients were assigned as meloncholic by the CORE measures. These patients produced lower levels of interferon-γ (compared with nonmelancholic depressed patients) and thiobarbuturic reactive substance (TBARS) and higher IL-6 than controls. Both depressed groups generated higher PCC score than controls, with no significant difference between melancholic and nonmelancholic patients, suggesting that a sign-based measure to rate melancholia can replicate and extend biological findings discriminating melancholic depression. Hence signs of psychomotor disturbance may be a useful diagnostic measure of melancholia.

Clinical Relavence of Depression

It is now known that depression is the primary cause of early morbidity and mortality. It is associated with almost all types of chronic illnesses such as cancer, chronic back pain, migraine, pre-menstrual syndrome, rheumatoid arthritis, fibromyalgia, post-traumatic stress disorder, post-operative patients, HIV/AIDs, progressive neurodegenerative disorders (Parkinson's disease, Alzheimer's disease, Huntington's disease, Frederick Ataxia, Multiple Sclerosis, Amyotrophic Lateral Sclerosis, Neuropsychological Disorders including Schizophrenia, Oligophrenia, Catalepsy, Epilepsy, Chronic Drug Addiction including; Alcoholism, Cocainism, Methamphetamine (METH) addiction, Morphine, Heroine, and Nicotine. Particularly, hypothyoid patients suffer severely from depression. In general, women suffer more than men as its incidence is almost double in women. The incidence of depression is 8% among men and 16% among women in the US. Although the incidence of depression is higher among women, the number of suicides particularly among 85 years or older males is higher as compared to females. Alcohol and other substance abuse have been been linked to it. It is known that almost 750,000 persons attempt suicide every year in the US. Out of which 30,000 succeed to take away their own lives. Many international terrorists and acts of violence have been directly and indirectly associated with substance abuse and severe depression and anxiety. Hence it is highly significant to understand and treat disease and gender-specific depression for better quality of life and world peace. One of the several approaches could be through dietary manipulations in addition to other therapeutic interventions as described in this book. General behavioral manifestations of depression are:

Agitation. This condition referes to a situation where depression and restlessness co-exist. The patient finds it difficult to sit or lie still. These patients are always on the go, and often irritable, angry, frustrated, and impulsive with risks of suicide, and other forms of self-mutilation, or violence towards those who may be perceived as the cause.

Hibernation. Even healthy persons may refuse invitations or making excuses to avoid social contact particularly during the winter when long nights, short days and lack of exposure to sun light leave them feeling fatigued, depressed, anxious, and irritable also known as seasonal affective disorder (SAD), some investigators consider SAD to be an evolutionary hangover.

Lethargy. Some patients with depression find their motivation going down. They slow down, speak slowly, and move as if carrying a weight on their shoulders and/or dragging weights around their ankles. A mild depression appears in facial expressions and gestures, not to do anything such as: getting out of bed, getting washed, eating, and even drinking.

Procrastination. There are things one can do to elevate mood but pessimism directs it isn't worth it which provokes procrastination. If someone is already prone to putting things off, depression will increase it further. It provides relief that he/she does not need to make an effort. It fuels depression and can add to guilt.

Diet. Some patients do not take food when their mood is down and others desire comfort foods. It is unusual during depression to find that diet isn't affected, even if it's the choice of preferred foods.

Sleep. About 80% of patients with depression have sleep problems. Lack of sleep has negative impact on mood. However sleep pattern vary and some patients find themselves experiencing problems getting to sleep or waking too early in the morning. Antidepressants have positive benefits not only in treating depression but also for chronic pain like fibromyalgia, migraines, PMS, and even urinary symptoms. The weight gain is an adverse side effect associated with antidepressants. Unfortunately, many people are unaware of weight gain when they start taking their medications - physicians may not mention it. It remains unknown that all of a sudden one can't stop eating chips, bagels, or ice cream, or instructed to eat a low-carb, high protein diet to lose weight. Hence dietary interventions to alleviate depression seem promising to majority of patients with depression as discussed in this book.

References

American Psychiatric Association (1968). "Schizophrenia" (PDF). *Diagnostic and statistical manual of mental disorders: DSM-II*. Washington, DC: American Psychiatric Publishing, Inc. pp. 36–37, 40. Retrieved 2008-08-03.

American Psychiatric Association (2000a). *Diagnostic and statistical manual of mental disorders, Fourth Edition, Text Revision: DSM-IV-TR*. Washington, DC: American Psychiatric Publishing, Inc. p. 345

Barlow DH; Durand VM (2005). *Abnormal psychology: An integrative approach (5th ed.)*. Belmont, CA, USA: Thomson Wadsworth. Cite uses deprecated parameters (help)

Beck, Aaron T.; Rush J, Shaw BF, Emery G (1987) [1979]. *Cognitive Therapy of depression*. New York, NY, USA: Guilford Press. Cite uses deprecated parameters (help)

Berrios GE (September 1988). "Melancholia and depression during the 19th century: A conceptual history". *British Journal of Psychiatry* 153 (3): 298–304. Cite uses deprecated parameters (help)

Blair RG (October 2004). "Helping older adolescents search for meaning in depression". *Journal of Mental Health Counseling* 26 (4): 333–347. Retrieved 2008-11-06. Cite usesdeprecated parameters (help)

Boeree, CG (1998). "Abraham Maslow: Personality Theories" (PDF). Psychology Department, Shippensburg University. Retrieved 2008-10-27.

Bolwig, Tom G.; Shorter, Edward (2007). "Melancholia: Beyond DSM, beyond neurotransmitters. Proceedings of a conference, May 2006, Copenhagen, Denmark". *Acta Psychiatrica Scandinavica Suppl* 115 (433): 4–183.

Carhart-Harris RL, Mayberg HS, Malizia AL, Nutt D (2008). "Mourning and melancholia revisited: Correspondences between principles of Freudian metapsychology and empirical findings in neuropsychiatry". *Annals of General Psychiatry* 7 (1): 9. doi:10.1186/1744-859X-7-9.

Daly, RW (2007). "Before depression: The medieval vice of acedia". *Psychiatry: Interpersonal & Biological Processes* 70 (1): 30–51.

Davison, K (2006). "Historical aspects of mood disorders". *Psychiatry* 5 (4): 115–18..

Fink M, Bolwig TG, Parker G, Shorter E (2007). "Melancholia: Restoration in psychiatric classification recommended". *Acta Psychiatrica Scandinavica* 115 (2): 89–92.

Frankl VE (2000). *Man's search for ultimate meaning*. New York, NY, USA: Basic Books. pp. 139–40.

Freeman, Epstein & Simon 1987, pp. 64,66.

Freud, S (1984). "Mourning and Melancholia". In Richards A *(ed.). 11.On Metapsychology: The Theory of Psycholoanalysis*. Aylesbury, Bucks: Pelican. pp. 245–69.

Geppert CMA (May 2006). "Damage control". *Psychiatric Times*. Retrieved 2008-11-08.Cite uses deprecated parameters (help)

Gruenberg, A.M., Goldstein, R.D., Pincus, H.A. (2005) Classification of Depression: Research and Diagnostic Criteria: DSM-IV and ICD-10 (PDF). Wiley.com. Retrieved on October 30, 2008.

Haque A (2004). "Psychology from Islamic perspective: Contributions of early Muslim scholars and challenges to contemporary Muslim psychologists". *Journal of Religion and Health* 43 (4): 357–377 [366].

Healy, David (1999). *The Antidepressant Era*. Cambridge, MA: Harvard University Press. p. 42.

Hergenhahn BR (2005). *An Introduction to the History of Psychology* (5th ed.). Belmont, CA, USA: Thomson Wadsworth.

Hippocrates, *Aphorisms*, Section 6.23.

Jackson SW (July 1983). "Melancholia and mechanical explanation in eighteenth-century medicine". *Journal of the History of Medical and Allied Sciences* 38 (3): 298–319. Citeuses deprecated parameters (help)

Jacquart D. "The Influence of Arabic Medicine in the Medieval West" in Morrison & Rashed 1996, pp. 980

Kent, Deborah (2003). *Snake Pits, Talking Cures & Magic Bullets: A History of Mental Illness*. Twenty-First Century Books. , p. 55.

Lewis, AJ (1934). "Melancholia: A historical review". *Journal of Mental Science* 80 (328): 1–42.

Mapother, E (1926). "Discussion of manic-depressive psychosis". British Medical Journal 2 (3436): 872–79. doi:10.1136/bmj.2.3436.872. ISSN 0959-8138.

Maslow A (1971). *The Farther Reaches of Human Nature*. New York, NY, USA: Viking Books. p. 318.

Merkel, L. (2003) The History of Psychiatry PGY II Lecture (PDF) Website of the University of Virginia Health System. Retrieved on 2008-08-04.

Online Etymology Dictionary. Retrieved June 30, 2008, from Dictionary.com Parker 1996, p. 11.

Parker G (2000). (abstract) "Classifying depression: Should paradigms lost be regained?". *American Journal of Psychiatry* 157 (8): 1195–1203. doi:10.1176/appi.ajp.157.8.1195.

Parker, Gordon; Dusan Hadzi-Pavlovic, Kerrie Eyers (1996). *Melancholia: A disorder of movement and mood: A phenomenological and neurobiological review*. Cambridge: Cambridge University Press.

Philipp M, Maier W, Delmo CD (1991). "The concept of major depression. I. Descriptive comparison of six competing operational definitions including ICD-10 and DSM-III-R". *European Archives of Psychiatry and Clinical Neuroscience* 240 (4–5): 258–65. doi:10.1007/BF02189537.

Radden, J (March 2003). "Is this dame melancholy? Equating today's depression and past melancholia". *Philosophy, Psychiatry, & Psychology* 10 (1): 37–52.Cite uses deprecated parameters (help)

S Safavi-Abbasi, LBC Brasiliense, RK Workman (2007), The fate of medical knowledge and the neurosciences during the time of Genghis Khan and the Mongolian Empire, *Neurosurgical Focus* 23 (1), E13, p. 3.

Schildkraut, JJ (1965). "The catecholamine hypothesis of affective disorders: A review of supporting evidence". *American Journal of Psychiatry* 122 (5): 509–22. doi:10.1176/appi.ajp.122.5.509.

Schneider, K (1920). "Zeitschrift für die gesante". *Neurol Psychiatr* 59: 281–86.

Seidner, Stanley S. (June 10, 2009) "A Trojan Horse: Logotherapeutic Transcendence and its Secular Implications for Theology". *Mater Dei Institute*. pp 14-15.

Spanemberg L, Caldieraro MA, vares EA, Aguiar BW, Anna MKS, Galvao E, Parker G, Fleck MP (2014) Biological differences between melanchilic and nonmelancholic depression subtypes by the CORE measure. Neuropsychiatric Disease & Treatment. 10:1523-1531.

Spitzer RL, Endicott J, Robins E (1975). "The development of diagnostic criteria in psychiatry" (PDF). Retrieved 2008-11-08.

"The Anatomy of Melancholy by Robert Burton". *Project Gutenberg*. 1 April 2004. Retrieved 2008-10-19.Akiskal HS, McKinney WT (1975). "Overview of recent research in depression: Integration of ten conceptual models into a comprehensive clinical frame". *Archives of General Psychiatry* 32 (3): 285–305.

Wolpert, L. "Malignant Sadness: The Anatomy of Depression". *The New York Times*. Retrieved 2008-10-30.

Chapter 2

Dietary Requirements and Depression

Abstract

Our diet is composed of numerous essential ingredients including carbohydrates, proteins, minerals, (calcium, chromium, iron, lithium, selenium, zinc, and iodine), vitamins (folate, cyanocobalamine), omega-3 fatty acids which can significantly influence our mood. Dietary status of various minerals can be quantitatively assessed by atomic absorption spectrophotometery and/or inductively-coupled plasma mass spectrometry. Other physiological factors, psychological factors, and moderate exercise can also influence our mood. In addition, the modulatory role of aspartame is described which can also influence our mood. Hence a balanced diet is extremely important to remain free from any overt symptom of depression and remain healthy. In this chapter essential ingredients in our diet have been discussed which can directly or indirectly alleviate various symptoms of depression.

Keywords: Dietary ingredients, Spectrophotometry, B-Vitamins, Essential Fatty acids, Mood, Aspartame

It is now known that around 19 million adults are affected by depression each year, yet this disease is misunderstood or misdiagnosed globally. There are several treatment options that can alleviate depression. Although the relationship between nutritional deficiencies and physical health is well-known, a definite physiological link between nutrition and depression is known to limited number of people. It is generally held that depression is primarily neurochemically-based or emotionally-linked. However nutrition can play a pivotal role in the onset, severity, and duration of depression. Several dietary patterns are known to precede depression, including: poor appetite, inadequate meals, and craving for simple carbohydrate foods. It has been emphasized that nutritional factors are associated with cognition, behavior, and emotions. The most prevalent mental disorders are depression, bipolar disorder, schizophrenia, and obsessive-compulsive disorder (OCD) (Murray and Lopez., 1996). The dietary pattern of several Asian and Americans is generally deficient in nutrients, especially essential vitamins, minerals, and omega-3 fatty acids (American Psychiatric: Diagnostic and statistical manual of mental disorders-2000). The severity of deficiency of these nutrients is high among patients suffering from mental disorders. It has been reported that daily supplements of these nutrients are effective in attenuating patients' symptoms (Lakhan and Vieira, 2008). Particularly amino acids are known to reduce symptoms of depression, as these are converted to neurotransmitters which alleviate depression and other mental disorders (Lakhan and Vieira, 2008). Nutritional supplements can be utilized for therapeutic interventions of neurobehavioral disorders including depression, bipolar disorder, schizophrenia, eating disorders, anxiety disorders, attention deficit disorder/attention deficit hyperactivity disorder (ADD/ADHD), autism, and drug addiction (Lakhan and Vieira, 2008). Most prescription drugs, including antidepressants cause adverse effects, which is the primary cause of non-compliance in psychiatric patients those are at a higher risk for committing suicide or being institutionalized. Because these drugs have low margin of safety, chronic use of increasing doses may result in life-threatening neurotoxicity (Lakhan and Vieira, 2008). An alternate and effective way to overcome the noncompliance is to familiarize these patients about alternative or complementary nutritional therapies. Although further research is needed to determine the most appropriate doses of nutritional supplements that can be recommended; these doses can be adjusted based on the results obtained by closely watching the changes in the patient.

Indeed the diet of depressed patients is inadequate. Their poor dietary habits may even contribute to more depression. A recent study suggested a relationship between low levels of serotonin and suicide (http:/diet.hajimeru.biz/category/health/nutrition). Reduced levels of 5-HT can lead to insensitivity to future consequences, triggering risky, impulsive and aggressive behavior which may result in aggretion and suicide. Depression is associated with sadness, anxiety, loss of appetite, depressed mood, and a lack of interest in pleasurable activities. If remained untreated, depression can lead to deleterious consequences.

Incidentally depression is not simply an impairment of brain region-specific serotonin deficiency, it is a complex neuronal abnormality, which may have several unknown causes and consequences, which require further investigations. Depression is associated with the deficiency of several neurotransmitters including: serotonin, dopamine, noradrenaline, and γ-aminobutyric acid (GABA) (Brown et al., 1982; Rush, 2007; NIMH, 2000; Diehl and Gershon, 1992; Stockmeier, 1997; Van Praag 1983; Firk et al., 2007). Usually, patients suffering from depression exhibit suicidal tendency and hence are treated with antidepressants and/or psychotherapy (Brown et al., 1982). In addition brain derived growth factors (BDNF) and hormones may be involved in the etiopathogenessis of depression. There are several studies supporting that the amino acids tryptophan, tyrosine, phenylalanine, and methionine are helpful in treating depression (Firk and Markus, 2007; Leonard, 1997; Petty, 1995; McLean et al., 2004; Agnoli et al., 1976; Agnoli et al., 1976; Bourre, 2005).

Tryptophan. Tryptophan, as precursor of serotonin, is converted to serotonin by tryptophan hydroxylase and pyrodoxal phosphate (Vitamin B_6)-dependent enzyme, 5-HTP decarboxylase respectively. Hence, tryptophan can induce sleep and tranquility, suggesting that restoring serotonin can alleviate depression induced by serotonin deficiencies, whereas tyrosine and sometimes its precursor phenylalanine are converted to dopamine and norepinephrine (Hoes, 1982). Dietary supplements containing phenylalanine and/or tyrosine cause alertness and arousal (increased vigilance). Methionine along with ATP produces S-adenosylmethionine (SAM), which enhances the synthesis of neurotransmitters in the CNS (Buist, 1983; Maurizi, 1990; Ruhe et al., 2007; DeLeo, 1987). Hence the daily supplements of these nutrients should be consumed to accomplish antidepressant effects. Adequate consumption of omega-3 fatty acids from fish and other sources like flax seeds may also lead to reduced incidence of MDD (Janicak, 1988). The two omega-3 fatty acids, eicosapentaenoic acid (EPA) which the body converts into docosahexanoic acid (DHA), in fish oil, exert antidepressant effects. This conversion involves neurotransmitters. The antidepressant effects could be due to conversion of EPA to leukotrienes, prostaglandins, and other neurochemicals in the CNS. Both EPA and DHA influence signal transduction by activating peroxisomal proliferator-activated receptors (PPARs), inhibiting G-proteins and protein kinase C, in addition to sodium, potassium, and calcium ion channels. Epidemiological data and clinical studies demonstrated that omega-3 fatty acids can treat depression (Hibbeln, 1998).

In mammals, nicotinamide (Nam) is synthesized from L-tryptophan (L-Trp). The enzymes involved in the initial step of the L-Trp→Nam pathway are L-Trp-2,3-dioxygenase (TDO) and indoleamine-2,3-dioxygenase (IDO). Terakata et al., (2013) determined whether tdo-knockout (tdo(-/-)) mice fed a diet without niacin can synthesize Nam to sustain optimum growth. Wild-type (WT) and tdo(-/-) mice were fed 20% casein diet with or without niacin (30 mg nicotinic acid/kg) for 28 d. Body weight, food intake, and liver NAD concentrations did not differ among the groups. Mice fed the niacin-free diet, urinary concentrations of the metabolites kynurenine, kynurenic acid, xanthurenic acid, and 3-hydroxyanthranilic acid were higher in the tdo(-/-) mice than in the WT mice, while quinolinic acid and Nam and its catabolites were lower in the tdo(-/-) mice than in the WT mice, suggesting that the kynurenine formed in extrahepatic tissues by IDO and enzymes can be metabolized to 3-HA, but not into QA. However, the tdo(-/-) mice sustained growth even when fed the niacin-free diet for 1 month, suggesting that they can synthesize Nam from L-Trp, because the liver can import blood kynurenine formed in extrahepatic tissues and metabolize it into Nam via NAD and the resulting Nam is then distributed back into extrahepatic tissues.

A daily consumption of dietary supplements of omega-3 fatty acid that contain 1.5-2 g of EPA enhanced mood elevation in depressant patients. However, doses of omega-3 higher than 3 g did not exhibit better effects than placebos and may be contraindicated in those taking anti-thrombotic drugs (Adams et al., 1996). In addition to omega–3 fatty acids, vitamin B (e.g., folate) and magnesium deficiencies are associated with depression (Grubb, 1990; Bell et al., 1991; Young, 2007). Randomized trials involving folate and vitamin B_{12} suggested that patients treated with 0.8 mg of folic acid/day or 0.4 mg of vitamin B_{12}/day exhibited reduced depressive symptoms (Young, 2007). In case controlled studies where patients were treated with 125-300 mg of magnesium (as glycinate or taurinate) induced recovery from MDD within 7 days. Earlier studies have provided association between nutritional deficiencies and mental disorders (Janicak et al., 1988; Hibbeln, 1998; Adams et al., 1995; Eby et al., 2006; Wurtman et al., 1989; Chouinard et al., 1985; Reis et al., 2006). The most common nutritional deficiencies in patients with mental disorders are of omega–3 fatty acids, B vitamins, minerals, and amino acids that are precursors to neurotransmitters (Maurizi, 1990; Kanicak et al., 1988; Hibbeln 1998; Young, 2007; Bell et al., 1991; Wurtman et al., 1989; Tanskanen et al., 2001). Furthermore, demographic studies suggested a relationship between high fish consumption and low incidence of mental disorders; as a result of omega–3 fatty acid intake (Janicak et al., 1988; Chouinard et al., 1985; Reis and Hibbeln, 2006). A daily intake of 1-2 gram of omega-3 fatty acids is adequate for healthy individuals, but for patients with mental disorders, up to 9.6 g has been reported to be safe and effective (Rudin, 1981; Eritsland, 2000; Von Schacky, 2006). Asian diets also lack in fruits and vegetables, which may lead to mineral and vitamin deficiencies. The significance of these nutrients in mental health, with special relevance to depression is explained below.

Carbohydrates. Carbohydrates are polysaccharides that play an important role in structure and function of an organism. In human, carbohydrates influence mood and behavior. Eating a meal rich in carbohydrates augments the release of insulin in the body. Insulin acts as a carrier to let blood sugar into cells for energy and facilitates the entry of tryptophan to brain through blood brain barrier. Tryptophan in the brain affects the levels of serotonin and melatonin is implicated in mood alleviation and sleep regulation. Consumption of diets low in carbohydrate can augment depression, since the production of CNS serotonin and tryptophan that promote the feeling of well-being, is triggered by carbohydrate rich foods. Low glycemic index (GI) diets such as some fruits and vegetables, whole grains, pasta, etc. can provide a moderate but lasting effect on brain chemistry, mood, and energy than the high GI foods - mainy sweets - that tend to provide immediate but temporary relief.

Proteins. Proteins are composed of amino acids and are the structural and functional building blocks of life. At least 12 amino acids are synthesized in the body itself and remaining 8 (*essential amino acids*) have to be supplemented through diet. A high quality protein diet contains all essential amino acids. Foods rich in high quality protein include meats, eggs and dairy products. Plant proteins such as beans, peas, and grains may be low in one or two essential amino acids. Protein intake and the individual amino acids can affect the brain functioning and mental health. Many of the neurotransmitters in the brain are synthesized from amino acids. The neurotransmitter dopamine is synthesized from tyrosine and serotonin from tryptophan (http:/diet.hajimeru.biz/category/health/nutrition). Lack of any of these two amino acids, can reduce the synthesis of respective neurotransmitters, resulting in anxiety and depression. The excessive synthesis and buildup of amino acids may also induce neurodegeneration and mental retardation. For instance, increased accumulation of phenylalanine in patients with phenylketonuria can cause neurodegeneration and mental retardation.

Essential Omega-3 fatty acids. The brain has the second highest levels of lipids, which form structural and functional components of neuronal cell membranes. It has been estimated that gray matter contains 50% fatty acids that are polyunsaturated (about 33% belong to the omega-3 family), and have to be supplemented through diet. The omega-3 fatty acids (especially α-linolenic acid, ALA) are the member to take part. Lowering plasma cholesterol by diet and medications increases depression. The quantity and ratio of omega-3 and omega-6 PUFA affect serum lipids and alter the physicochemical properties of cell membranes. It has been proposed that long chain PUFAs, especially DHA, may alleviate depression (Stoll et al., 1999). The structural and functional components of membrane in brain cells, include phospholipids, spingolipids, and cholesterol. The glycerophospholipids in brain consist of PUFA derived from the essential fatty acids (EFAs), linoleic acid and α-linolenic acid. The main PUFA in the brain are DHA, derived from the omega-3 fatty acid α-linolenic acid, arachidonic acid (AA) and docosa tetraenoic acid, both derived from omega-6 fatty acid, linoleic acid. It has been reported that diets lacking omega-3 PUFA may lead to disturbance in neural function (Sinclair et al., 2007). Despite their abundance in the CNS; DHA and AA cannot be synthesized by mammals *de novo* and hence these or their precursors have to be supplied through the diet and transported to the brain. During late gestation and the early postnatal period, neurodevelopment occurs at accelerated rates, which makes the supply of PUFAs, particularly DHA, highly essential to ensure neurite outgrowth in addition to appropriate development of brain and retina (Marszalek and Lodish, 2005). In earlier studies, Bruinsma and Taren (2000) explored the involvement of dieting-related psychological factors as potential confounders. They emphasized that lowering plasma cholesterol by diet and medications contributes to depression. An imbalance in the ratio of the EFAs, namely the omega-6 and omega-3 fatty acids, and/or a deficiency in omega-3 fatty acids, may induce depressive symptoms associated with low plasma cholesterol. These relationships may explain the inconsistency in the results of trials on cholesterol-lowering interventions and depression. On similar grounds, dieting has been associated with mood fluctuations (Anita et al., 1998). Dietary omega-3 fatty acids play a significant role in the prevention of depression. Their deficiency can accelerate cerebral aging by preventing the renewal of membranes. However, the roles of the vascular component where the omega-3s are active, and the cerebral parenchyma remains unknown. The clinical significance of omega–3 in certain diseases such as dyslexia and autism has been suggested. Experiments were carried out on ex-*vivo* cultured brain cells, then on *in vivo* brain cells, on physicochemical, biochemical, physiological, neurosensory, and behavioral parameters. The results of this study indicated that the PUFAs (in particular omega–3) in formula milks determine the visual, cerebral, and intellectual capabilities in infants (Agnoli et al., 1976).

B-Complex Vitamins. Neurobehavioral studies provided evidence that nutrition and depression are intimately linked (Benton et al., 1995). Supplementation of nine vitamins, 10 times in excess of normal RDA for 1 year improved mood in both men and women. These changes in mood occurred even though the blood status of these vitamins reached a plateau after 3 months. The mood alleviation was associated with improved vitamin B_2 and B_6 status. In women, baseline vitamin B_1 status was associated with poor mood and an improvement after 3 months was associated with alleviation of mood. Thiamine improved cognitive performance particularly in the geriatric population (Bourre, 2006).

Vitamin B_{12} (Cynocobalamin). Vitamin B_{12} delays the onset of dementia (and blood abnormalities), if it is administered in a propoer clinical timing window, before the onset of the first symptoms. Cobalamin enhances cerebral and cognitive functions in the elderly; promotes the functioning of the frontal lobe, in addition to the language function of patients with cognitive disorders. Adolescents with borderline level of vitamin B_{12} deficiency develop symptoms of cognitive impairments (Bourre, 2006).

Folate. Depressive symptoms are the most common neuropsychiatric manifestation of folate deficiency (Alpert and Fava, 1997). It remains uncertain whether poor nutrition causes folate deficiency or primary folate deficiency produces depression and its symptoms. Patients with depression have blood folate levels 25% lower than healthy controls (Coppen and Bailey, 2000). Low levels of folate have also been detected as a predisposing factor of poor prognosis of antidepressant therapy. Folic acid enhanced the effectiveness of antidepressant medication (Abou-Saleh and Coppen, 2006).

Minerals

Calcium. Selective serotonin uptake inhibitors (SSRIs) inhibit absorption of calcium into bones. As a consequence one can be a victim of osteoporosis. In addition to this, the SSRIs can lower BP, resulting in falls which may lead to bone fractures. Indiscriminate prescription of SSRIs by patients at risk of depression or other mental health problems may put them at increased risk of fractures. Aging subjects and those already taking other medications may also predispose to osteoporosis (Golzman, 2007).

Chromium. Several studies on the association of chromium in depression have been reported suggesting the significance of this micronutrient in mental health (Davison et al., 2003; Docherty et al., 2005).

Iodine. Iodine plays an important role in mental health. The iodine from the thyroid hormone (T_3 and T_4) ensures the energy metabolism of the neuronal cells. During pregnancy, the dietary reduction of iodine can induce cerebral dysfunction, leading to cretinism.

Iron. Iron is necessary for oxygenation to produce energy in the CNS (through cytochrome oxidase), and for the synthesis of neurotransmitters and myelin. Iron deficiency is found in children with ADHD. Iron levels in the umbilical artery are critical during the development of the fetus, and in relation with the IQ in the child; infantile anemia with iron deficiency is associated with disturbance in the development of cognitive functions (Bourre et al., 2006). Twice as many women as men are clinically depressed. This gender difference starts in adolescence and becomes more pronounced among married women aged 25-45, with children. Moreover, women of childbearing age experience more depression than during other times in their lives indicating the importance of iron in the etiology of depression since its deficiency is known to cause fatigue and depression. Iron deficiency anemia is associated with apathy, depression, and fatigue (Bourre et al., 2006).

Zinc. Zinc participates in gustation (taste perception). Zinc levels are lower in those with clinical depression (Levenson, 2006). Oral zinc can influence the effectiveness of antidepressant therapy (Nowak et al., 2005). Zinc also protects the neuronal cells against the damage by serving as free radical scavenger. The genetic potential of the child for physical and mental development may be compromised due to deficiency of micronutrients including zinc. When children and adolescents with poor nutritional status are exposed to alterations of mental and behavioral functions, they can be corrected by dietary measures to a certain extent. Nutrient composition of diet and meal pattern can have beneficial or adverse, immediate or long-term effects. Dietary deficiencies of antioxidants and nutrients (trace elements, vitamins, and micronutrients such as polyphenols) particularly during early development and aging may precipitate neurodegenerative diseases due to compromised antioxidant mechanisms against free radicals.

Selenium. Low selenium intake is associated with depressed mood (Benton, 2002). Selenium improves mood and diminishes anxiety (Shor-Posner, 2003; Duntas et al., 2003).

Lithium. Lithium, as a monovalent cation, is a drug of choice for bipolar disorder with antimanic, antidepressant, and antisuicidal properties. The therapeutic use of lithium also includes its usage as an augmenting agent in depression, scizoaffective disorder, aggression, impulse control disorder, eating disorders, ADHDs, and in alcoholism (Mohandas and Rajmohan, 2007). But adequate care has to be taken while using lithium, as a mood stabilizer, in the mentally ill. Lithium can be used in patients with cardiovascular, renal, endocrine, pulmonary, and dermatological comorbidity. The toxicity of lithium has to be taken in to consideration during pregnancy and lactation, in pediatric and geriatric population.

Physiological and Psychological Factors. The diet and depression involves old age, which is vulnerable period to weight loss associated with increased morbidity and premature death. Anorexia of aging may play an important role in precipitating morbidity and premature death, by either reducing food intake directly or in response to adverse factors as age-associated reductions in sensory perception (taste and smell), poor dentition, multiple prescription drugs, and depression (Robert, 2000). Malnutrition can occur in the elderly due to refusal to eat (Marcus and Berry 1998). Physiologic changes associated with aging, mental disorders such as dementia and depression, and medical, social, and environment as causative factors. Presently patients are following the alternative and complementary medical (CAM) interventions to combat depression. CAM therapies are defined by the National Center for Complementary and Alternative Medicine as a group of medical and health systems, practices, and products that are not currently considered to be a part of conventional medicine (National Center for Complementary and Alternative Medicine NIH 2002). The patients with bipolar disorder might use CAM interventions. Some clinicians consider these interventions to be effective and safe alternatives, or adjuncts to conventional psychotropic medications (Andreescu et al., 2008). Recent research in psychoneuroimmunology and neurochemistry indicates the possibility of communication pathways that can provide a better understanding of the association between nutritional intake, CNS, and immune function thereby influencing an individual's psychological health status. These findings may lead to more acceptance of the therapeutic value of dietary intervention addressing depression and other psychological disorders.

Exercise. A study in 1981 highlighted that regular exercise can improve mood in people with mild to moderate depression. It may also play an important role in treating severe depression. 156 men and women with depression were divided into three groups. One group took part in an aerobic exercise program, another took the SSRI Sertraline (Zoloft), and a third did both. At the 16-week, depression alleviated in all three groups. About 60%–70% of the people in all three groups had no major depression. Group scores on two rating scales of depression were similar, suggesting that for those who wish to avoid drugs, exercise is a substitute for antidepressants. The fastest response occurred in the group taking antidepressants, and that it is difficult to stay motivated to exercise when someone is depressed. The exercise's effects lasted longer than those of antidepressants. People who exercised regularly, regardless of which treatment they were on, were less likely to relapse into depression. Walking fast for about 35 minutes a day five times a week or 60 minutes a day thrice a week had a significant influence on mild to moderate depression. Walking fast for only 15 minutes a day five times a week or doing stretching exercises three times a week did not help significantly for a 150 pound person. (*Longer exercise times apply if we weigh more, while the opposite is true if we weigh <150 pounds*). Exercise boosts the action of circulating endorphins which improve immunity and mood, and reduce pain perception. In addition, exercise stimulates norepinephrine, which can alleviate mood. Regular exercise offers other health benefits, such as lowering BP, protecting against heart disease and cancer, and augmenting self-esteem. How often or intensely we need to exercise to alleviate depression remains unknown, however for general health, 0.5-1 hr of moderate exercise, such as brisk walking every day is adequate. *(Modified from the Special Health Report from Harvard Medical School* "Understanding Depression". *For more information or to order, please go to* www.health.harvard.edu/UD.).

Aspartame. Aspartame is a low-calorie sweetener, and has been used in carbonated drinks since the 1980s. In 1981, the FDA approved aspartame in soft drinks only after extensive studies and 15 years after aspartame had been discovered. Some studies associate Aspartame to various adverse symptoms and conditions, including neurological effects such as blurred vision, headaches, dizziness, seizures and severe depression. Others claimed that aspartame is safe and doesn't cause side effects or illness. However, a doctor should be consulted before consuming any food items that contain aspartame in the diet. A 1993 study published in the "Biology of Psychiatry" reported that individuals who had a history of depression showed increased symptoms when Aspartame (30 mg/kg body weight/day) was administered for 7 days. However, the study was terminated because the group suffered severe adverse effects. Hence it remained determined if individuals who did not have mental illness developed symptoms of depression because of Aspartame. A 2002 review in the journal "*Regulatory Toxicology and Pharmacology*" discussed the safety of Aspartame in studies that had labeled it to be unsafe. The Aspartame has been tested and no evidence exists that this food additive is linked to severe depression or to other adverse reactions. It was stated that when people use Aspartame as intended, it is safe and has no toxic effects.

References

Abou-Saleh, M.T; Coppen, A. (2006) Folic acid and the treatment of depression., *J Psychosom Res*. 61, 285–287.

Adams, P.B; Lawson, S; Sanigorski, A; Sinclair AJ. (1996) Arachidonic acid to eicosapentaenoic acid ratio in blood correlates positively with clinical symptoms of depression., *Lipids*. 31, S157–161.

Agnoli, A; Andreoli, V; Casacchia, M; Cerbo, R. (1976). Effects of s-adenosyl-l-methionine (SAMe) upon depressive symptoms., *J Psychiatr Res*. 13, 43–54.

Alpert, J.E; Fava, M. (1997) Nutrition and depression: The role of folate., *Nutr Rev*. 55, 145–149.

American psychiatric A: Diagnostic and statistical manual of mental disorders. 4th ed. Washington DC: 2000.

Andreescu, C; Mulsant, B.H; Emanuel, J.E. (2008) Complementary and alternative medicine in the treatment of bipolar disorder: A review of the evidence., *J Affecrt Disord.* May 2;

Anita, S.W; Nicholas, W.R; Jonathan, D.E; Laugharne, Ahluwalia, N.S. (1998) Alterations in mood after changing to a low-fat diet, *Br J Nutr.* 79, 23–30. Available from: http:/diet.hajimeru.biz/category/health/nutritionj/

Beardsley. B Depression and nutrition from:http://www.healingwell.com/LIBRARY/depression/beardsley/.asp.

Bell, I.R; Edman, J.S; Morrow, F.D; Marby, D.W; Mirages, S; Perrone, G. et al. (1991) B Complex vitamin patterns in geriatric and young adult inpatients with major depression., *J Am Geriatr Soc*. 39, 252–527.

Benton, D; Haller, J; Fordy, J. (1995) Vitamin supplementation for one year improves mood. 32, 98–105.

Benton, D. (2002) Selenium Intake, mood and other aspects of psychological functioning., *Nutr Neurosci*.5, 363–374.

Bourre, J.M. (2005) Dietary omega-3 Fatty acids and psychiatry: Mood, behavior, stress, depression, dementia and aging., *J Nutr Health Aging*. 9, 31–38.

Bourre, J.M. (2006) Effect of nutrients (in food) on the structure and function of the nervous system: Update on dietary requirements for brain, Part 1: Micronutrients., *J Nutr Health Aging*. 10, 377–385.

Brown, G.L; Ebert, M.H; Gover, P.H; Jimerson, D.C; Klein, W.J; Bunney, W.E; et al. (1982) Aggression, suicide and serotonin: Relationships to CSF amine metabolites., *Am J Psychiatry*. 139, 741–746.

Bruinsma, K.A; Taren, D.L. (2005) Dieting, essential fatty acid intake and depression., *Nutr Rev*. 58, 98–108.

Buist, R. (1983) The therapeutic predictability of tryptophan and tyrosine in the treatment of depression., *Int J Clin Nutr Rev*. 3, 1–3.

Chouinard, G; Young, S.N; Annable, L. (1985) A controlled clinical trial of L-tryptophan in acute mania., *Biol Psychiatry*. 20, 546–547.

Coppen, A; Bailey, J. (2000) Enhancement of the antidepressant action of fluoxetine by folic acid: A randomized placebo controlled trial., *J Affect Disord*. 60, 121–130.

Davison, K; Abraham, K.M; Connor, McLeod, MN. (2003) Effectiveness of chromium in atypical depression: A placebo-controlled trial., *Bio Psychiatry*. 53, 261–264.

DeLeo, D. (1987) S-adenosylmethionines an antidepressant: A double blind trial versus placebo., *Cut Ther Res*. 41, 865–870.

Diehl, D.J; Gershon, S. (1992) The role of dopamine in mood disorders., *Comp Psychiatry*. 33, 115–120.

Docherty, J; Sack, D.A; Roffman, M; Finch, M; Komorowski, J.R. (2005) A double-blind, placebo-controlled exploratory trial of chromium picolinate in atypical depression: Effect on carbohydrate craving. J Psychiat Pract. 11, 302–314.

Duntas, L.H; Mantzou, E; Koutras, E.A. (2003) Effects of a six month treatment with selenomethionine in patients with autoimmune thyroiditis., *Eur J Endocrinol. 148*, 389–393.

Eby, G.A; Eby, K.L. (2006) Rapid recovery from major depression using magnesium treatment., *Med Hypotheses*. 67, 362–370.

Eritsland, J. (2000) Safety considerations of polyunsaturated fatty acids., *Am J Clin Nutr*. 71, 197S–201S.

Firk, C; Markus, C.R. (2007) Serotonin by stress interaction: A susceptibility factor for the development of depression?., *J Psychopharmacol*. 21; 538–544.

Golzman, D. (2007) Canadian study: SSRI increase Bone fracture risk., *Arch Intern Med*. 167, 188–194.

Grubb, B.P. (1990) Hypervitaminosis a following long-term use of high-dose fish oil supplements., *Chest*. 97,1260.

Hibbeln, J.R. (1998) Fish consumption and major depression., *Lancet*. 351, 1213.

Hoes, M.J. (1982) L-tryptophan in depression., *J Orthomolecular Psychiatry*. 4, 231.

Janicak, P.G; Lipinski, Davis, J.M; Comaty, J.E; Waternaux, C; Cohen, B. et al. (1988) S-adenosylmethionine in depression: A literature Review and preliminary report., *Ala J Med Sci*. 25, 306–313.

Lakhan, S.E; Vieira, K.F. (2008) Nutritional therapies for mental disorders. *Nutr Jr.*;7, 2.

Leonard, B.E. (1997) The role of noradrenaline in depression: A review., *J Psychopharmacol*. 11, S39–47.

Levenson, C.W. (2006) Zinc, the new antidepressant?., *Nutr Rev*. 6, 39–42.

Marcus; and Berry. (1998) Refusal to eat in the elderly., *Nutr Rev*. 56, 163–171.

Marszalek, Lodish HF. (2005) Docosahexanoic acid, fatty acid-interacting proteins and neuronal function: Breast milk and fish are good for you., *Annnu Rev Cell Dev Biol*. 21, 633–657.

Maurizi, C.P. (1990) The therapeutic potential for tryptophan and melatonin: Possible roles in depression, sleep, Alzheimer's disease and abnormal aging., *Med Hypotheses*. 31, 233–242.

McLean, A; Rubinsztein, J.S., Robbins, T.W., Sahakian, B.J. (2004) The effects of tyrosine depletion in normal healthy volunteers: Implications for unipolar depression., *Psychopharmacology*. 171, 286–297.

Mohandas, E; Rajmohan, V. (2007) Lithium use in special populations., *Indian J Psychiatry*. 49, 211–218.

Murray CJL, Lopez AD. The global burden of disease. *World Health Organization*. 1996:270.

National Center for Complementary and Alternative Medicine - National Institutes of Health. 2002.

National Institute of Mental Health: Depression. National Institute of Mental Health. 2000. (US Department of Health and Human Services, Bethesda (MD) [reprinted September 2002]

Nowak, G; Szewczyk, A. (2005) Zinc and depression, An update., *Pharmacol Rep*. 57, 713–718.

Petty, F. (1995) GABA and mood disorders: A brief review and hypothesis., *J Affect Disord*. 34, 275–281.

Rao, T.S.S; Asha, M.R; Ramesh, B.N; and Jagannatha Rao, K.S. (2008) *Indian J Psychiatry*. 50, 77–82.

Reis, L.C; Hibbeln, J.R. (2006) Cultural symbolism of fish and the psychotropic properties of omega-3 fatty acids., *Prostaglandin Leukot Essent Fatty Acids*. 75, 227–236.

Roberts, S.B. (2000) Energy regulation and aging: recent findings and their implications., *Nutr Rev*. 58, 91–97.

Rudin, D.O. (1981) The major psychoses and neuroses as omega-3 fatty acid deficiency syndrome: Substrate pellagra., *Biol Psychiatry*. 16, 837–850.

Ruhe, H.G; Mason, N.S; Schene, A.H. (2007) Mood is indirectly related to serotonin, norepinephrine and dopamine levels in humans: A meta-analysis of monoamine depletion studies. *Mol Psychiatry*.12, 331–359.

Rush, A.J. (2007) The varied clinical presentations of major depressive disorder,. *J Clin Psychiatry*. 68, 4–10.

Shor-Posner, G.R; Lecusay, Miguez, M.J; Moreno-Black, G; Zhnag, G; Rodriguez, N; et al. (2003) Psychological burden in the era of HAART: Impact of selenium therapy., *Int J Psychiatry Med*. 33, 55–69.

Sinclair, A.J; Begg, D; Mathai, M; Weisinger, R.S. (2007) Omega-3 fatty acids and the brain: review of studies in depression., *Asia Pac J Clin Nutr*. 16, 391–397.

Stockmeier, C.A. (1997) Neurobiology of serotonin in depression and suicide., *Ann N Y Acad Sci*.836, 220–232.

Stoll, A.L; Severus, W.E; Freeman, M.P; Rueter, S; Zboyan, H.A; Diamond, E; et al. (1999) Omega 3 fatty acids in bipolar disorder: A preliminary double-blind, placebo-controlled trial., *Arch Gen Psychiatry*. 56, 407–412.

Tanskanen, A; Hibbeln, J.R; Hintikka, J; Haatainen, K; Honkalampi, K; Viinamaki, H. (2001) Fish consumption, depression, and suicidality in a general population., *Arch Gen Psychiatry*. 58, 512–513.

Van Praag, H.M. (1983) Depression, suicide and the metabolism of serotonin in the brain., *J Affect Disord*.4, 275–290.

Von Schacky, C.A. (2006) Review of omega-3 ethyl esters for cardiovascular prevention and treatment of increased blood triglyceride levels., *Vasc Health Risk Manag*. 2, 251–262.

Wurtman, R; O'Rourke, D; Wurtman, J.J. (1989) Nutrient imbalances in depressive disorders: Possible brain mechanisms., *Ann NY Acad Sci*. 575, 75–82.

Young, S.N. (2007) Folate and depression: A neglected problem., *J Psychiatry Neurosci*. 32, 80–82.

Chapter 3

Tryptophan-Rich Diet and Depression

Abstract

Amino acids are the structural and functional building blocks of proteins in our body. Out of 20 amino acids, 12 can be synthesized, where as the rest 8 cannot be synthesized. Hence these are called essential and need to be taken from natural or synthetic sources. Tryptophan is an essential amino acid and naturally less-abundant. There are specific types of diets that are rich in tryptophan. Tryptophan is a neutral amino acid and is a precursor for the synthesis of serotonin (5-HT) in the brain. Serotonin is involved in regulating appetite, mood, and motivation. Depletion of brain region-specific serotonin can induce depression and anxiety. Although there are diets rich in serotonin; as such it does not cross the blood brain barrier (BBB). However its precursor tryptophan can easily enter CNS and synthesizes serotonin. Tryptophan is converted to 5-hydroxy tryptophan (5-HTP) by a rate limiting enzyme; tryptophan hydroxylase. 5-HTP is converted to 5-HT by 5-HTP decarboxylase in the presence of a coenzyme, pyridoxal phosphate (PLP), derived from dietary vitamin B_6. Serotonin is the precursor for the sleep-inducing hormone, Melatonin which is formed by the acetylation of serotonin. Melatonin regulates sleep-wake cycle and the circadian rhythm. Hence deficiency of tryptophan can induce mood alteration associated with anxiety and depression in addition to sleep disturbance. Mood is altered during sleep deprivation. Hence tryptophan-rich diet is essential to prevent and/or treat depression and enjoy proper sleep, which is impaired in chronic diseases and old age.

Keywords: Tryptophan, Serotonin, Pyridoxal phosphate, Melatonin, Depression, Sleep-wake cycle

Tryptophan is one of the eight essential amino acids required for the synthesis of cellular proteins. In addition to preventing niacin deficiency, tryptophan is the precursor for the synthesis of neurotransmitter, serotonin (5-HT), involved in relaxation, restfulness, and sleep. Tryptophan as an essential amino acid is the precursor of serotonin, melatonin, and niacin required for regulating mood and sleep-wake cycle. A small amount of the tryptophan from our diet (3%) is converted to niacin (vitamin B_3) which prevents the symptoms of niacin deficiency when dietary intake of vitamin is reduced. Niacin deficiency causes pellagra associated with diarrhea, dementia, dermatitis, and death. Tryptophan serves as a precursor for the synthesis of serotonin, which regulates appetite, sleep, and mood. Tryptophan has been used therapeutically in the treatment of depression, insomnia, and anxiety because it raises CNS serotonin levels. Many antidepressants improve mood by augmenting brain serotonin synthesis. Serotonin is involved in controlling appetite. The antidepressants can attenuate the appetite control of serotonin, hence are associated with an uncontrolled appetite and, eventually, weight gain. For patients on antidepressants, common weight loss strategies like keeping a food log, exercise, or trying a low-carb/high protein diet are less effective because these strategies do not address the fundamental issues of controlling appetite. However it is possible to raise brain regional serotonin by eating healthy foods. Carbohydrates allow brain to produce more serotonin which controls appetite. Wurtman showed that when carbohydrates are eaten and insulin is released into the bloodstream, serotonin synthesis is augmented. The "comfort foods" facilitate in making feel good and satisfying appetite. Grilled chicken and steamed broccoli, while delicious and healthy, are not the foods when we get food cravings or feel stressed. Mashed potatoes, oatmeal with brown sugar, pizza may be avoided. The problem with cutting down carbohydrates is that appetite becomes uncontroled and those eating the wrong carbohydrates, loaded with fat, feel sluggish and add undesirable calories. Levels of serotonin decline by afternoon and evening. So one should aim to eat carbohydrates like whole wheat pasta with vegetables for dinner, a granola bar as a late afternoon snack and protein-packed breakfasts and lunches during the day. With antidepressants, we can control appetite and lose weight. Gracida et al., (2013) reported that animals can thrive on variable food resources as a result of beneficial relationships with their gut microbes. Food intake elicits physiological changes, which are counteracted by systemic responses that maintain homeostasis in the organism. This integration of information occurs through nuclear receptors which modulate gene expression in response to specific cues. Given the importance of germline stem cells (GSCs), it is logical to assume that GSCs might be shielded from the negative influence of environmental perturbations. In the Caenorhabditis elegans somatic activity of the nuclear receptor nhr-114/HNF4 protects GSC integrity from dietary metabolites. In the absence of nhr-114 and on certain bacterial diets, normal animals accumulate germ cell division defects during development and become sterile. In nhr-114(-) animals, the induction of germline defects and sterility depend on bacterial metabolism with the tryptophan. These findings provide an animal-microbe interaction where nuclear receptor activity preserves the germline by buffering dietary metabolites, through a detoxifying response. These findings highlight evolutionarily-conserved, soma-to-germline axis that maintains reproductive intactness on variable foods.

Tryptophan and Maternal Undernutrition. It is known that maternal undernutrition programs metabolic adaptations are detrimental to adult. Nascimento et al., (2013) supplied L-tryptophan to manipulate the long-term sequelae of early-life programming by undernutrition and explored whether cultured cells acquire circadian clock dysregulation. Male rat pups from mothers fed on low protein (8%, LP) or control (18%, CP) diet were given, one hour before light off, an oral L-tryptophan (125 mg/kg) between Day-12 and Day-21 of age. Body weight, food intake, blood glucose along with the capacity of colonization of primary cells from biopsies were measured during the young (45-55 days) and adult (110-130 days) phases. Circadian oscillations were induced by a serum shock over 30 hours on near-confluent cell monolayers to follow PERIOD1 and CLOCK proteins by ELISA and period1 and bmal1 mRNA by RT-PCR. Cell survival in amino acid-free conditions were used to measure expression of MAP-LC3B, MAP-LC3B-FP and Survivin. Tryptophan did not alter body weight gain nor feeding pattern. The blood glucose sampling time was found significant during all phases. A significant interaction between Tryptophan, saline and diets (LP, CP) were found during young and adult phases. In adult phase, the capacity of colonization at seeding of primary cells was twice lower for LP rats. ANOVA of PERIOD1 perinuclear/nuclear immunoreactivity during young phase, found a significant effect of diets daily bolus and synchronizer hours. MAP-LC3B, MAP-LC3B-FP and Survivin were altered according to diets during young age. The early-life undernutrition and the effects of L-tryptophan can be monitored by circadian sampling of blood glucose and on the expression of PERIOD1 protein in primary cell lines. It was demonstrated that an increasing demand for calcium during pregnancy and lactation can result in both clinical and subclinical hypocalcemia during the early lactation period in the dairy cows.

Serotonin (5-HT) has been identified as a regulator of lactation and bone turnover. Laporta et al., (2013) determined whether supplementation of the diet with a 5-HT precursor would increase maternal bone turnover and calcium mobilization to maintain appropriate circulating concentrations of ionized calcium during lactation. Female Sprague-Dawley rats were fed either a control diet or a diet supplemented with the 5-HT precursor 5-hydroxytryptophan (5-HTP) from day 13 of pregnancy through day 9 of lactation. Maternal serum and plasma (day 1 and day 9 of lactation), milk and pup weight (daily), mammary gland and bone tissue (day 9 of lactation) were collected for analysis. The 5-HTP diet elevated circulating 5-HT on day 1 and day 9 of lactation and parathyroid hormone related-protein (PTHrP) on day 9 of lactation. In addition, 5-HTP increased total serum calcium concentrations on day 1 of lactation and milk calcium concentration on day 9 of lactation. Supplementation of 5-HTP did not alter milk yield, body weight, mammary gland structure, or pup litter weights. 5-HTP also increased concentrations of mammary 5-HT and PTHrP, as well as mRNA expressions of tryptophan hydroxylase 1 and Pthrp on day 9 of lactation. 5-HTP increased mRNA expression of mammary calcium transporters and resorption of bone in the femur, indicated by increase osteoclast number and diameter as well as mRNA expression of biomarkers of bone resorption on day 9 of lactation suggesting that increasing 5-HT biosynthesis during the transition from pregnancy to lactation could be a potential therapeutic target for the prevention of hypocalcemia associated with severe depression.

Valproic acid (VPA) is a short-chained, branched fatty acid that is generally used as an anticonvulsant and mood stabilizer, and increases the liver nicotinamide (NAD) concentration. Shibata et al., (2013) investigated the effects of VPA on the conversion of tryptophan to nicotinamide. Rats were fed diets containing VPA (0, 0.5, and 1.0% in the diets) for 14 d; 24-h urine samples were collected, and tryptophan and its catabolites were measured. The conversion of tryptophan to NAD was increased by feeding a diet containing VPA. During the conversion of tryptophan to NAD, the tryptophan to 3-hydroxyanthranilic acid step was not affected by the administration of VPA, while metabolites as quinolinic acid, NAD, and its catabolites were increased. Furthermore, Coppola et al., (2013) described association of branched-chain amino acids (BCAA) and aromatic amino acids (AAA) with obesity and insulin resistance. These authors investigated the impact of BCAA on behavioral activity. Supplementation of either a high-sucrose or a high-fat diet with BCAA induced anxiety-like behavior in rats. These behavioral changes were associated with decreased tryptophan (Trp) and serotonin in brain tissues without any difference in the synaptic serotonin function. The anxiety-like behavior and decreased Trp in the brain of BCAA-fed rats were reversed by Trp but not by fluoxetine, a selective serotonin reuptake inhibitor, suggesting that the behavioral changes are independent of the serotonergic pathway of Trp metabolism. Instead, BCAA lowered the brain Trp-derived metabolite, kynurenic acid, and these levels were normalized by Trp, suggesting that high-energy diets with BCAA cause neurobehavioral impairment. Elevation of BCAA in obesity, suggests a potential mechanism for explaining the association of obesity and mood disorders.

Depression is a common disorder in elderly, especially in those institutionalized. Nutrition could play a pivotal role in the onset and/or progression of depression, since the intake of carbohydrates with a high glycemic index (GI) or diets with a high glycemic load (GL) may increase the insulin-induced brain serotonin secretion. The brain serotonin (5-HT) and dopamine (DA) play a crucial role in behavioral and neuroendocrine responses to challenges, and comparative models suggest common mechanisms for dietary modulation of transmission by these signaling molecules in vertebrates. Previous studies in teleosts demonstrate that 7 d of dietary administration with L-tryptophan (Trp), suppresses the endocrine stress response. Basic et al., (2013) investigated how long the suppressive effects of a Trp-enriched feed regimen, at doses corresponding to two, three or four times the Trp levels in commercial diet, last in juvenile Atlantic cod (Gadus morhua) when these are reintroduced to a diet with standard amino acid composition. These authors also explored Trp induced changes in brain monoaminergic system in the forebrain structures innervated by DA and 5-HTergic neurons, by measuring DA and 5-HT in the lateral pallial regions (Dl) of the telencephalon and nucleus lateralis tuberis (NLT) of the hypothalamus. Dietary Trp caused a dose-dependent suppression in plasma cortisol among fish exposed to confinement stress on the first day following experimental diet; however, such an effect was not observed at 2 or 6 d after Trp treatment. Feeding the fish with moderate Trp increased DA and 5-HT-ergic activity, suggesting that these neural circuits within the NLT and Dl may be involved in regulating the acute stress response.

Dysregulation of the stress axis is a hallmark of MDD in human patients. However, it remains unknown how glucocorticoid signaling is linked to affective disorders. Ziv et al., (2013) recently reported that upon binding to cortisol, the glucocorticoid receptor (GR) regulates the transcription of specific target genes, including those that encode the stress hormones corticotropin-releasing hormone (CRH) and adrenocorticotropic hormone (ACTH). These researchers used a zebrafish mutant in which the negative feedback on the stress response was disrupted, due to abolition of transcriptional activity of GR. As a consequence, cortisol was elevated, but unable to signal through GR. When placed into an aquarium, mutant fish became immobile, demonstrated reduced exploratory behavior and did not habituate to this stressor upon repeated exposure. Addition of the antidepressant fluoxetine in the water and social interactions restored normal behavior, followed by correction of cortisol levels. Fluoxetine did not affect the transcription of CRH, the mineralocorticoid receptor (MR), the serotonin transporter (Serta) or GR. However, it suppressed the stress-induced upregulation of MR and Serta in both wild-type fish and mutants, suggesting a protective role of glucocorticoid signaling in the regulation of behavior and molecular mechanism of how chronic stress influences neurophysiology and behavior. Hence the zebrafish may be used as a high-throughput drug screening model for the development of new classes of antidepressants.

Serotonin and Depression. Serotonergic medications can mitigate the negative affective biases in disorders such as depression or anxiety, however the basic neural mechanism remains unknown. In line with recent advances demonstrating that negative affective biases may be driven by specific medial prefrontal-amygdala circuitry, Robinson et al., (2013) investigated whether serotonin manipulation can alter affective processing within dorsal medial prefrontal-amygdala circuit: the human homologue of the rodent prelimbic-amygdala circuit or 'aversive amplification' circuit. The subjects performed a forced-choice face identification task with word distractors in an fMRI scanner over two separate sessions. On one session subjects received dietary depletion of the tryptophan while on the other session they received a balanced diet. Dorsal medial prefrontal response was elevated in response to fearful relative to happy faces under depletion but not placebo. The negative bias was accompanied by increase in positive dorsal medial prefrontal-amygdala functional connectivity suggesting that serotonin depletion engages prefrontal-amygdala circuit during fearful processing relative to happy face stimuli. The same 'aversive amplification' circuit was also engaged during anxiety induced by shock anticipation, suggesting that serotonergic projections may inhibit engagement of the 'aversive amplification' circuit and dysfunction in this projection may contribute to the negative affective bias in mood and anxiety disorders. These findings thus provided an explanation for the role of serotonin and serotonergic medications in the neurocircuitry of negative affective bias.

Recently we reported that depression causes severe symptoms for several weeks, and dysthymia, which may cause chronic, low-grade symptoms (Shabbir et al., 2013). Treatment of depression involves psychotherapy, medications, or phototherapy. Clinical and experimental evidence indicates that an appropriate diet can reduce symptoms of depression. The neurotransmitter, serotonin (5-HT), synthesized in the brain, plays an important role in mood alleviation, satiety, and sleep regulation. Although certain fruits and vegetables are rich in 5-HT, it is not easily accessible to the CNS due to blood brain barrier. However the serotonin precursor, tryptophan, can readily pass through the blood brain barrier. Tryptophan is converted to 5-HT by tryptophan hydroxylase and 5-HTP decarboxylase, respectively, in the presence of pyridoxal phosphate, derived from vitamin B_6. Hence diets poor in tryptophan may induce depression as this essential amino acid is naturally less abundant even in protein-rich foods. Hence tryptophan-rich diet is essential in patients susceptible to depression such as certain females during pre and postmenstrual phase, post-traumatic stress disorder, chronic pain, cancer, epilepsy, PD, AD, schizophrenia, and drug addiction. Carbohydrate-rich diet triggers insulin response to enhance the bioavailability of tryptophan in the CNS which is responsible for increased craving of carbohydrate diets. Although selective serotonin reuptake inhibitors (SSRIs) are prescribed to obese patients with depressive symptoms, these are incapable of precisely regulating the CNS serotonin and may cause life-threatening adverse effects in the presence of monoamine oxidase inhibitors such as Selegiline, Raslgine, Tranylcypromine, and Phenalzine. However, CNS serotonin synthesis can be controlled by proper intake of tryptophan-rich diet. We highlighted the clinical significance of tryptophan-rich diet and vitamin B_6 to enhance serotonergic neurotransmission in depression in various neurodegenerative diseases. However pharmacological interventions to modulate serotonergic neurotransmission in depression, remains clinically significant. Several other molecular mechanisms may be involved in the etiopathogenesis of depression about which very limited information as yet available.

Serotonergic Antidepressants and Body weight Both chronic stress and antidepressant medications have been associated with changes in body weight. In a study, mechanisms by which stress and antidepressants interact to affect meal patterns were investigated. Kumar et al., (2013) subjected mice to the chronic social defeat stress model of major depression followed by fluoxetine treatment and analyzed food intake using metabolic cages. Chronic social defeat stress increased food intake, an effect that was reversed by fluoxetine treatment. To determine mechanism involved in alterations in meal patterning induced by stress and fluoxetine, fasting serum samples were collected every 4h over a 24-h period, and acyl-ghrelin, leptin, and corticosterone levels were estimated. Chronic stress induced a peak in acyl-ghrelin prior to the onset of the dark phase, which was shifted in mice treated with fluoxetine suggesting that stress increases food intake by decreasing satiation which can reverse changes in meal patterns.

Melatonin and Depression. Chrononutrition is a field that establishes consuming foods at times of the day when they are more useful for health, improvement, biorhythms, and physical performance. Melatonin and serotonin rhythms, which exhibit a close association with the endogenous circadian component of sleep, are attenuated with increasing age. This decrease is linked to sleep alterations in the elderly. Bravo et al., (2013) analyzed whether the consumption of cereals rich in tryptophan, the precursor of both serotonin and melatonin, may help in the regulation of the sleep/wake cycle and counteract depression and anxiety in 35 middle-aged/elderly (aged 55-75 year) volunteers. These investigators collected data for 3 weeks. The control participants consumed cereals (22.5 mg tryptophan in 30 g cereals per dose) at breakfast and dinner; for the treatment, cereals enriched with a higher dose of tryptophan (60 mg tryptophan in 30 g cereals per dose) were eaten at both breakfast and dinner; the post treatment volunteers consumed usual diet. Each participant wore a wrist actimeter that logged activity during the whole experiment. Urine was collected to analyze melatonin and serotonin metabolites to measure total antioxidant capacity. The intake of cereals containing the higher dose in tryptophan increased sleep efficiency, actual sleep time, immobile time, and decreased total nocturnal activity, sleep fragmentation index, and sleep latency. Urinary 6-sulfatoxymelatonin, 5-HIAA levels, and antioxidant capacity also increased after tryptophan-enriched cereal ingestion improving symptoms of anxiety and depression. Hence cereals enriched with tryptophan may be useful as a chrononutrition for alterations in the sleep/wake cycle. Recently Agomelatine as an antidepressant has been developed which acts as an MT1/MT2 melatonin receptor agonist/5-HT2C serotonin receptor antagonist. Agomelatine resolves the abnormalities of circadian rhythms associated with mood disorders, including abnormalities of the sleep/wake cycle. Mairesse et al., (2013) examined the effect of chronic Agomelatine treatment on sleep architecture and circadian rhythms of motor activity using prenatal restraint stress (PRS) as a model of depression. PRS was delivered to the mothers during the last 10 d of pregnancy. The adult progeny ('PRS rats') showed a reduced duration of slow wave sleep, an increased duration of rapid eye movement (REM) sleep, an increased number of REM sleep events and motor activity before the beginning of the dark phase of the light/dark cycle. In addition, adult PRS rats showed an increased expression of *c-Fos*, in the hippocampus prior to the beginning of the dark phase. These changes were reversed by Agomelatine. The effect of Agomelatine on sleep was attenuated by treatment with the MT1/MT2 melatonin receptor antagonist, S22153, which caused PRS-like sleep disturbances. These data provided the evidence that Agomelatine corrects sleep architecture and restores circadian homeostasis in depression and supports its therapeutic potential as a novel antidepressant that resynchronizes circadian rhythms under pathological conditions.

Clinical Symptoms of Tryptophan Deficiency In general, the dietary deficiency of tryptophan can cause protein deficiency symptoms, including weight loss and impaired growth in infants and children. Tryptophan deficiency may lead to reduced serotonin synthesis associated with depression, anxiety, irritability, impatience, impulsiveness, inability to concentrate, weight gain, hyperphagia, carbohydrate cravings, poor dream recall, and insomnia. Tryptophan deficiency along with niacin deficiency in the diet can also cause pellagra, characterized by: *Dementia, Diarrhea, Dermatitis, & Death as discussed above.* However pellagra is rare in the US and may not occur simply because of only tryptophan deficiency.

Toxicity Symptoms. Increased dietary intake of tryptophan is unknown to cause any overt clinical symptoms of toxicity. Tryptophan has been given therapeutically as a prescription or dietary supplementation in doses exceeding 5 g per day with no adverse effects. However in 1989, its use was blamed for the development of eosinophilia-myalgia syndrome (EMS), which caused muscle and joint pain, fever, weakness, swelling of arms and legs, shortness of breath in >1000 people, In addition, >30 deaths were attributed to EMS caused by tryptophan supplements. Although it was discovered that the EMS was caused by a contaminant in one batch of tryptophan and occurred only in small number of susceptible individuals, the FDA announced that high doses of tryptophan were unsafe. Since 1989, tryptophan has not been available as a dietary supplement in the US. Hence tolerable upper limit (TUL) for tryptophan intake has not yet been established.

Factors Affecting Deficiency of Tryptophan. Vitamin B6 is required for the conversion of tryptophan to both niacin and serotonin. Hence dietary deficiency of vitamin B6 may result in reduced serotonin levels and/or impaired conversion of tryptophan to niacin. Various dietary, lifestyle, and health factors reduce the conversion of tryptophan to serotonin, including cigarette smoking, high sugar intake, and alcohol abuse, excessive intake of protein, hypoglycemia, and diabetes.

Effect of Cooking, Storage, and Processing. No report on the deleterious effects of cooking, storage, or processing on tryptophan levels in food is available.

Nutrient Interactions. It is known that vitamin B_6, vitamin C, folic acid, and magnesium are required for the normal metabolism of tryptophan. In addition, tyrosine and phenylalanine compete with tryptophan for the intestinal absorption. Therefore some physicians believe that food sources of tryptophan does not cause significant increase in blood levels to produce therapeutic results, and that tryptophan may be taken as a supplement to increase circulating levels. Anxiety, depression, headaches, insomnia, nightmare, obesity, obsessive/compulsive disorders, pain, premenstrual syndrome, senile dementia, and Tourette's syndrome may require tryptophan supplementation.

Food Sources of Tryptophan. Tryptophan occurs in all most all natural foods that contain protein, but in small amounts compared to the other essential amino acids. *Red meat, dairy products, nuts, seeds, legumes, soybeans and soy products, tuna, shellfish, and turkey are particularly rich sources of tryptophan.*

Nutrient Rating Chart. In order to identify foods that contain a high concentration of nutrients for the calories, a Food rating system has been created by the *George Meteljan Foundation (whfoods.org)* as follows. The world's healthiest foods are excellent, very good, or good sources of tryptophan with FDA guidelines as illustrated below:

Healthiest Foods as Quality Sources of Tryptophan

Food	Serving Size	Cals	Amount(G)	DV%	Nutrient Density	Food Rating
Chicken	4 oz wt	187.1	0.41	128.12	12.3	Excellent
Soybeans	1 Cup Coked	297.6	0.39	121.9	7.4	Excellent
Turkey	4 Onz	153.1	0.38	118.75	14	Excellent
Tuna	4 Onz	153.1	0.38	118.75	13.6	Excellent
Salmon	4 Onz	244.9	0.35	109.38	8	Excellent
Lamb	4 Onz	229.1	0.35	109.38	8.6	Excellent
Halibut	4 Onz	158.8	0.34	106.25	12	Excellent
Shrimp	4 onz	112.3	0.33	103.25	16.5	Excellent
Cod	4 onz	119.3	0.29	90.62	13.7	Excellent
Sardines	3.20 onz	188.7	0.25	78.12	7.5	Excellent
Tofu	4 onz	86.2	0.14	43.75	9.1	Excellent
Spinach	1 cup	41.4	0.07	21.8	9.5	Excellent
Asparagus raw	1 cup	26.8	0.04	12.5	8.4	Excellent

Healthiest Foods as Quality Sources of Tryptophan

Food	Serving Size	Cals	Amount(G)	DV%	Nutrient Density	Food Rating
Chicken	4 oz wt	187.10	0.41	128.12	12.3	Excellent
Soybeans	1 Cup Coked	297.6	0.39	121.90	7.4	Excellent
Turkey	4 Onz	153.1	0.38	118.75	14.0	Excellent
Tuna	4 Onz	153.1	0.38	118.75	13.6	Excellent
Salmon	4 Onz	244.9	0.35	109.38	8.0	Excellent
Lamb	4 Onz	229.1	0.35	109.38	8.6	Excellent
Halibut	4 Onz	158.8	0.34	106.25	12.0	Excellent
Shrimp	4 onz	112.3	0.33	103.25	16.5	Excellent
Cod	4 onz	119.3	0.29	90.62	13.7	Excellent
Sardines	3.20 onz	188.7	0.25	78.12	7.5	Excellent
Tofu	4 onz	86.2	0.14	43.75	9.1	Excellent
Spinach Cooked	1 cup	41.4	0.07	21.8	9.5	Excellent
Asparagus raw	1 cup	26.8	0.04	12.50	8.4	Excellent
Dried peas	1 cup	231.3	0.18	56.25	4.4	Very Good
Kidneys	1 cup	224.5	0.18	56.25	4.1	Very Good

Beans					
Pinto Beans 1cup	254.5	0.18	56.25	4.0	Very Good
Navy Beans 1 Cup	254. 8	0.18	56.25	41.	Very Good
Black Beans 1 Cup	227.0	0.18	56.25	4.5	Very Good
Lima Beans 1 cup	216.2	0.17	53.12	4.4	Very Good
Pumpkins 0.25 cup Seeds	180.3	0.17	53.12	4.4	Very Good
Lentils 1 cup	229.7	0.16	50.0	3.9	Very Good
Wheat 1 cup Cooked	151.1	0.09	28.12	3.4	Very Good
Cow's Milk 4 onz	74.4	0.09	28.12	6.8	Very Good
Eggs 1 each	77.5	0.08	25.00	5.9	Very Good
Cheese 28.35 g	114.2	0.08	25.00	3.9	Very Good
Collard 1 cup Greens	49.4	0.05	15.62	5.7	Very Good
Meso 1tbs	34.2	0.03	9.38	4.9	Very good
Turnip © 1 cup	35.0	0.03	9.38	15.6	Very Good
Soy Sauce 1 ts	10.8	0.03	9.38	4.9	Very Good
Swiss 1 cp Chard Cooked	35.0	0.03	9.38	4.8	Very Good
Brussels 1cup Sprouts	37.8	0.03	9.38	8.0	Very Good
Mustard 1cup Green	21.0	0.03	9.38	4.5	Very Good
Brocolli 1cup	30.9	0.03	9.38	5.5	Very Good
Kale 1 cup	36.4	0.03	9.38	4.6	Very Good
Cauliflower 1 cup	26.8	0.02	6.25	4.2	Very Good
Geen Beans 1cup	31.0	0.02	6.25	3.6	Very Good
Garbanzo Bean 1 cup	269	0.14	43.75	2.9	Good
Barley 270	0.12		37.50	2.5	Good
Sesame 0.25 cup	206.3	0.12	37.50	3.3	Good
Sunflower 0.25	204.4	0.10	31.25	2.8	Good
Cashews 0.25 cup	189.5	0.09	28.12	2.7	Good
Peanuts 0.25 cup	206. 9	0.09	28.12	2.4	Good
Buckwehat 1 cup	154.6	0.08	25.0	2.9	Good
Almonds 0.25 cup	206	0.07	21.8	1.9	Good
Yogurt 1 cup	154.3	0.07	21.88	2.6	Good
Millet 1 cup	207.1	0.07	21.88	1.9	Good
Quinoa 42.5 g	156.4	0.07	21.88	2.50	Good
Potatoes 1 each	160.9	0.07	21.8	2.4	Good
Rye 1 each	188.5	0.07	18.7	1.8	Good
Brown Rice 1 cup	216.4	0.06	18.75	1.8	Good
Green Pea 1cup c	115.7	0.05	15.62	2.7	Good
Sweet peas 1cup c	102.6	0.05	15.60	2.7	Good
Flax seed 2 tbs	74.8	0.04	12.50	3.0	Good
Winter Squash 1 cup	75.8	0.03	9.38	2.2	Good
Beets 1 cup	58.5	0.03	9.38	2.9	Good

(Continued)

Onions	1cup	64	0.02	6.25	1.8	Good
Basil	2tsp	7.0	0.01	3.12	8.0	Good
Apricot	1 each	16.8	0.01	3.12	3.3	Good
Bell pepper	1cup	28.5	0.01	3.12	2.0	Good
Romaine Lettuce	2 cups	16.0	0.01	3.14	3.5	Good
Celery	1cp	16.2	0.01	3.12	3.5	Good
Oregano	2tsp	9.5	0.01	3.12	5.9	Good
Mustard seed	2 tsp	20.3	0.01	3.12	2.8	Good
Cucumber	1cup	15.6	0.01	3.12	3.6	Good
Garlic	1oz	26.8	0.01	3.12	2.1	Good
Plum	1 each	30.4	0.01	3.12	1.9	Good
Eggplant	1 cup	19.7	0.01	3.12	2.9	Good
Thyme	1cup	7.7	0.01	3.12	7.3	Good
Summer Squash	1 cup	18.1	0.01	3.12	3.1	Good
Cabbage	1cup	17.5	0.01	3.12	3.2	Good
Sea Vege	0.25	8.6	0.01	3.12	6.5	Good
Tomatoes	1cup	32.4	0.01	3.12	1.7	Good

Healthiest Food Rating

Excellent	DV>=75% or,Density >=7.6 and DV>=10%
Very Good	DV>=50% Or,Density>=3.4 and DV >=5%
Good	DV>=25%, Density>=1.5% and DV>=2.5%

Health Recommendations for Tryptophan. The National Academy of Sciences (NAS) has established a general principle for tryptophan intake. All individuals 1 year of age or greater consume 7 mg tryptophan/gram of food protein. The recommendation for each age and gender group, assuming RDA-level protein intake for each group:

S.No	Subjects	Age	Tryptophan (mg)
1	Children	1-3 years	91
2	Children	4-8 Years	133
3	Males	9-13 Years	238
4	Males	14-18 Years	322
5	Males	19 Years or Older	392
6	Felames	9-13 Years	238
7	Females	14 Years	322
8	Pregnant or Lactating female		497

Source: The Dietary Reference Intakes for Energy, Carbohydrate, Fiber, Fat, Fatty Acids, Cholesterol, Protein, and Amino Acids (Macronutrients), National Academies Press, 2005.

Tryptophan-Rich Foods to alleviate Depression

Milk and milk products (Yogurt, Soy Milk); **Meat** (Mutton, Venison, Beef Liver, Calf liver, Chicken Breast, Turkey Breast; **Fish** (Halibut, Cod Tjuna, Shrimp, Meackerel, Salmon, Snapperm Scallops; **Cheese:** Cheddar processed cheese, cottage cheese, Tofu, Gruyere; **Fruits:** Apples, Bannas, Blue Berries, Strawberries, Avocados, Pine aple, Peaches; **Vegetables**: Spinach, mustard greens, asparagus, Eggplant, Winter Squash, Green peas, kelp, broccoli, onions, tomatoes, cabbage, cauliflower, mushrooms, cucumber, potatoes; **Nuts:** Walnuts, peanuts, cashews, pistachios, chestnuts, almonds; **Seeds:** Ground flax, season, pumpkin, fenugreek, sunflower seeds (Roasted); **Legumes:** Mung beans, soybeans, kidneys beans, lima beans, chick peas; **Grains:** Wheat, Brown rice, red rice, barely, corn, oats. Tryptophan in food is protein-bound and is not freely available.

Tryptophan Content per 100 g of Food

Food	Total Protein	Tryptophan	Tryptophan% of Protein
Soybeans	36.50%	590 mg	1.60%
Sugar-free	19.60%	283 mg	1.50%
Coca Powder	19.60%	283 mg	1.50%
Cashews	18.20%	287 mg	1.60%
Raw Chicken Breast	21.20%	267 mg	1.30%
Dried peas	24..6%	266 mg	1.10%
Raw Pork	21%	220 mg	1.10%
Raw Salmon	20.40%	209 mg	1%
Oats	13.20%	182 mg	1.40%
Walnuts	15.20%	170 mg	1.10%
Chicken eggs	12.60%	167 mg	1.30%
Brown Rice	7.90%	101 mg	1,3%
Corn flour	6.90%	49 mg	0.70%
Cow Milk	3.30%	46 mg	1.40%

Generally adult consumes 3.5-6 mg of L-tryptophan/Kg of body weight/day. There is variation of how much a particular individual will require. This will depend on the sources of diet with different tryptophan content. Deficiency of tryptophan can induce liver damage or inflammatory GI disorders, limiting the ability to absorb the nutrients properly particularly in aging. As described earlier, tryptophan is an essential amino acid that plays crucial role in the synthesis of serotonin (5-HT). Tryptophan is a precursor of 5-HTP or serotonin which is obtained from the dietary sources. Tryptophan in the presence of coenzyme, pyridoxal phosphate, transforms into serotonin and niacin in the liver to improve blood circulation, enhance memory, and lower cholesterol, making it an essential amino acid to improve overall health. Vitamin B_6 (pyridoxine) is converted to pyridoxal by an enzyme pyridoxine oxidase, whereas pyidoxal is converted to pyridoxal phosphate (PLP) by an enzyme, pyridoxal kinase. Pyridoxal phosphate (PLP) serves as a coenzyme for the decarboxylation of several CNS neurotransmitters including serotonin, dopamine, and GABA, involved in mood regulation.

Benefits of Tryptophan-Rich Diet

Sleep. Generally sleep aids contain tryptophan as 1g of tryptophan can increase sleep and decreases the amount of time it requires to fall asleep. Patients with insomnia experience improvement in asleep duration when they increase their tryptophan intake.

Premenstrual Syndrome. (PMS) can cause physical, mental, and emotional symptoms that can be resolved by consuming 6 mg doses of tryptophan/day which is helpful in alleviating mood during the period before the menstrual cycle.

Seasonal Affective Disorder. This disorder causes symptoms of depression during winter. These symptoms are consistent. Consuming 3 g of tryptophan for two weeks can reduce depression.

Depression and Anxiety. As tryptophan is essential for providing with adequate levels of serotonin; those who do not get adequate tryptophan in their diet may be prone to depression. Increasing dietary tryptophan can improve symptoms of depression without potential side effects associated with antidepressants.

Clinical Application of Tryptophan. Consuming tryptophan may improve the effectiveness of antidepressant drugs. Additional 2-5 g of tryptophan/day can improve the symptoms of fluoxetine without increasing the tryptophan dose.

Increasing Tryptophan Levels. Tryptophan deficiency can lead to weight loss in children and infants and pellagra that can occur by concomitant vitamin B-3 deficiency, which can be caused by malnutrition or alcoholism. Pellagra causes a defect that limits the body's ability to convert tryptophan into niacin leading to mental disorders, erythema, GIT disturbances, and neurological disorders. A drop in serotonin levels may cause difficulty concentrating, irritability, and mood swings (anxiety and depression). To alleviate these symptoms we can increase foods rich in tryptophan, by consuming those foods or by consulting the physician about tryptophan supplements. Consuming tryptophan-rich diet causes insulin release that clears other amino acids from the system so that the brain can easily access tryptophan. Hence consuming tryptophan-rich diet can improve serotonin and niacin levels to relax, sleep, and regulate appetite. Moreover tryptophan-rich diets regulate appetite, sleep, and alleveate mood.

Clinical Conditions Requiring more Tryptophan There are several clinical conditions which require increased levels of tryptophan such as depression, anxiety, irritability, impatience, impulsive behavior, inability to concentrate, weight gain, or unexpected weight loss (anorexia nervosa), retarded growth in children, overeating and or carbohydrate cravings (bulimia), poor dream recall, and insomnia. *The important food sources of tryptophan include red meat, dairy products, nuts, seeds, legumes, soybeans products, tuna, shellfish, and turkey as presented below*:

Tryptophan-Rich Foods		(Healthiest Foods)
Food	Cals	% Daily Value
Chicken	187	128%
Soybeans	298	121.80%
Turkey	153	118.80%
Tuna	158	118.70%
Lamb	129	109.30%
Sardines	245	109.30%
Halibut	159	106.20%
Shrimp	112	103.10%
Cod	119	90.60%
Sardines	189	78.10%

The Nutrient Rating Chart may be referred to determine the serving size (Source: www.Med-Health.Net.).

References

Basic, D; Schjolden, J; Krogdahl, A; von Krogh, K; Hillestad, M; Winberg, S; Mayer, I; Skjerve, E; Höglund; E. (2013) Changes in regional brain monoaminergic activity and temporary down-regulation in stress response from dietary supplementation with l-tryptophan in Atlantic cod (Gadus morhua)., *Br J Nutr.* 109, 2166-2174.

Bravo, R; Matito, S; Cubero, J; Paredes, S.D; Franco, L; Rivero, M; Rodríguez, A.B; Barriga, C. (2013) Tryptophan-enriched cereal intake improves nocturnal sleep, melatonin, serotonin, and total antioxidant capacity levels and mood in elderly humans., *Age (Dordr).* 35, 1277-1285.

Coppola, A; Wenner, B.R; Ilkayeva, O; Stevens, R.D; Maggioni, M; Slotkin, T.A; Levin, E.D; Newgard, C.B. (2013) Branched-chain amino acids alter neurobehavioral function in rats., *Am J Physiol Endocrinol Metab.* 304, E405-413.

Gracida, X; Eckmann, C.R. (2013) Fertility and germline stem cell maintenance under different diets requires nhr-114/HNF4 in C. elegans., *Curr Biol.* 23, 607-613.

Kumar, J; Chuang, J.C; Na, E.S; Kuperman, A; Gillman, A.G; Mukherjee, S; Zigman, J.M; McClung, C.A; Lutter, M. (2013) Differential effects of chronic social stress and fluoxetine on meal patterns in mice., *Appetite.* 64; 81-88.

Laporta, J; Peters, T.L; Weaver, S.R; Merriman, K.E; Hernandez, LL. (2013) Feeding 5-hydroxy-l-tryptophan during the transition from pregnancy to lactation increases calcium mobilization from bone in rats., *Domest Anim Endocrinol.* 44, 176-184.

Mairesse, J; Silletti, V; Laloux, C; Zuena, A.R; Giovine, A; Consolazione, M; van Camp, G; Malagodi, M; Gaetani, S; Cianci, S; Catalani, A; Mennuni, G; Mazzetta, A; van Reeth, O; Gabriel, C; Mocaër, E; Nicoletti, F; Morley-Fletcher, S; Maccari, S. (2013) Chronic agomelatine treatment corrects the abnormalities in the circadian rhythm of motor activity and sleep/wake cycle induced by prenatal restraint stress in adult rats., *Int J Neuropsychopharmacol.* 16, 323-338.

Nascimento E, Guzman-Quevedo O, Delacourt N, da Silva Aragão R, Perez-Garcia G, de Souza SL, Manhães-de-Castro R, Bolaños-Jiménez F,Kaeffer B. Long-lasting effect of perinatal exposure to L-tryptophan on circadian clock of primary cell lines established from male offspring born from mothers fed on dietary protein restriction. PLoS One. 2013;8(2):e56231.

Robinson, O.J; Overstreet, C; Allen, P.S; Letkiewicz, A; Vytal, K; Pine, D.S; Grillon, C. (2013) The role of serotonin in the neurocircuitry of negative affective bias: serotonergic modulation of the dorsal medial prefrontal-amygdala 'aversive amplification' circuit., *Neuroimage.* 78, 217-223.

Shabbir, F; Patel, A; Mattison, C; Bose, S; Krishnamohan, R; Sweeney, E; Sandhu, S; Nel, W; Rais, A; Sandhu, R; Ngu, N; Sharma, S. (2013) Effect of diet on serotonergic neurotransmission in depression., *Neurochemistry International.*, Volume 62, 324-329.

Shibata, K; Kondo, R; Sano, M; Fukuwatari, T. (2013) Increased conversion of tryptophan to nicotinamide in rats by dietary valproate., *Biosci Biotechnol Biochem.* 77, 295-300.

Ziv, L; Muto, A; Schoonheim, P.J; Meijsing, S.H; Strasser, D; Ingraham, H.A; Schaaf, M.J; Yamamoto, K.R; Baier, H. (2013) An affective disorder in zebrafish with mutation of the glucocorticoid receptor. *Mol Psychiatry.* 18, 681-691.

Chapter 4

Natural Diets and Depression

Abstract

There are several foods which contain flavonoids as antioxidants. The antioxidants serve as free radical scavengers. In addition fruits and vegetables are rich sources of B vitamins including folate and B_{12}. Mediterrean diet utilizes olive oil and fish those are rich in omega-3 PUFA, including eicosapentanoic acid (EPA), and docosaheptanoic acid (DHA). However, augmenting intake of certain essential nutrients may help prevent depression, alleviate symptoms, and/or improve the effectiveness of antidepressant medication. There are numerous options for the alleviation of depression from the natural sources. The healthy lifestyle, diet, digestive and psychological causes are highly significant for long-term benefit. Using St. John's wort, saffron, 5-hydrotryptophan (5-HTP) or S-adenosyl methionine (SAMe) can be effective as a part of recovering from depression. In this chapter, natural diets have been described with their beneficial effect due to their antioxidant, anti-inflammatory, and anti-apoptotic properties in alleviating depression. In addition, major side effects of antidepressants are described.

Keywords: Flavonoids, Antioxidants, Omega-3 Polyunsaturated fatty acids (n-3 PUFA), Saint John's wort, 5-HTP, Saffron, SAMe

While any one may experience "the blues" from time to time, depression can affect ability to live effectively and enjoy life. Depression impacts about 120 million people worldwide, with about 6% of men and 9.5% of women. It is frequently misdiagnosed in elderly people, and has negative impacts on quality of life. The WHO predicts depression to become the second most burdensome disease by 2020, which means it will cost, in terms of medical care, sickness and days lost from work, more than other clinical condition except cardiovascular diseases. Antidepressants are the major category of psychiatric drugs. According to Dr. Mercola, every year, 230 million prescriptions are filled, making them one of the most prescribed drugs in the US. The psychiatric industry is a $330 billion industry. Despite all of these prescriptions, more than one in 20 Americans are depressed, according to the recent statistics from the Centers for Disease Control and Prevention (CDC). Of those depressed Americans, 80% report they have some level of functional impairment, and 27% report their condition makes it worst to do routine tasks for daily living, and getting along with others. The use of antidepressant drugs for depression has doubled from 13.3 million in 1996 to 27 million in 2005. Over 160 million antidepressant prescriptions are written annually, despite the fact that a 2010 study in the *Journal of the American Medical Association* (JAMA) revealed antidepressants to be no more effective than placebos (sugar pills) in most cases of depression. These drugs *don't work at addressing the underlying cause.* Anti-depressants are helpful in the minority of severely depressed cases, and should be used for these cases after consulting the physician. Moreover antidepressants can cause sexual side effects, infertility, increased weight gain, diabetes risk, BP problems, increased heart attack risk, heart defects in unborn children, and increased tendency to commit suicide. Antidepressants have numerous side effects, some of which are life threatening. About 750,000 people attempt suicide each year in the US, and ~30,000 of those succeed. Psychiatric drugs kill 42,000 people every year i.e. 12,000 successfully commit suicide due to depression. Unfortunately, antidepressant drugs are no more effective than sugar pills. Sugar pills may produce better results than antidepressants. Both pills work via the placebo effect, but the sugar pills produce fewer adverse effects. In addition, since most of the treatment focus is on drugs, many safe and natural dietary treatment options have been ignored.

The reason why antidepressants do not work is because these agents target only Unitarian aspect of this complex condition: neurotransmitters. When neurotransmitters like dopamine, epinephrine and serotonin are low, artificially raising the levels with the drugs may help in severe cases. Unfortunately, depression is a multi-factorial complex disorder. Therefore, a holistic therapeutic approach could be more successful in the treatment of depression. For instance, a thorough examination of the thyroid function, vitamin D, B_{12}, iron, essential fatty acids, positive attitude, and proper nutrient absorption are highly significant. In general, 100 mg of 5-HTP twice a day, acupuncture, and prevention of negative thoughts may help alleviate depression. A well-trained holistically-minded physician explores all these interventions for personalized treatment of depression.

Of those depressed Americans, 80% report they have some level of functional impairment, and 27% reported their condition makes it difficult to do every day work, activities of daily living, and getting along with others. The use of antidepressant drugs for depression has doubled in just one decade, from 13.3 million in 1996 to 27 million in 2005. It has been shown that antidepressant drugs are no more effective than sugar pills. Some studies have even found that sugar pills may produce better results than antidepressants. Both pills work via the placebo effect, but the sugar pills produce fewer adverse effects. In addition, since most of the treatment focus is on drugs, many safe and natural treatment options are being ignored. Unfortunately about two-thirds of people with depression remain undiagnosed. Untreated depression is the primary cause of suicide. *If you think someone is suicidal, do not leave him or her alone.* Seek immediate help from doctor or the nearest hospital emergency room, or call 911. Eliminate access to firearms or other potential suicide aids, including unnecessary access to medications. Besides straight forward or "sideways" comments about not wanting to live any longer, some of the warning signals a person has a high risk for self-harm include: acquiring a weapon, hoarding medication, no plan for the future, putting affairs in order, making or changing a will, giving away personal belongings, mending grievances, checking on insurance policies, withdrawing from people. The suicide risk is higher if someone has experienced any of the following stressful life situations: loss of a relationship or death of a loved one, diagnosis of a terminal illness, loss of financial security or livelihood, loss of home or employment, early childhood abuse, rape or other serious emotional trauma.

People sometimes become more suicidal as they begin to recover from depression, as antidepressant drugs can increase suicide risk. As lethargy (*common in depression*) lifts, one can easily find the energy for a suicide plan. These patients with MDD might feel more in control and therefore at peace with situation once decision is made to end his/her own life.

Diagnosis of Depression Untreated depression is the major cause of suicide. Unfortunately, about two-thirds of people with depression remain undiagnosed. The diagnostic clues establish that someone might be suffering from this illness. One set of diagnostic criteria to assess depression is known as "SIGECAPS," which stands for *sleep, interest, guilt, energy, concentration, appetite, psychomotor and suicide*. If four or more of these symptoms exist, it suggests MDD. However, it is important to watch for symptoms besides mood changes, considering relevant information from family and friends as well. If someone has been feeling down for two weeks or more and have lost interest in activities once enjoyed, he/she may consider the treatment options for healing depression as opposed to resorting to antidepressant drugs. Most suicide attempts are expressions of extreme distress. The Clinical diagnosis and treatment of depression is described at the end of this book. Although the exact etiopathogenesis of depression remains unknown the most important risk factors have been described below:

1. Genetically-Modified Foods. Genetically-modified foods contain toxic herbicides, and because they are yet unexplored, we are now beginning to understand how they do damage, and the relevance of the gut to mental health. The modification of plant genes using animal, insect, and bacterial DNA is unpredictable that: disrupts that plant's natural development (lowers its nutritional content and raises its allergy content); introduces proteins, antibiotic resistance genes and the potential for transfer of genes to gut bacteria. These plants are modified so that they can withstand more and more glyphosate-containing herbicide. This chemical (a) kills beneficial bacteria through its interference with the "shikimate" pathway, (b) the interference with this bacteria promotes "dysbiosis" and the generation of inflammatory compounds from tryptophan; (c) When it is broken down by the gut, produces ammonia; (d) blocks an enzyme that converts testosterone to estrogen, aromatase; (e) chelates calcium, magnesium, zinc, iron, and cobalt; (f) interferes with sulfate availability, critical to cholesterol metabolism and cellular function; and (g) interferes with liver enzymes responsible for breaking down other toxins.

2. Gluten. Often processed with genetically-modified oils, gluten is a brain and body poison. It promotes intestinal permeability through a compound called zonulin. Local inflammation precedes systemic inflammatory responses accompanied by antibodies to the different components of gluten (gliadin, glutenin), complexes with enzymes called transglutaminase, and to tissue in the brain, GIT, and thyroid through molecular mimicry. The gluten intolerance include depression, seizures, headaches, multiple sclerosis/demyelination, anxiety, ADHD, ataxia, and neuropathy. Independent of the brain effects, gliadin peptides may enter the blood stream and can stimulate opiate receptors in the brain, resulting in the formation of gliadorphins, causing withdrawal symptoms.

3. Sugar. Clinically, dysglycemia or sugar imbalance can look like depression, panic disorder, and even bipolar. Sugar triggers insulin that drop sugar low and leave feeling jittery, edgy, tired, foggy, and anxious; binds to proteins forming inflammatory compounds called advanced glycation products; promotes insulin resistance in the body and brain, which means that sugar can't be used for fuel and hangs outside the cells causing damage and it is addictive. Rats preferred it to cocaine. Hence pesticide-free shopping, avoiding genetically-modified foods, and gluten free-diet may alleviate symptoms of depression.

Seekatz et al., (2013) proposed that in the treatment of chronic back pain a multiple target approach to reduce pain; pain-related fear and avoidance behavior and depressive symptoms should be considered. The interference of biological, social, and psychological factors of the patient, as the biopsychosocial perspective, plays a significant role in the chronification of postsurgical pain. These investigators performed a pilot study to detect whether patients suffering from chronic pain to a recent operation differ from chronic pain patients whose pain exists since operation and was related with it in these factors. The analysis of patients with chronic pain was conducted via a questionnaire in which mental state, pain, fear, and depression [Hospital Anxiety and Depression Scale – Deutsche Version (HADS-D), Chronic Pain Grade Questionnaire (CPGQ, von Korff), SF-12, McGill Pain Questionnaire (sensoric/affective)] were surveyed. Twenty nine months postoperatively, 113 chronic pain patients were analyzed. A comparison between the CPSP group (with chronic postsurgical pain) and the group CP (with chronic pain) was conducted. Both groups showed reductions of SF-12 data compared to normals, but normal results regarding depression in the HADS-D and a moderately limiting, highly pain-related limitation in the CPGQ (von Korff III). No significant differences in the sensory and affective parameters of the McGill Pain Questionnaire were noticed. Compared with the CPSP group, the CP group demonstrated higher pain intensities. There were no group differences between psychological and social factors in chronic pain with or without postsurgical pain (Seekatz et al., 2013). Although the efficacy of functional restoration programs for the treatment of chronic back pain is well documented, a few trials have been conducted to demonstrate that implementing such programs in clinical settings with large numbers of patients is as effective as in a research setting. Heinrich et al., (2013) examined whether the positive effects of such programs can be observed in the context of a standardized day clinic treatment regimen. A total of 681 back pain patients were examined at 4 measurement points (before and immediately after the program, as well as 6 and 12 months after treatment) using a questionnaire on perceived pain and symptoms of anxiety and depression, as well as the work situation. A significant improvements in back pain, pain-related impairment and degree of chronification were observed, as well as a high return-to-work rate after treatment.

HIV-1 Infection and Depression. Due to improved antiretroviral therapy (HAART), HIV-1 infection has evolved from a lethal to a chronic disease. Hence health-related quality of life (HRQoL) has become an important concern. Degroote et al., (2013) identified socio-economic, behavioral, (neuro) psychological and clinical determinants of HRQoL among people living with HIV (PLHIV). These investigators admistered validated self-report questionnaires to collect socio-demographic data, to assess HRQoL (Medical Outcomes Study-HIV), depressive symptoms (Beck Depression Inventory-II) and adherence to HAART (*Short Medication Adherence Questionnaire*) and to screen for neurocognitive dysfunction. A total of 237 subjects participated, among whom 187 were male. Mean age was 45.8+/-10.7 years and 144 participants were homosexual. Median physical and mental health score (PHS, MHS) were 55.6 (IQR 48.2-60.6) and 52.0(IQR 44.2-57.9), respectively. Regression analysis revealed that incapacity to work, depressive symptoms, neurocognitive complaints (NCCs), dissatisfaction with the patient-physician relationship and non-adherence were negatively associated with HRQoL. Socio-economic (work status), behavioral (adherence) and neuropsychological (depressive symptoms, NCCs) determinants impacted HRQoL. This study concluded that clinical parameters (viral load, CD4 cell count) were not associated with HRQoL.

Recently the prescription of antidepressants has increased since the introduction of SSRIs, while depressive symptoms may remain untreated. Midlov et al., (2013) examined whether depression among residents in nursing homes is treated adequately. 429 participants from 11 Swedish nursing homes were selected and were assessed with the Cornell Scale for Depression in Dementia (CSDD) and using medical records and drug prescription data. For 256 participants a follow-up assessment was performed after 12 months. The prevalence of depression was 9.1%, and CSDD score of >/=8 was 7.5%. Depression persisted in more than 50% of cases at the 12-month follow-up. Antidepressants were prescribed to 33% of the participants without a diagnosis of depression or with a CSDD score of <8. 14% of the participants without a diagnosis of depression or with a CSDD score of <8 had psychotropic polypharmacy. 15.2% of all participants had psychotropic polypharmacy, which persisted at the 12-month follow-up in three-quarters of cases. The prescription of antidepressants in elderly was extensive and without clear indication suggesting that there is a need for systematic drug reviews, paying special attention to the aging subjects on antidepressants.

Sleep Disorders and Agomelatine. Sleep disorders are generally associated with depression that, in the absence of a diagnosis of depression should be made with caution. Insomnia may occur in 60%–80% of depressed patients. Depressive symptoms are risk factors for insomnia, and depression is comorbidity in patients with chronic insomnia. Certain commonly prescribed drugs for the treatment of depression may worsen insomnia and impair recovery. Sleep disturbances during depression include pavor nocturnus, nightmares, hypersomnia, and insomnia; circadian sleep disturbances; and treatment could be by manipulation of the sleep-wake rhythm (chronotherapy, phototherapy, sleep cycles, and manipulation of the sleep-wake rhythm itself). A case report of a 65-year-old Caucasian woman suffering from insomnia associated with depression was treated with sleep deprivation. Furthermore, Agomelatine is a novel antidepressant that acts as a melatonin MT1 and MT2 receptor agonist and serotonin 5-HT2C receptor antagonist, reversing circadian rhythm disruption in MDD and promoting neurogenesis in animal models of depression. It may be an alternative to antidepressants due to its improved tolerability. Macisaac et al., (2013) conducted the PubMed database search for randomized controlled trials (RCTs) evaluating the efficacy of Agomelatine, and its tolerability and safety in the treatment of MDD. These investigators showed that Agomelatine is a multi-modal agent with novel mechanisms of action, suggesting its efficacy and tolerability profile for MDD treatment. However, the clinical significance of agomelatine has been questioned, requiring further investigations in evaluation of its effectiveness. Of major concern are transient elevations in transaminases and liver reactions. In a pilot study, Byrne et al., (2013) demonstrated that a blended mindfulness and skills-based childbirth education was essential for women and was associated with improvements in confidence in giving birth. Previous findings that low self-efficacy and high childbirth fear are linked to greater labor pain, stress reactivity, and trauma suggest that improvements in these variables have important implications for maternal mental health and child health outcomes. Another study identified predictors of postpartum sexual activity and functioning in a heterogeneous population of women using the Sexual Health Outcomes in Women Questionnaire (SHOW-Q). Although a relationship between mode of birth and SHOW-Q scores did not emerge, a trend toward lower SHOW-Q scores among women who underwent cesarean compared with those giving birth vaginally was noticed.

Multiparty and younger age predict early resumption of sexual activity, whereas depression and breastfeeding were associated with poorer postpartum sexual functioning. However the relationship between mode of birth and resumed sexual activity or postpartum sexual function is yet to be established.

Depressive symptoms of midlife Latinas. Immigrant Latinas have different cultural attitudes toward menopause and aging, and experience higher levels of distress associated with adaptation to new environment. A study was performed to describe the frequency of depressive symptoms in premenopausal Latinas (40–50 years of age) living in the US and compare Latinas born in the US with immigrant Latinas on stress and sociodemographic factors that influence depressive symptoms. Analysis was conducted on 94 Latinas who completed the Center for Epidemiological Studies-Depression (CES-D) scale for 6 months. Immigrant Latinas had a higher CES-D than US-born Latinas. There was no difference in age, BMI, self-report of general health, or perceived stress. Higher BMI, work-related stress, and insufficient income were associated with depressive symptoms in immigrant Latinas. In addition, high BMI and less education were associated with depression in the US-born Latinas.

Nutrition. Foods have significant impact on our body and brain, and eating whole foods support mental and physical health. Avoiding sugar (particularly fructose) and grains helps normalize insulin and leptin levels. Sugar causes chronic inflammation, which disrupts body's normal immune function and can impair CNS function. Sugar also suppresses BDNF, which promotes brain neurons and involved in memory. BDNF levels are significantly reduced in patients with depression.

Dietary Interventions to treat Depression. Diets can be divided into two major categories—the fad diet of the day and the traditional standbys. The fad diets may include eating three protein-fortified cookies a day, cleansing of the colon. Quick weight loss, the chance to talk about the diet at a dinner party, and ultimately abandonment after a few weeks. Conventional diets, such as the American Heart Association plan or Weight Watchers, offer a way of staying on a weight-loss program for many weeks with the chance to change permanently eating and exercise patterns. The point system of Weight Watchers, which allows the dieter to devise his or her individual food plan, stresses the consumption of vegetables and fruits. They allow the points to be used for protein, starchy carbohydrates, dairy products, and fats. Conventional diets such as Weight Watchers pose a problem for people whose weight gain is caused by their antidepressant or mood stabilizing medications. These drugs diminish will power and leave feeling hungry even though enough food has been eaten to meet the calorie requirements.

Natural Antidepressants. While antidepressants are the answer for some with clinical depression, others may seek natural methods in addition to or as an alternative to taking medication. While there is no definite cure for all kinds of depression, there is research supporting several natural options that may help alleviate mind as well as spirit. Water is one of the best natural antidepressants. Dehydration causes fatigue, which in turn, causes body to not feel so great. People who don't feel well physically, have a tendency to not feel well mentally, as well. Drink at least one ounce of water per pound of body weight daily to help feel less depressed. Spinach is a very good source of folic acid for maintaining physical and mental health. A lack of folic acid causes the body to not produce enough serotonin. Spinach is a natural antidepressant. Oranges and other citrus fruits have vitamin C essential to synthesize dopamine. It also keeps RBCs count normal. Red pepper has more vitamin C than citrus fruit. Whole wheat can act as a natural antidepressant. It's loaded with complex carbohydrates that will produce adequate amounts of serotonin. A sandwich on whole wheat bread with spinach and red peppers, with a glass of water and some orange juice will provide antidepressant effect. This combination of sandwich has all five of these natural antidepressants in one meal. Many other foods also act as natural antidepressants by eating healthy. As long as a food is good and rich in vitamins, it will help fight depression.

Amino Acids. Tryptophan is involved in the synthesis of serotonin, which regulates mood. It is difficult to obtain sufficient tryptophan from food alone, so tryptophan-rich foods (like peanuts, fish, milk, dates, and even chocolate) in the diet may be included. We can also help body synthesize its own tryptophan by eating meats and soy protein. Turkey is good source of tryptophan as well as B-vitamins, iron, selenium, zinc, and other nutrients to alleviate depression. Tryptophan is critical to production of the neurotransmitter serotonin, which regulates mood. Taking 1g of tryptophan thrice a day helps improve mood. By aiming to include more tryptophan-rich foods (like peanuts, fish, milk, dates, and even chocolate) in the diet, we can help our body make its own tryptophan by eating meats and soy protein.

B Vitamins in Diets. Research has focused on folate (or folic acid), B_6, and B_{12} because these vitamins are inadequate among people with depression. Between 15-38% of people with depression are folate-deficient. While it's uncertain whether this causes depression, or the lack of folate can delay symptom relief from antidepressants. Women who take birth control pills or hormone replacement therapy can also be low in vitamin B_6 (possibly why women's depression rates are twice than those of men). Also, vitamin B_{12}-deficiencies are common among vegans who don't eat animal proteins. It is yet to be established whether B vitamins can prevent or treat depression, though it's believed that it benefits brain health. Most research has focused on folate, vitamin B_6, and vitamin B_{12} because these have inadequate supply among people with depression. Between 15 and 38% of people with depression are folate-deficient. While it's uncertain whether this causes depression, lack of folate can delay symptom relief from antidepressants.

Vitamin B_6. We require 1.3 to 1.5 mg vitamin B_6 daily. A serving (100 gr/3.5 oz) of tuna or a cup of chickpeas will be sufficient. Buckwheat flour is another good source. Vitamin B_{12}: 2.4 μg daily can be obtained from a serving of beef or eggs. Folate: 400 μg daily can be obtained from a cup of cooked lentils, as is a cup of cooked spinach with a glass of orange juice. Asparagus and avocado are also good sources of folate.

Complex Carbohydrates. Carbohydrates indirectly help synthesize serotonin. Simple carbohydrates like sugary and starchy foods and those made with white flour boost serotonin levels, too, that is why we have craving for them when we feel depressed. But these foods cause blood sugar to rise quickly and then fall quickly. When blood sugar levels fall, so do our moods. Swings in blood sugar that come from eating high amounts stress the adrenal glands, which causes fatigue and depression. However, complex carbs, found in whole-grain products (breads, rice, and pasta), fruits, vegetables, and legumes, boost and maintain serotonin levels without spiking blood sugar. Seven to ten servings of fruits and vegetables per day are beneficial in addition to three servings of whole grains. Eating a bowl of high-fibre cereal in the morning and making sandwich for lunch of whole-grain bread. Up to 25% of people taking antidepressants gain weight, at least ten pounds, while on the medication. Caracoglia, a naturopathic doctor emphasizes that regular exercise can be as effective as antidepressants and psychotherapy. Consuming omega-3 PUFAs can have a positive impact on brain neurotransmitters and is critical for normal CNS function. Salmon and walnuts are rich sources of omega-3 PUFAs in addition to a daily dose of vitamins such as vitamin B_{12}, folic acid, vitamin D_3 and tyrosine. Foods like fish, oysters, beans, nuts, whole grains, leafy vegetables and dairy products are rich in these essential nutrients. Acupuncture is beneficial and may be comparable in effectiveness to prescription anti-depressant medications. During treatment, pressure points are stimulated with either fingertips, heat or needles to release tension. Bright light in the morning is also effective on mood. Along with natural sunshine, trials have been conducted using phototherapy and can have a positive effect. Carbohydrates, caffeine, alcohol and dairy can cause mood alleviation. "In some cases, blood testing, skin testing, endoscopic biopsy (for gluten sensitivity), and elimination diets may be required in diagnosing food sensitivities. Irritability and mood swings can induce lack of sleep. Eight hours a night is adequate but most people get less. Breakfast is important to set the mood for the day. Carbohydrates and proteins are required to promote stable blood sugar. Add sliced almonds cereal or peanut butters on toast. In addition, meditation and yoga can offer benefits. Meditation (moment-to-moment nonjudgmental awareness of breathing, physical sensations, emotions, and thoughts), can alleviate mood and can change brain activation patterns in a positive way. St. John's Wort is a remedy for mild to moderate depression. Gingko biloba is another option for older patients who are having circulatory problems. It is important to consult a physician before starting an herbal regime as many may have adverse interactions with other medication.

Omega-3 Fatty Acids in Diet. Studies have shown that long chain omega-3 polyunsaturated fatty acids (n-3 PUFA) may be useful in the clinical management of depression. N-3-PUFA are involved in mood disorders, yet clinical trials have shown mixed results. It is now recommended to take a high-quality, animal-based omega-3 fat, like krill oil. This is the single most important nutrient for optimal brain function, thereby preventing depression. Taking a high-quality, animal-based omega-3 fat may be the most important nutrient for optimal brain function to prevent depression. DHA is one of the Omega-3 fatty acids in fish and krill oil. Reduced DHA levels have been associated with depression, memory loss, Schizophrenia, and AD. DHA is one of the Omega-3 fatty acids in fish and krill oil, and brain is highly dependent on it. Women who rarely eat fish have more than twice the risk of depression compared to those who eat "fin food" quite often. Although it's difficult to consume enough omega-3s to treat depression through food alone (Between 1 and 3 grams of omega-3s a day is required to alleviate mood), eating fish, such as sardines, may help prevent depression. Eating at least two fish meals a week is beneficial. If someone does not like fish, a teaspoon (5 ml) of ground flaxseed to cereal, yogurt, or salads may be added. A study was performed to determine whether n-3 PUFA improves depression in elderly patients, and whether the blood fatty acid pattern is correlated with these changes. The severity of depressive symptoms according to the Geriatric Depression Scale (GDS), blood fatty acid composition, and erythrocyte phospholipids were analyzed in 46 depressed females aged 66-95y according to DSMIV, as a randomized, double-blind, placebo-controlled trial. Twenty two depressed females were included (2.5 g/day of n-3 PUFA for 8 weeks), and 24 in the placebo group. These investigators also measured CD2, CD3, CD4, CD8, CD16, CD19 and cytokines (IL-5, IL-15). The mean GDS score and AA/EPA ratio, in whole blood and RBC membrane phospholipids, were lower after 2 months supplementation with n-3 PUFA. A correlation between the amelioration of GDS and the AA/EPA ratio with some immunological parameters, such as CD2, CD19, CD4, CD16 and CD4/CD8 ratio, was also observed. Omega-3 did not improve the immunological functions however ameliorated symptoms of depression. The n-3 PUFA may be monitored by determining whole blood AA/EPA ratio, anxiety- and depression-like behavior. Vans et al., (2012) assayed plasma n-3 and omega-6 (n-6) that are involved in the biosynthesis and processing of plasma membranes, to affect brain function and mood. These investigators used lipomic technology to assay plasma levels of n-3 and n-6 fatty acids from 40 bipolar and 18 control subjects to investigate the severity of disease biomarkers, neuroticism, global assessment of function (GAF), and mood (Hamilton Depression Scale : HAM-D) and found the levels of dihomo-γ-linolenic acid (DGLA) to correlate positively with neuroticism and HAM-D scores and negatively with GAF scores; and HAM-D to correlate negatively with linoleic acid (LA) and positively with fatty acid desaturase 2 (FADS2) activity, an enzyme involved in converting LA to γ-linolenic acid (GLA). Hence n-6 fatty acids and the enzymes that control their biosynthesis may be used as biomarkers of MDDs. People suffering from depression have lower circulating levels of omega-3 fatty acids. One study showed that the lower the level of EPA, the more severe the clinical depression. Fish oil reduced suicidal tendencies and improved helath when 40 people were given fish oil or placebo for 12 weeks (*Hallahan, Hibbeln, and Davis - British Journal of Psychiatry*). Fish oil can be found in raw and cooked fish and can also be taken as a dietary supplement. Zebra Organics is a rich source for high quality, organic fish oil supplements. According to Johnson, in countries where fish consumption is high, such as Japan, Taiwan, and Finland; rates of depression tend to be low. Conversely, in areas where fish consumption is low, like North America and Europe; depression rates are much higher (as much as 10 times higher) as illustrated in Figure 1.

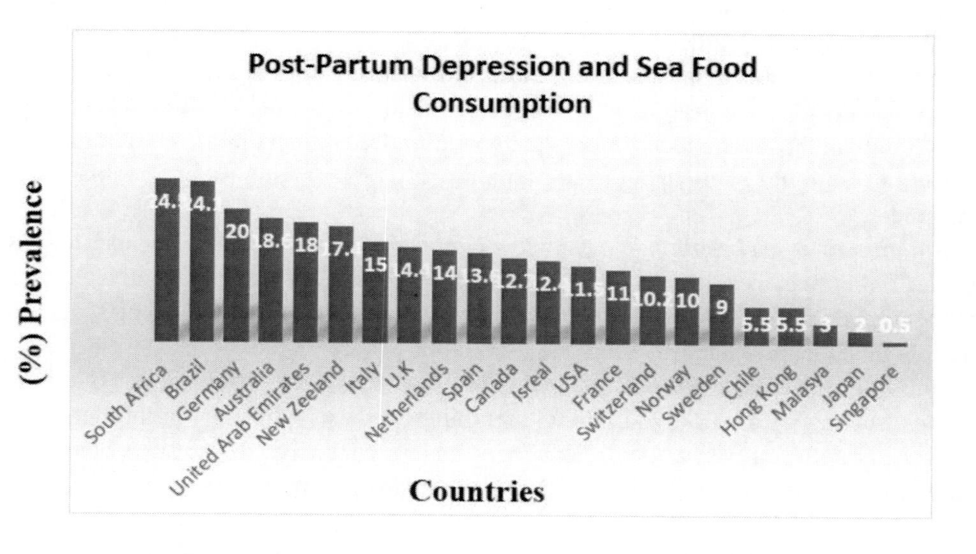

Figure 1. A histogram representing minimum prevalance of post-partum depression among women living in regions where sea food consumption was maximum and vice versa for those who were living in regions where meat is the primary component of diet such as South Africa, Brazil, Germany Australia as compared to Hongkong, Malasya, Japan and Singapore.

Exercise. Regular exercise is *as good as antidepressants for helping people who are depressed.* It works by normalizing insulin levels while augmenting the endorphins (feel good hormones) in the brain. *Physical exercise changes the brain regional serotonin and increases endorphin levels. Exercise can increase the number of cells in the hippocampus". These* *studies were first done on animals, and are significant because in depression, there are fewer of those cells in the hippocampus. But we can change our brain with exercise.* People who regularly exercise benefit from positive effect on mood and reduced risk of depression. When we exercise, the body releases endorphins that initiate positive feelings in the body and mind, while the use of refined sugar is linked to depression. Dr. Dufty suggests avoiding sugar in his book "Sugar Blues". Another interesting book is "Sugar Shock", by Drs. Bennett and Sinatra. Natural sweeteners such as Agave (*sweet cactus nectar*) and maple syrup (*a sweetener made from the sap of maple trees*) may be used as alternatives to refined sugar. Vitamin D has been shown to increase serotonin in the brain. People who were suffering from depression, particularly those with seasonal affective disorder (SAD), tended to improve as their levels of vitamin D increased. The recommendation is to allow limited, unprotected sun exposure in the early morning and late afternoon (no >15 minutes for light-skinned individuals, 40 minutes for darker skin). Vitamin D is also available as a dietary supplement. Laughter combats depression by reducing stress hormones. The positive results of laughter may encourage people to relax and alleviate the stress that causes depression. Reading the comics, watching sitcom, or listening to a comedian may be a prescription for happiness and alleviate depression. Dr. Keedwell emphasizes that depression is not a human defect at all, but a defense mechanism that can force a healthy reassessment of personal circumstances. We experience difficult events in our lives and while it is recommended to see a professional to alleviate clinical depression, changes in diet and lifestyle can go a long way in the clinical management of depression. Some foods are natural antidepressants. Hence eating a natural healthy diet can help to cure depression. We can save lot of money by including foods that are natural antidepressants rather than spending money on expansive medication.

Sun Shine. Getting safe sun exposure, allows body to produce vitamin D for mood alleviation. People with the lowest levels of vitamin D were 11 times more prone to depression than those who received adequate vitamin D. We can optimize vitamin D either by exposure to sunlight, or by using a safe tanning bed, or by taking a high-quality vitamin D3 supplement.

Emotional Housekeeping. We can view depression as a sign that body and life are out of balance, rather than as a disease. We need to regain balance addressing negative emotions that may be trapped in our level of awareness. Emotional Freedom Technique (EFT), is a form of psychological acupressure. If someone is having severe depression, it would be best to consult with a mental health professional. There are alternative effective stress-management methods, such as meditation, journaling, breathing exercises, yoga, or sharing feelings with a friend. Although it is easy to learn EFT and far less expensive to use, it is better to seek a professional to perform EFT as it is an art that takes many years of refined practice to maximize its effectiveness.

Gardening and Meditation. It is known for its meditative, relaxing, and grounding effects. Friendly bacteria in soil affects the brain similar to antidepressants by increasing the release of serotonin. Meditation reduces stress and has an effect on the brain. Professor Williams, indicates that meditation reduces depression by over 50%. He suggests to people that they begin to see all their thoughts as just thoughts, whether they are positive, negative or neutral. Incense has long been used in rituals across the globe to create a peaceful environment. It has been discovered how burning frankincense (*resin from the Boswellia plant*) activates ion channels in the brain that alleviate depression. Floracopeia provides organic frankincense as incense and essential oil.

Prescriptions. Feeling depressed is never pleasant, and we want to escape it as quickly as possible. Hence it is easy to become attracted into thinking a pill might relieve pain, especially when the prescription is coming from a physician. But drugs should be last choice, and antidepressants are no exception. We wouldn't want to expose to the risks these drugs present with limited therapeutic benefits. Implementing the healthy dietary strategies may provide better clinical outcome.

Limitation of Antidepressants Drugs. A study in the January 2010 issue of *JAMA* concluded that there is little evidence that SSRIs (*antidepressants including; Prozac, Paxil, Zoloft and others*) have any benefit to people with mild to moderate depression, and they work no better than a placebo. SSRIs are 33% effective as a placebo. And a study presented at the Neuroscience conference in 2009 had similar findings. It was concluded that (1) Antidepressant drugs were not invented for depression. Researchers used certain drugs to manipulate the behavior of stressed animals, and concluded that these drugs would be "*antidepressants*." But chronic stress does not cause the same molecular changes that depression does, making the hypothesis incorrect. So, antidepressants were actually designed to treat stress, rather than depression. (2) An imbalance of neurotransmitters in the brain may not trigger depressive symptoms; that is generally held. Instead, the biochemical events that lead to depression appear to start in the development and functioning of neurons. The antidepressants focus on the *effect of depression* and miss the real cause. In reality a single drug solution may not be the answer. In 2008, a study published in PLoS Medicine concluded that the difference between antidepressants and placebo pills is negligible, and that both are ineffective for many depressed patients. Only the most *severely depressed* showed minimal response to antidepressants. The use of antidepressant drugs may actually result in more relapses back into depression in the long run. In other words, these drugs may be turning depression into a more chronic condition. Antidepressant drugs may convert people from unipolar depression into bipolar; meaning, fluctuating between mania and depression, with a poor prognosis. 75% of the response to antidepressants could be duplicated by placebo. Many antidepressants may make "mental illness" worse.

Side Effects of Antidepressant Drugs. Antidepressants are associated with serious health risks: (i) Diabetes**:** The risk for type 2 diabetes is two to three times higher if we take antidepressants. (ii) Problems with immune system: SSRIs cause serotonin to remain in synaptic terminals longer, interfering with immune cell signaling and T cell growth; (iii) Suicidal thoughts and feelings of violent behavior : the risk for suicide may be twice as high if we take SSRIs; seven out of twelve school shootings were by children who were either on antidepressants or withdrawing from them; (iii) Stillbirths: A Canadian study of 5,000 mothers found that women on SSRIs were twice as likely to have a stillbirth, and a premature or low birth weight baby; another study showed a 40% increased risk for birth defects, such as cleft palate; (iv) Women on antidepressants have a 30% higher risk of spinal fracture and a 20% high risk for all other fractures; (v) the risk for stroke could be 45% higher if someone is on antidepressants, related to how the drugs affect blood clotting (vi) Overall death rates have been found to be 32% higher in women on antidepressants. Diabetes or stroke could be fatal, but suicide is much quicker. The link between suicide and antidepressants is so strong that these drugs have suicide warnings. One of the psychotropic medications that is prescribed for depression is Abilify (also called *aripiprazole*). Abilify is used for the treatment of bipolar disorder, schizophrenia, autism, and MDD to augment the effects of the antidepressants. Abilify has several side effects. Andy Behrman, a former spokesman for Abilify, stopped taking the drug to avoid the deleterious side effects such as coma and death. Doctors haven't delineated a specific reason why antidepressants can cause weight gain. Many experts suspect the drugs have an effect on metabolism, slowing the process that allows to burn food as energy before it becomes fat. Others point out that an increase in well-being often leads to an increase in appetite. Some patients lose weight or maintain a lower weight due to their depression, and antidepressants remove that mental block against robust eating. Or, as life itself becomes more pleasurable, so does food.

Several theories have been put forward to explain why antidepressants induce weight gain. Antidepressants may contribute to increased body weight: stimulation of appetite (TCAs), increased carbohydrate cravings (TCAs), interference with CNS functions that regulate energy balance, changes in the Resting Metabolic Rate (TCAs, SSRIs, MAOIs), interaction with a genetic predisposition to weight gain, counteracting the action of the 5-HT2 receptors), increases appetite, interference with the production of NE. Appetite regulation and weight gain or loss, are complex reactions which are influenced by several hormones and compounds, all of which may be negatively affected by antidepressants (Westmore 2010). The patient is required to discuss any changes in body weight when being treated with antidepressants with the doctor who may be able to adjust dosage or change prescription to another antidepressant which is better suited to unique metabolism and requirements. If someone is turning to food as 'comfort', doctor will suggest better methods of coping with depression. Consult a dietitian to assist with a balanced slimming diet. Do as much cardio or aerobic exercise as possible. The exercise not only help control weight and promote weightless by stimulating metabolism, but it has positive effect on psychological makeup. Daily exercise is also an expression of taking back control of life despite being depressed. Never stop antidepressants without discussing with the doctor. It could be dangerous and even fatal to stop taking antidepressants suddenly if someone suffers from MDD because the danger of suicide is increased if medication is abruptly stopped. Do not take over-the-counter slimming pills or fat-burners or any other herbal or pharmaceutical agent as a solution to rapid weight loss because these can interfere with antidepressant treatment and even counteract the antidepressants effects leading to deleterious side-effects. Do not use starvation diets to accomplish rapid weight loss because very-low-energy diets have been linked to an increase incidence of depression. Never take antidepressants for just losing weight.

Avoid Antidepressants. Professor Davis wrote an excellent article about SSRIs in the January 2010 issue of *Psychology Today*. He emphasized that physicians usually prescribe not one, but two or three SSRIs and psychopharmacological drugs in combination—with no studies to substantiate the beneficial effects. Physicians who engage in "polypharmacy" are hoping that if one didn't work, may be two or three will. *"Doctors are performing uncontrolled experiments on their patients, hoping that in some scattershot way they might hit on a solution. But of course drugs have dangerous interactions and most physicians are shooting in the dark with all the dangers that attend such bad marksmanship."* It is generally believed that depression is caused by a chemical imbalance of neurotransmitters, mainly serotonin, dopamine and norepinephrine. Scientists can't even decide on what "normal" serotonin level is. Infact some depressed subjects have high serotonin levels, while many normal healthy subjects have low ones. Our brain is exceedingly complex for this simplistic explanation. Moreover "psychiatric diseases" could be considered "*lifestyle disorders*": Of the 297 mental disorders, none can be measured by empirical tests. Because writing a prescription is much faster approach for the conventional model. There are five important strategies to consider if a person is facing depression. These strategies have positive impact and are inexpensive to implement. Depression can be serious and often requires professional help or sometimes medication. However, increasing intake of certain essential nutrients may help prevent depression, alleviate symptoms, or improve the effectiveness of antidepressant medications. There are many options for depression from the natural sources. Addressing underlying lifestyle, diet, digestive and psychological causes is important for long-term results. Using St. John's wort, saffron, 5-HTP or SAMe can be a helpful in alleviating depression. Some important life style interventions can also help alleviating depression such as adopting healthy diets and saying no to drugs of abuse, alcohol consumption, and cigarette smoking.

Nutrients and Herbs for Depression. Depression is a multi-factorial disorder. The reason why antidepressants do not work is because these drugs target only one aspect of this complex condition: neurotransmitters. When neurotransmitters such as dopamine, epinephrine and serotonin are low, artificially raising the levels with the drugs can help to a certain extent in the minority of severe cases. While conventional medicine focuses only on neurotransmitters, naturopathic and holistic medicines are at an advantage to treat several factors that contribute to depression: sleep and lifestyle issues, lack of exercise, poor diet choices and poor digestion, inflammation in the body and the brain, hormonal imbalances and spiritual issues, nutrients, healthy oil deficiencies, and environmental toxicity. There are many safe nutrients and herbs that can help with low mood. A few nutrients are beneficial to help patients who are suffering from depression. If we overlook many factors described earlier to address the underlying causes of depression, these nutrients or herbs alone may not be effective. Also, if we are taking antidepressant medications, we should check with the doctor before changing medication dosage, or using these supplements along with other medications. While antidepressants could be used for some patients with clinical depression, others may seek natural methods or as an alternative medication. While there is no cure for all types of depression, there is research supporting natural options that may help boost minds as well as spirits. Some of these natural antidepressants are desctribed below:

St. John's Wort. St. John's wort *Hypericum perforatum* means "above a ghost" and the plant was used to get rid of evil spirits. St. John's wort is useful in treating mild to moderate depression as it works like a weak version of an antidepressant drug. Current research suggests that it has many effects on both the brain and the body. It is known to help digestion, act as an antiviral, has anti-inflammatory properties and supports thyroid function. It also balances the neurotransmitters GABA, NE, 5-HT, and DA. Those who have chronic depression called dysthymia often do the best with this herb. If we can get out of bed and function at a job, but are just still low in mood, self-esteem and zest for life, this may be a good choice. We can take St. John's wort in capsule, as a tea, or as a liquid extract in capsule form at 900 mg to 1800 mg a day in divided doses. St. John's wort can influence the effectiveness of other medications. It can help Plavix work better for whom it is not initially effective. It can lower the effects of contraceptive pills and immune suppressants.

Saffron. Saffron is a well-known spice to help the digestive system. Because most neurotransmitters are made in the digestive tract; this might be the reason saffron has been shown to elevate low mood. It is high in carotenoids and B-vitamins. Saffron has been compared to both Prozac and Imipramine, and work as well, or better, with less side effects. While the petal is expensive, we can also take capsules of the stigma, which is less expensive, but possesses the mood-enhancing ingredients. A dose of 15 mg twice a day is usually adequate. No toxicity has been reported when taking saffron in therapeutic amounts or in cooking.

5-HTP for Depression with Anxiety. 5-Hyrdroxytryptophan (5-HTP) is found in low amounts in foods like turkey and bananas. 5-HTP is required to synthesize serotonin (5-HT), a molecule that helps elevate mood. While many antidepressants inhibit the production of enzymes that breakdown serotonin, 5-HTP facilitates to synthesize serotonin as it can cross the blood brain barrier to achieve alteration in brain regional neurochemistry. In general, 5-HTP is used in patients suffering from both depression and anxiety. It is also an effective option for people who have insomnia. It has beneficial effect with weight loss. Some patients may experience nausea with 5-HTP. Hence it is advised to take it with carbohydrate which facilitates its absorption as well. It is prescribed as 100 mg twice a day, up to 200 mg three times a day.

S-Adenylyl Methioneine. S-adenosylmethionine is a naturally occurring chemical based on the amino acid methionine; it enhnces the activity of number of neurotransmitters. SAMe also facilitates nerve conduction. It is helpful in patients who have arthritis and joint pain. SAMe tends to work quickly, alleviating mood within days, whereas most other supplements and drugs take longer. It has been shown to be useful for PD patients with depression, it may be beneficial in the aging population as well. It is safe for children and in pregnancy. Usually, 200 mg twice daily, for the first day, then 400 mg twice daily on day three, then to 400 mg three times daily on day 10, and finally to the full dose of 400 mg four times daily are prescribed.

Reducing Medications. There are options to consider if we want to avoid anti-depressant induced weight gain. The most popularly prescribed drugs, SSRIs, are also associated with weight gain. There are antidepressant drugs that are not associated with weight gain, but are not commonly prescribed. Among the more weight-friendly drugs are: Nefazodone, Venlafaxine, Duloxetine and Bupropion. Effexor, Serzone and Wellbutrin that have less incidences of weight gain, although many who take them still claim to put on weight. Not all antidepressants work for all people, and there is a chance more figure-friendly drugs will not provide psychiatric help. If we are concerned about weight gain, we should ask the doctor if a different class of antidepressants might work. Another option is to discuss the possibility of reducing the medication to the minimal effective dose. The lessening of the dose might also lessen the side-effects, including weight gain.

Antidote Medications. There are medications that can be prescribed to those on antidepressants to counteract the tendency of weight gain. These drugs have serious side effects, and there is controversy as to their efficacy. The doctor will be able to tell the most recent information and safety issues of weight-gain antidote medication. We should not use over-the-counter diet pills to fight weight gain from anti-depressants without consulting a doctor. Many weight-loss pills can have dangerous to fatal interactions with prescription antidepressants.

Diet and Exercise. Exercise is the safest and cheapest way for weight loss. This is the least complicated and most efficient option for combating the weight gain associated with antidepressants. Even the smallest amount of exercise, as simple as a walk to the mailbox, can have positive effect. Exercise is not only useful for combating weight gain, but has also been proven to have anti-depressant effects of its own. Although the benefit of taking the proper antidepressant can be much greater than the detriment of weight gain, excess fat is not a healthy option. Consider increasing physical activity before seeking out medical intervention..

(i) Food Log (ii) Activity Track help lose weight. There are health promotion parameters such as avoiding smoking and drinking, maintaining <25 Kg/m2 BMI, regular moderate physical exercise, adhering to recommended dietary intake. Maintaining total cholesterol <200 mg/dL, BP <120/80 mm Hg, and fasting blood glucose <100 mg/dL for normal healthy life free from mood fluctuations (anxiety and depression) as Figure 2 illustrates.

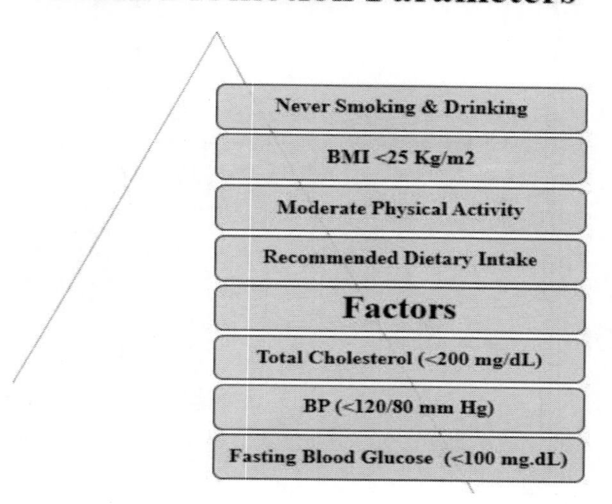

Figure 2. A diagram illustrating healthier life styles and depression risk management. There are primarily four types of risk factors. Risk factors associated with life style include body mass Index (BMI), waist circumference, physical activity, Mediterranean diet score, smoking, and Fish, fruits and vegetables consumption. Psychological component include anxiety, depression scale, and quality of life indices in addition to total cholesterol (HDL nd LDL) dietary fibers intake. The medical risk factors include: increased BP, lipids, and glycemic index.

Different antidepressants and their effects. Weight gain can occur in up to 25% of patients taking antidepressants". The tricyclic antidepressants (TCAs) and monoamine oxidase inhibitors (MAOIs) as antidepressant medications can cause weight gain, while selective serotonin reuptake inhibitors (SSRIs) are less likely to have this negative effect on weight. In some cases, patients using SSRIs may lose a small amount of weight initially during their treatment (usually only about 0.5 kg), but then gain, rather than lose weight. Some patients suffering from severe depression lose lot of weight, so that when they receive treatment with antidepressants and gain some weight, this may actually be a sign of an improvement in their clinical picture. But the majority of patients with MDD gain more weight than desired. Various factors: seeking comfort in food which leads to overeating; the effects of antidepressants such as TCAs which stimulate appetite and increased carbohydrate cravings cause gains between 0.57 to 1.37 kg per month during treatment (Westmore, 2010).

In general there are four types of risk factors. The risk factors associated with life style include BMI, waist circumference, physical activity, Mediterranean diet score, smoking, Fish intake, fruits and vegetables consumption. In addition, psychological component include anxiety, depression scale, and quality of life indices in addition to total cholesterol (HDL and

LDL) dietary fibers intake. The medical risk factors include: increased BP, lipids, and glycemic index as illustrated in Figure 3.

Healthier Life Styles and Depression Risk Management

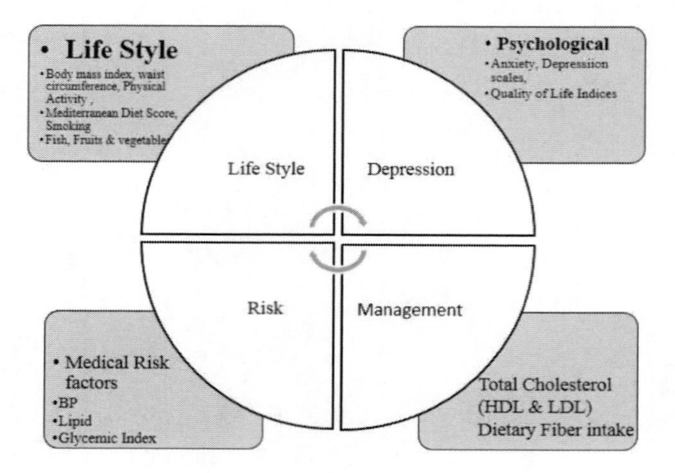

Figure 3. A flow diagram illustrating healthy life style to alleviate depression by remaining socially active, selecting a diet that is low in saturated fat, with fruits and vegetables, smoking and alcohol cessation, and prevention of head injury with loss of consciousness.

A healthy life style to alleviate depression by remaining socially active, selecting a diet that is low in saturated fat, with fruits and vegetables, cessation of smoking and alcohol, and prevention of head injury with loss of consciousness as Figure 4 illustrates.

Healthy Life Style Alleviates Depression

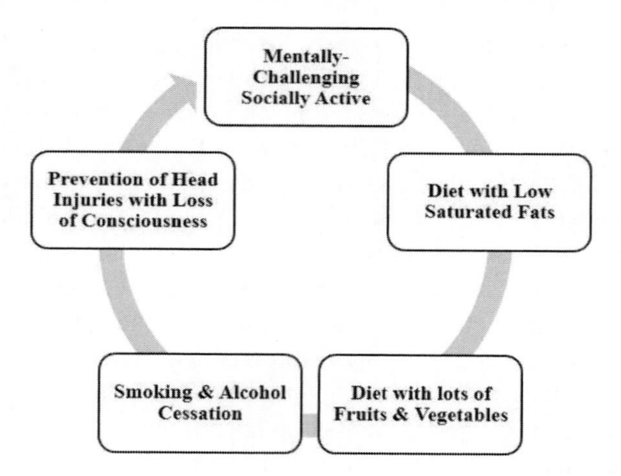

Figure 4. A diagram illustrating various health promotion paramters such as never smoking and drinking, maintaining <25 Kg/m2 BMI, regular moderate physical exercise, adhering to recommended dietary intake. In addition, maintaining total cholesterol <200 mg/dL, BP <120/80 mm Hg, and fasting blood glucose <100 mg/dL are highly significant to enjoy normal healthy free from mood fluctuations (anxiety and depression).

Healthy Diets. A healthy, balanced low-fat, adequately-energy-reduced diet that includes food groups will ensure that we can either prevent further weight gain or achieve weight loss despite taking antidepressants. Certain patients benefit from using a low-fat, low-glycemic index (GI) diet to control their weight. If some patient is not losing weight on a standard low-fat diet ask doctor to check insulin resistance. Patients with insulin resistance respond more readily to a combination of low-fat and low-GI foods. Even when losing weight, one need to eat some foods from each one of the foods catagories to avoid deficiencies which can make feel even more depressed: Low-fat dairy products (milk, yoghurt, cottage cheese) are the best source of calcium in the diet. Calcium is essential for bone health and nerve impulse conduction. Have 3 servings a day. 1 serving = 1 cup of milk/yoghurt/mass; ½ cup cottage cheese. Fresh fruit and vegetables are rich in phytonutrients and dietary fiber which protect against a variety of diseases and keep digestion regular. Have at least 5 servings a day. 1 serving = ½ to 1 fruit, ½ cup cooked vegetables/salad. Low-GI grains and cereals (e.g. low-GI breads, high-fiber breakfast cereals, whole-wheat crackers, brown rice and whole-wheat pasta) are low in fat and high in fiber and B-vitamins (these are essential for CNS). Have 4-5 servings a day. 1 serving = 1 slice of bread; ½ cup dry or cooked cereal/rice/pasta; 3 crackers. Lean meat, fish, eggs and legumes (dry, cooked or canned beans, peas, lentils and soya) are rich in protein and minerals like iron (to prevent anemia) and zinc (to boost immunity). Have 2-3 servings a day. 1 serving = 30g meat/fish; 1 egg; ½ cup cooked legumes. "Good" fats and oils like soft margarine made with mono- or polyunsaturated fats, and oils rich in monounsaturated and omega-3 fatty acids (olive, canola, flax seed and avocado oils) are beneficial to the CNS and prevent cardiovascular diseases. Have 2 servings a day. (1 serving = 1 tablespoon). In general adherence to a diet including: vegetables, fruits, whole grains, fish, and legumes protect against the development of depression in old age as illustrated in Figure 5. (Source: Dry IV van Heerlen, October 2010). A healthier life style prevents depression prophylactically).

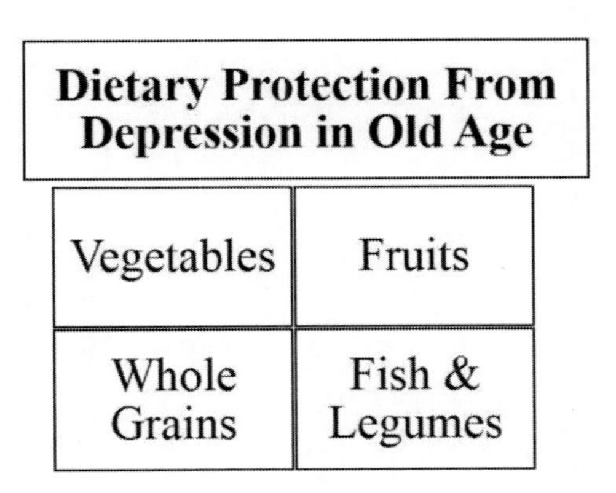

Figure 5. A diagram illustrating adherence to a diet comprised of vegetables, fruits, whole grains, fish, and legumes may protect against the development of depressive symptoms in older age.

References

Byrne, J; Hauck, Y; Fisher, C; Bayes, S; Schutze, R. (2013) Effectiveness of a Mindfulness-Based Childbirth Education Pilot Study on Maternal Self-Efficacy and Fear of Childbirth. *J Midwifery Womens Health*. Dec 10.

Degroote, S; Vogelaers, D.P; Vermeir, P; Mariman, A; De Rick, A; Van Der Gucht, B; Pelgrom, J; Van Wanzeele, F; Verhofstede, C; Vandijck, D.M, (2013) Socio-economic, behavioural, (neuro)psychological and clinical determinants of HRQoL in people living with HIV in Belgium: a pilot study. *J Int AIDS Soc.* 16, 18643.

Heinrich, M; Muller, G; Maritz, U; Mallwitz, J; Klinger, R. (2013) [Effects of interdisciplinary functional restoration treatment with cognitive behavior therapy in patients with chronic back pain: Healthcare research in the context of selective contracts]. *Schmerz*. 27, 566-576.

Macisaac, S.E; Carvalho, A.F; Cha, D.S; Mansur, R.B; McIntyre, R.S. (2014) The mechanism, efficacy, and tolerability profile of agomelatine., *Expert Opin Pharmacother*. 15, 259-274.

Midlov, P; Andersson, M; Ostgren, C.J; Molstad, S, (2014) Depression and use of antidepressants in Swedish nursing homes: a 12-month follow-up study., *Int Psychogeriatr.* 26, 669-675.

Seekatz, B; Meng, K; Faller, H. (2013) Depressivity as mediator in the fear-avoidance model: A path analysis investigation of patients with chronic back pain]. Schmerz. 27, 612-618.

Westmore, I (2010) Weight gain caused by antidepressants., Medical Chronical. *The Doctors Newpaper*. Published in Psychiatry Aug 2010.

Chapter 5

Diet, Exercise, and Depression

Abstract

Although studies on the association of nutrition with depression and anxiety are limited, existing evidence support significant links between diet and depression. Nutritional deficiencies of vitamins and minerals can also induce depression. Nutrients particularly important in relation to depression are: omega-3 fatty acids, folate, vitamin B_{12}, iron, and zinc. Antioxidant nutrients are potentially beneficial dietary factors that could be further explored. Body weight issue may be related to depression and anxiety in a complex manner. Above all dietary interventions to prevent and/or treat depression are inexpensive with reduced risk of adverse effects; hence warrant future research and clinical applications as discussed in this chapter.

Keywords: Viamins, Minerals, Omega-3 Fatty Acids, Iron, Zinc

The past century has experienced a global shift in lifestyle. Dietary intake has altered, with a significant increase in consumption of sugar, snacks, and nutrient-deficient foods, while the consumption of nutrient-dense foods is gradually diminishing. Industrialization and urbanization has a significant impact on physical activity and more than 30% of global population is inadequately physically active. According to WHO report chronic lifestyle-driven non-communicable diseases are the major contributor to early mortality in developed and developing countries. Particularly, depression imposses extensive burden of illness in middle income countries. (*WHO: Global status report on noncommunicable diseases 2010. Geneva*). Jaca et al., (2012) reported that unhealthy lifestyle is posing a significant burden of chronic non-communicable diseases such as depression are one of the most common non-communicable diseases globally. *Poor diet (rich in high energy drinks) and lack of exercise are primarily responsible for the genesis of depression*. Although studies examining dietary improvement as potential therapeutic approach in depression is as yet unavailable, recent epidemiological studies supports poor quality of diet as a major risk factor of depression. Exercise has been reported to be an effective treatment strategy for depression. But increased physical activity is inadequately encouraged during the clinical management of depression. Improved diet, physical activity and cigarette smoking cessation should be encouraged to patients with depression. Recommendations may be focused primarily on following national guidelines for healthy eating and regular exercise. Life style changes to diet and exercise will be highly significant to aging population as non-drug, easy-to–follow intervention with no adverse effect, would make promising potential therapy. There are several clinical conditions that are associated with minor to major depression. Most vulnerable include: severe undernutrition, immunocompromized persons, chronic drug addicts, psychotics, HIV/AIDs patients, cancer patients, astronauts, war-wounded soldiers with post-traumatic stress disorder, post-operational patients, post-partum women and several other clinical conditions. These victims develop typical anorexia and have aversion for any healthy diet. These patients have special dietary requirements such as radapertized or redurized diet (*Gamma-sterilized diet at cryogenic temperature*) as Figure 6 illustrates.

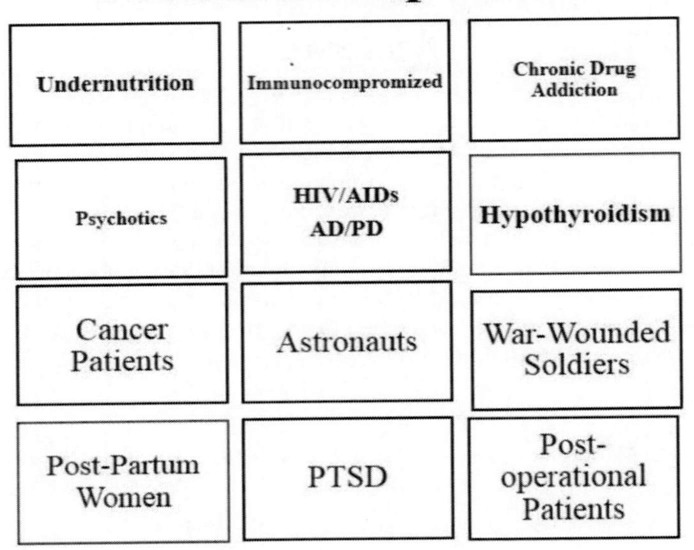

Figure 6. A diagram illustrating undernutrition: immunocompromized, chronic drug addicts, psychotic, HIV/AIDs patients, cancer patients, astronauts, war-wounded soldiers with post-traumatic stress disorder, post-operational patients, post-partum women and several other clinical conditions. These patients have special dietary requirements such as radapertized or Redurized diet (Gamma-sterilized diet at cryogenic temperature).

Experimental studies have demonstrated that 12 consecutive day exercise in aging rats could help preserve improve function due to changes in dopamine, suggesting that exercise could reverse the slowed movements that are hallmarks of old age. Yoga or meditation enhance body/mind awareness particularly in persons with paralysis. Long-term exercise in aging rats improved memory as well as enhanced vascular angiogenesis in the white matter of their brains. Increased blood flow may explain why exercise can help preserve memory. Hence exercise could be an important treatment for depression in adolescents. A calorie restricted diet in middle age onward protected rats against the effects of aging on movement. Thus dietary interventions can help preserve movement in a manner similar to exercise.

Indeed exercise has a significant impact in healthy aging. Hence diet, meditation and exercise can help accomplish wellness in body and brain as as function of aging.

Sanheeza et al., (2013) recently reviewed the association between dietary variables and the risk of depression. The participants in the age range 18-97 years and the sample size was in the range of 526-27111 with a follow up from 2-13 years. The variables inversely associated with depression risk were the consumption of nutrients including folate, omega-3 fatty acids, and monounsaturated fatty acids, olive oil and fish; and diet rich in fruits, vegetables, nuts, and legumes. Some of these associations varied with sex and some exhibited a nonlinear association. This study revealed conflicting evidence for relationship between diet and depression. Moreover these analyses were prone to subjectivities in these meta-analyses. Although diet may influence the risk of depression, the evidence is yet inconclusive. However encouraging healthy-dietary patterns may have a benefit. Further studies are needed to determine the association between diet and the risk of depression. There are three major risk factors of depression such as *(i) smoking, (ii) physical inactivity, and (iii) improper dietary habits.* A study provided limited evidence of the association between the Mediterranean and Norwegian diets as protective factors from depression. Twenty five studies with a total of 53,770 participants were undertaken in USA (11 studies), Japan (3), Spain (2) and countries in Europe, Asia and Australasia (one from each country). Most studies pointed out factors such as age, sex, education, income, and physical activity as important variables using traditional regional diets: Mediterranean study provided limited evidence of an association between increased adherence to this diet and reduced likelihood of depression. Japanese study also showed conflicting evidence: one study showed association between adherence to a Japanese diet and reduced depressive symptoms, where as the other showed no association. Norwegian study showed limited evidence. One study found a positive association in line with above diets for men but not for women. Healthy diets involving low-calorie or balanced meals or whole food diets): showed conflicting evidence with six studies demonstrating that healthy diet reduces the likelihood of depression whereas six showed no association. The western or less healthy diets: also showed a conflicting evidence: Three studies reported positive association between consumption of a Western diet (including processed and take-away foods, and foods high in sugar and or fat content) and incidence of depression. Seven studies showed no association. Depression as predictor of diet quality: exhibited conflicting evidence: Two studies found that depressive symptoms predicted the consumption of an unhealthy diet. Due to conflicting results and heterogeneity, including the measurement and definitions of dietary quality, depression assessment and study samples, the authors concluded that to elucidate whether a true causal relationship exists between diet and depression, further research is needed. Hence, longitudinal studies are required to determine the role of diet in the development of mental disorders across the life span. No study examined a comparison of diets between countries, which may elucidate greater variation. It was uncertain whether the conflicting evidence is the result of heterogeneity between studies, difference in statistical methods, or the difficulty in controlling for all potential confounding socio-economic variables. In order to develop a better understanding of the relationship between diet and depression, more research is needed to determine the exact functional association between diet and depression.

Dietary Pattern and Depression. Melanson (2007) has written an excellent review on the influence of diet on depression and anxiety. Recently Quirk et al., (*2013)* reported that diet modifies various biological factors associated with the development of depression. However, association between diet quality and depression are poorly understood. These investigators performed a review to evaluate evidence regarding the association between diet quality and depression. To accomplish evidence-based analysis, a computer-aided literature search was conducted using Medline, CINAHL, and PsycINFO from Jan 1965 to Oct 2011. Twenty five studies from nine countries met eligibility criteria. The analysis found limited evidence to support an association between traditional diets (Mediterranean or Norwegian diets) and depression. A conflicting evidence for association between (i) traditional Japanese diet and depression (ii) a healthy diet and depression (iii) a Western diet and depression, and (iv) individuals with depression and likelihood of eating a less healthy diet. This was the first study to provide evidence regarding diet quality, dietary pattern, and depression. Studies of single nutrients on depression have generated inconsistent results, and have failed to consider the complex interactions between nutrients. Several studies are now investigating the association of overall dietary patterns and depression. Lai et al., (2014) recently reviewed the current literature and performed meta-analyses to determine the association between dietary pattern and depression. The healthy dietary pattern was associated with reduced odds of depression. No significant association was observed between the western diet and depression, however studies were limited to estimate this effect, suggesting that high intake of fruits, and vegetables, fish, and whole grains may be associated with a reduced depression risk.

In general diets can be divided in three major classes (i) Class-1 diet includes dominance of fruits and vegetables and low SB, intake of sweets, soft drinks, chips, and fries; Class-2 diet is composed of high SB and high intake of sweets, soft drinks, and fires; Class-3 diet is composed of low PA, low fruits and vegetables intake, low intake of sweets, chips and fries (milk and dairy products; meat, fish, and eggs; cereals and derivatives; fruit and vegetables) as illustrated in Figure 7. These kinds of diets can be derived from three dietary patterns including (i) plant food and fish, (ii) Fish intake and (iii) Western diet (predominantly meat) as an important ingredient as Figure 7 illustrates.

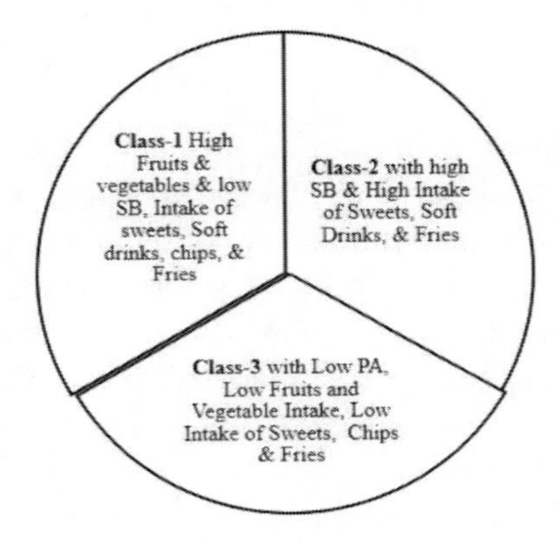

Figure 7. A pie chart illustrating primarily three types of diets. (i) Class-1 diet includes dominance of fruits and Vegetables and low SB, intake of sweets, soft drinks, chips, and fries; Class-2 diet is composed of high SB and high intake of sweets, soft drinks, and fires; Class-3 diet is composed of low PA, low fruits and vegetables intake, low intake of sweets, chips and fries. *(milk and dairy products; meat, fish, and eggs; cereals and derivatives; fruit and vegetables).*

Dietary Patterns and Depression

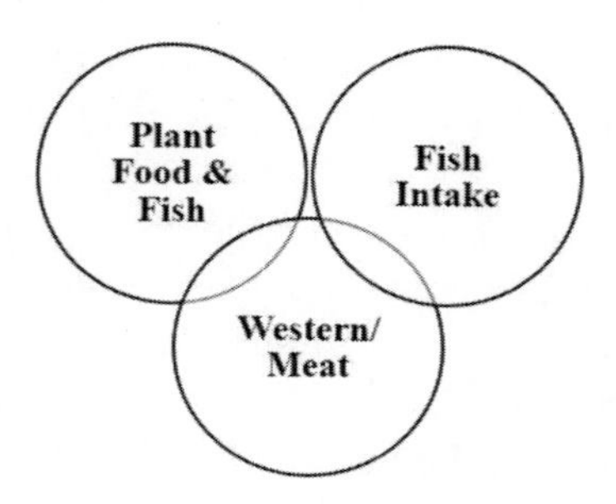

Figure 8. A diagram illustrating primarily three dietary patterns including (i) plant food and fish, Fish intake and (iii) Western diet predominantly meat as an important ingredient.

Folic Acid and Depression. Recently Reynolds (2014) wrote an excellent review on folic acid and its combined role with vitamin B_{12} in regulating CNS and hematopoietic development. Folic acid and vitamin B_{12} metabolism are closely linked because deficiency of either leads to megaloblastic anemia. The neurological manifestations of folate and vitamin B_{12} deficiency overlap and include cognitive impairments, dementia, depression, peripheral neuropathy and degeneration of the spinal cord. There is often dissociation between the psychiatric and hematological manifestations. A similar association exists between in born errors of folate and vitamin B_{12} deficiency. Reduced folate and increased homcysteine levels are major risk factors for dementia, including AD and depression. Clinical response to treatment with folate is usually slow due to blood brain barrier for the vitamin and is related to excitatory properties of folate derivatives. Inappropriate administration of folic acid in the presence of vitamin B_{12} deficiency may lead to both neurologic and hematological relapse. Imapired maternal folate intake and status increases the risk of neural tube defects. Periconceptual prophylactic administration of the vitamin reduces, but not eliminates the risk of neural tube defects even in the absence of folate deficiency. Folate and vitamin B_{12} play a central role in the CNS function at all ages, especially in purine, thymine nucleotide, and DNA synthesis, genomic and nongenomic methylation and, therefore, in tissue growth, differentiation and repair. Folate is an important B vitamin which plays a significant role not only in the DNA synthesis but also in the methylation reactions in the cells. Folate metabolism is influenced by dietary intake and the polymorphism of the associated genes. Impaired folate metabolism impacts both methylation (epigenetic) as well as the DNA synthesis process, both of which have been implicated in the development of diseases including depression. Polymorphic genes have been implicated in the development of various diseases such as vascular diseases, Down's syndrome, neural tube defects, psychiatric disorders (Depression), and cancers (Nazki et al., 2014). These vitamins have role in prevention of disorders of CNS development, mood, and dementia, including AD, and aging.

Omega-3 Fatty Acids and Depression. Recently Hennebelle et al., (2014) reported that chronic stress causes the release of glucocorticoids, which influence the cerebral function, particularly the glutamatergic neurotransmission. The stress-induced changes in neurotransmission can be counteracted by increasing the consumption of n-3 PUFAs. Numerous studies have described that n-3 PUFAs protects glutamatergic neurotransmission from damage induced by stress and glucocorticoids, preventing the development of stress-related disorders such as depression and anxiety. The hippocampus possesses glucocorticoid receptors and is involved in learning and memory, which renders it more susceptible to stress. Hence stress can alter certain aspects of hippocampal function. n-3 PUFA may prevent the deleterious effects of chronic stress, particularly alterations of glutamatergic synapses in the hippocampus.

Dysmenorrhea and Depression. Dysmenorrhea is a general symptom for large proportion of women of reproductive age; however, severe pain limiting daily activities is less common. Dysmenorrhea improves with increased age, parity, and use of oral contraceptives and is positively associated with stress and family history. Ju et al., (2014) recently reported that dysmenorrhea is a common menstrual complaint with major impact on women's quality of life, work performance, and health-care. These investigators used fifteen primary studies published between 2002 and 2011 to determine the prevalence of dysmenorrhea, 16% to 91% in women of reproductive age, with severe pain in 2%-29%. Women's age, parity, and use of oral contraceptives were inversely associated with dysamenorrhea, and stress increased the risk of dysamenorrhea. The effect was generally modest to moderate, with odd ratios 1-4. Family history of dysamenorrhea increased its risk, with odd ratios 3.8- 20.7. Inconclusive evidence was obtained for modifiable factors such as cigarettes smoking, diet, obesity, depression, and substance abuse.

Obesogenic Risk Factors and Depression. Hoare et al., (2014) reported that adolescence is a transitional life phase that is associated with increased risk for two major health conditions-obesity and mental health problems. Given the established comorbidity of obesity and depression, further exploration was required to investigate the association between obesogenic risk and obesity in the maintenance of depression symptoms. These researchers evaluated the relationship between obesogenic risk factors (physical activity, sedentary behavior, and diet and weight status) and depression in adolescents. Relationships were found between lack of physical exercise, increased sedentary behavior, poor quality of diet, obese or overweight and repression in adolescence. However the finding that obseogenic risk factors are associated with poor adolescent mental health need to be interpreted with caution because these data were from non-representative samples with sub-optimal study design and methodology.

Eating Disorders and Depression. The exact relationship between eating disorders, mood, and anxiety disorders remains uncertain. Araujo et al., (2010) examined the previous studies that investigated the relationship between depression and binge eating disorders (BED). The findings of 14 studies showed an association between depression and binge eating disorder. Major depression is primarily observed in psychiatric disorders in women with anorexia nervosa. Anorexia nervosa occurs both before depression and vice versa, and several studies suggest depression may persist even after recovery from anorexia nervosa. The existence of anorexia nervosa increases the risk of an anxiety disorder. It is usually generalized anxiety disorder, obsessive compulsive disorder, or social phobia. More than 50% women with anorexia nervosa also have an anxiety disorder. Usually the onset of anxiety disorder precedes the onset of anorexia nervosa. Patients with bulimia-nervosa-associated MDD have different depressive features than those with depression. Depression may be present before bulimia nervosa and vice versa, and some patients with bulimia nervosa experience depression even after recovering from eating disorder. Women with bulimia nervosa and depression response to antidepressant medication. The most commonly noticed anxiety disorder in women with bulimia nervosa are social phobia and general anxiety disorder. The lifetime anxiety disorders exists in >50% of women with bulimia nervosa. Symptoms of anxiety disorders are usually seen before those of bulimia nervosa. Treatment for patients with eating disorders and depression and/or anxiety include: medication, nutritional rehabilitation, cognitive neurobehavioral therapy, family therapy, dialectical behavioral therapy, interpersonal therapy, psychotherapy and self-help. However limited evidence is as yet available about their effectiveness. There is limited information as to how to treat co-morbidity should be treated in patients with eating disorders. Weather eating disorders or the mood/anxiety disorders should be treated first or weather both disorders should be treated simultaneously remains unknown. The effective treatment should address the underlying cause of the eating disorder. However minimal effects of treatment can be expected if the patient is starved. The absorption of medication is a major issue, especially among purging patients. Cognitive therapies may be effective for depression in these patients. However there is no evidence to suggest that cognitive behavioral therapy is superior compared to pharmacological treatments. The effectiveness of treatment for anorexia nervosa, bulimia nervosa, and binge eating disorders varies in quality. Further studies may be conducted with improved research design, standardized measures, and appropriate statistical analyses.

References

Araujo, D.M.R; deSilva Santos, G.F; Nardi, A.E. (2010) Binge eating disorder and depression: a systemetic review. *The World Journal of Bilogical Psychiatry* 11, 199-207.

Hoare, E; Skouteris, H; Fuller-Tyszkiewicz, M; Millar, L; Allender, S. (2014) Association between obesogenic risk factors and depression among adolescents: a systematic review., Obes Res. 15, 40-51.

Jacka, F.N; Berk, M, (2012) Depression, diet and exercise. *MJA Open 1 Suppl* 4, 21-23.

Ju, H; Jones, M; Mishra, G.D. (2014) Premenstrual syndrome and dysmenorrhea: symptom trajectories over 13 years in young adults. *Maturitas.* 78, 99-105.

Lai, J.S; Hiles, S; Bisguera, A; Hure, A.J; McEyoy, M; Attia, J. (2014) A systematic review and meta-analysis of dietary patterns and depression in community-dwelling adults., *Am. J. Clin. Nutr.* 99, 181-197.

Melanson, K.J. (2007) Nutrition Review: Relationships Nutrition with Depression and Anxiety. *American Journal of Lifestyle Medicine* May 1, 171-174,

Nazki, F.H; Sameer, A.S; and Ganaie, B.A. (2014) Folate: metabolism, genes, polymorphism and related diseases. *Gene* 533; 11-20.

Quirk, S.E; Williams, L.J; O,Neil, A; Pasco, J.A; Jacka, F.N; Housden, S; Berk, M; Brenan, S.L. (2013) The association between diet quality, dietary patterns and depression in adults: a systematic review. *BMC Psychiatry* 13,175.

Reynolds, E.H. (2014) The neurology of folic acid deficiency., *Handbook Clin Neurol.* 120, 927-943.

Sanhueza, C; Ryan, L; Foxcroft, D.R.(2013) Diet and the risk of unipolar depression in adults: systematic review of cohort studies. *Journal of Human Nutrition & Dietetics.* 26, 56-70.

Chapter 6

Disease-Specific Antidepressant Diets

Abstract

Depression is a primary complaint of chronic degenerative diseases such as type-II diabetes. It is therefore highly significant to recommend a diabetes-specific antidepressant diet to these patients for their better quality of life. In this chapter disease-specific antidepressant diets have been described and recent literature information is provided to clinically manage patients with disease-specific MDD.

Keywords: Type II diabetes, Antidepressant Diets, MDD.

Type II diabetes mellitus (T2DM) and MDD are highly co-morbid, and there is a direct link between the two. Liu et al., (2013) described a mouse model of a depression-like and insulin-resistant (DIR) state induced by high-fat diet (HFD) and corticosterone (CORT) co-treatment. 5-Aminoimidazole-4-carboxamide-1-β-d- ribofuranoside (AICAR), a pharmacological agonist of AMP-activated protein kinase (AMPK), was used to improve insulin resistance (IR) as an antidepressant. AICAR prevented reduced insulin actions of skeletal muscle in HFD. Exercise also produced antidepressant effects suggesting that the effects of AICAR and exercise on DIR may enhance our understanding regarding association between diabetes and depression. Yu et al., (2013) investigated the association between depressive symptoms and diet quality, physical activity, and body composition. These researchers recruited 4511 men and women aged 35-69 years from 2009 through 2010. Depressive symptoms were assessed by using the Patient Health Questionnaire. Anthropometric indices and body composition were measured. Antidepressant use, dietary intake, physical activity, and potential confounders were analyzed. The depressive symptoms were positively associated with obesity indices. Compared with non-depressed individuals, those with mild and MDD had increased odd ratios for both obesity and abdominal obesity respectively. Depressed individuals were less likely to have a high quality diet or engage in high levels of physical activity compared with controls suggesting that depression is associated with obesity, poor diet, and physical inactivity.

Recently Mezuk et al., (2013) examined the association between prediabetes and Type 2 diabetes with depression and antidepressant medication. Analysis was performed on adults aged 30 and older (n = 3,183, Mean age = 52.1 year). Depression was measured by the Patient Health Questionnaire-9. Participants were categorized using fasting glucose levels as normoglycemic (glucose <100 mg/dL), undiagnosed prediabetes (glucose 100-125.9), clinically identified prediabetes (glucose 100-125.9 plus clinical diagnosis), undiagnosed Type 2 diabetes (glucose >126), and Type 2 diabetes (glucose >126 plus clinical diagnosis or use of antidiabetic medications). Health demotion behaviors included smoking, poor diet, alcohol abuse, and obesity. Health promotion behaviors included efforts to change diet, lose weight, and increase physical activity. Clinically diagnosed diabetes was associated with 4.3-fold greater odds of depression, but undiagnosed diabetes was not associated with depression. This relationship was more pronounced for prediabetes. Clinically identified diabetes was associated with 1.8-fold greater odds of antidepressant use, but undiagnosed diabetes was not associated with antidepressant use. Health behaviors were not related to depression. The relationship between diabetes and depression and antidepressant use was dependent on whether the diabetes was clinically diagnosed, suggesting that relationship between diabetes and depression may be attributable to factors related to disease management.

Omega-3 Fatty Acids and Depression. Persons et al., (2013) determined the relationship between the omega-3 fatty acids of RBC membranes, particularly DHA and EPA and depression in post-menopausal women. The association between dietary omega-3 fatty acid intake and depressive symptoms was characterized. These investigators included 7086 members of the Women's Health Initiative Memory Study (aged 63-81 years) who had an assessment of omega-3 fatty acid concentrations at the baseline. Depressive symptoms at baseline and follow-up were characterized using the Burnam eight-item scale for depressive disorders and inferred by antidepressant medication. In multivariable-adjusted models, primary exposure, RBC DHA + EPA, was not related to depressive symptoms at baseline or follow-up, nor were RBC omega-3, DHA, or EPA. Dietary intake of omega-3 was positively correlated with depressive symptoms, although this did not persist at follow-up, indicating no relationship between RBC omega-3 levels and depressive symptoms, and between dietary omega-3 and depressive symptoms. Thus omega-3 status was not related to risk of depression in post-menopausal women.

PMS and Chromium. Premenstrual dysphoric disorder (PMDD) afflicts ~7% of women during reproductive-age resulting in impaired relationships, diminished quality of life, and disability-adjusted years lost just like other MDDs. Response to pharmacological treatment is inadequate in ~50% of women. Brownley et al., (2013) performed a study to determine the effects of short-term chromium supplementation-on menstrual cycle-related mood and physical symptoms. Five women were studied (2 of them were referred specifically for treatment-resistant menstrual-related symptoms); 6 women completed study of chromium plus placebo versus chromium plus Sertraline. Treatments were from mid-cycle to onset of menses in 1-month intervals. Symptom ratings were obtained by self-report, using daily symptom checklists, and by clinical assessment, using the Hamilton Psychiatric Rating Scale for Depression (HAM-D) and the Clinical Global Impressions (CGI) scale. Treatment with chromium was associated with reduced mood symptoms and improved overall health satisfaction. In some cases, chromium was associated with significant improvement; in others, chromium plus an antidepressant resulted in greater improvement than either chromium or an antidepressant alone, suggesting that chromium may be a useful therapy for women suffering from menstrual cycle-related symptoms.

Irritable bowel syndrome (IBS) and Depression. Fashner and Gitu (2013) reported that the diagnosis of IBS should be considered when patients have had abdominal pain/discomfort, bloating, and change in bowel habits for 6 months. Patients may experience variation between periods of constipation and diarrhea. When evaluating patients with IBS, physicians should be alert for symptoms, such as rectal bleeding, anemia, night time pain, and weight loss. Clinicians who are confident in diagnosing IBS based on symptoms do not need many tests unless the patient has symptoms. Various etiologic mechanisms have been proposed for IBS, including abnormal bowel motility, inflammation, altered mucosal permeability, genetic predisposition, and visceral hypersensitivity. Lack of certainty about the etiology makes it difficult to develop effective management approaches directed toward symptom relief. Dietary changes, such as avoiding fermentable carbohydrates, may benefit some patients, particularly those with bloating. Constipation-dominant IBS can be managed with antispasmodics, Lubiprostone, or Linaclotide, whereas diarrhea-dominant IBS can be managed with Loperamide or Alosetron, however it can cause ischemic colitis. For long-term therapy, TCAs or SSRIs are beneficial. Peppermint oil and probiotics may also be beneficial.

Polydypsia and Depression. Dyspepsia is caused by inflammation in the upper GIT, food sensitivity, or a change in gut microflora. Although the initial management is well established, managing those with continued symptoms is a challenge. Antidepressants and newer gastric motility agents show promise. Ford and Moayyedi (2013) reported that polydyspepsia affects up to 40% of the general population and reduces quality of life. A small proportion of patients have peptic ulcer disease which can be treated with Helicobacter pylori eradication therapy. Approximately 20% have gastro-oesophageal reflux disease (GERD) which can be treated with proton pump inhibitors. Patients who remain symptomatic may require an endoscopic examination, but most will have functional dyspepsia which remains a challenge. Tricyclic antidepressant (TCA) therapy may be effective in functional dyspepsia. A phase III randomized controlled trial reports that a new prokinetic, Acotiamide, diminishes symptoms in functional dyspepsia patients. Preliminary data suggest Buspirone, a drug that promotes gastric accommodation, is also effective in functional dyspepsia. Lucas et al., (2014) identified a dietary pattern that was related to plasma levels of inflammatory biomarkers (C-reactive protein, interleukin-6, TNF-α receptor 2), and analyzed the relationship of this pattern and depression risk among participants in the Nurses' Health Study. A total of 43,685 women (aged 50-77) without depression were followed. Dietary information was obtained from food frequency questionnaires and computed as cumulative average of dietary intakes with a 2-year latency. These investigators used a strict definition of depression that required both self-reported physician-diagnosed depression and use of antidepressants, and a broader definition that included women who reported either clinical diagnosis or antidepressants. During the follow-up, 2594 cases of depression using the stricter definition and 6446 using the broader definition was recorded. After adjustment for BMI and other confounders, relative risks comparing extreme quintiles of the inflammatory dietary pattern were 1.41 for the broader definition of depression. The inflammatory dietary pattern was associated with a higher depression risk suggesting that chronic inflammation may underlie the association between diet and depression.

Several studies indicate the antidepressant effects of mGlu5 receptor antagonists such as 3-[(2-methyl-1,3-thiazol-4-yl)ethynyl]-pyridine (MTEP). The explanation for the mechanism of these effects might be crucial in finding novel antidepressant drugs (AD). Pałucha-Poniewiera et al., (2013) investigated the role of the serotonergic system in the antidepressant-like activity of MTEP in the tail suspension test (TST) in C57BL/6J mice, using selected serotonergic receptor antagonists and by applying two different methods of serotonin (5-HT) depletion. The mGlu5 receptor antagonist, MTEP, similar to the fluoxetine did not induce antidepressant-like effects in mice pretreated with tryptophan hydroxylase inhibitor, para-chlorophenylalanine, whereas, MTEP worked as an AD in the TST in mice fed on a tryptophan-free (TRP-free) diet for 3 weeks. However, fluoxetine, which was used as a reference control was also active, suggesting that a TRP-free diet was not effective in reducing the 5-HT level. Furthermore, these investigators showed that the 5HT2A/2C antagonist, Ritanserin, yet not the 5-HT1A antagonist, WAY100635, 5HT1B antagonist, SB224289 or 5HT4 antagonist, GR125487, reversed the antidepressant-like effects of MTEP. A sub-effective dose of MTEP co-administered with a sub-effective dose of Citalopram induced an antidepressant-like effect suggesting the involvement of serotonergic activation in the antidepressant-like effects of the mGlu5 antagonist, MTEP, in the TST.

Dietary Zinc and Depression. Zinc is an important immunomodulatory trace element and beneficial in enhancing antidepressant therapy. Recent studies suggest an association between low dietary zinc and depression. Preclinical and clinical studies have suggested a relationship between dietary zinc intake and depressive symptoms. Młyniec et al., (2013) determined whether zinc deficiency alters the response to antidepressants with a different mechanism of action. These researchers examined whether these changes are related to activity of the HPA axis. Male CD-1 mice were assigned to groups according to diet and antidepressant administration. To evaluate animal behavior, the immobility time in the forced swim test (FST) and locomotor activity were measured. Antidepressants administered to zinc-deprived mice induced an altered response in the FST compared to animals fed with an adequate diet. There were no changes in locomotor activity. Animals subjected to a zinc-deficient diet showed a significant reduction in serum zinc levels, which was normalized by antidepressant treatment. An increase in serum corticosterone levels in mice fed with a zinc-deficient diet and treated with antidepressants was observed. Reduced levels of zinc contribute to activation of the HPA axis and a diet with a reduced zinc alters antidepressant action, associated with a reduction in the serum zinc level and rise in the corticosterone level, indicating the involvement of zinc deficiency in the pathogenesis of depression. Another study examined the association between dietary zinc intake and depression in healthy men during a 20-year follow-up. Lehto et al., (2013) performed a population-based Kuopio Ischemic Heart Disease Risk Factor (KIHD) Study on 2317 Finnish men aged 42-61 years. Zinc intake was assessed at baseline by a 4-d food record. Baseline depression severity was recorded with the Human Population Laboratory Depression Scale. The depression was defined as having received a hospital discharge diagnosis of unipolar depressive disorder. 60 individuals received a hospital discharge diagnosis of depression. In Cox regression analysis adjusted for age, baseline depression severity, smoking, alcohol use, physical exercise and the use of dietary supplements, belonging to the lowest tertile of energy-adjusted zinc intake was not associated with an increased risk of depression suggesting that a low dietary zinc intake may not precede depression. Hence dietary zinc intake may be irrelevant for the prevention of depression in middle-aged men with a sufficient dietary zinc intake.

Mediterranean Diet and Depreesion. Skarupski et al., (2013) tested the association between a Mediterranean dietary pattern and depressive symptoms. Models were adjusted for age, sex, race, education, income, widowhood, antidepressant use, total calorie intake, BMI, smoking, alcohol consumption, number of self-reported medical conditions, cognitive function, and physical disability. Community-dwelling participants (n=3502) of the Chicago Health and Aging Project aged 65+ years (59% African American) who had no evidence of depression at the baseline were selected in this study. Adherence to a Mediterranean-dietary pattern was assessed by the MedDietScore. Dietary evaluation was performed with a food frequency questionnaire at baseline and related to depression as measured by the presence of four or more depressive symptoms. Adherence to a Mediterranean diet was associated with a reduced depressive symptoms. The annual rate of depressive symptoms was 98.6% lower among persons in the highest tertile of a Mediterranean dietary pattern compared with persons in the lowest tertile group supporting the hypothesis that adherence to a diet including vegetables, fruits, whole grains, fish, and legumes may protect against the development of depressive symptoms in older age. Furthermore, Perveen et al., (2013) performed a study to examine the antidepressant and anxiolytic effects and their neurochemical basis following repeated administration of extravirgin olive oil in male albino Wistar rats at the dose of 0.25 mL/kg daily for 4 weeks. Control rats received equal volume of water. Elevated-plus maze (EPM) test and forced swim test (FST) were performed for the assessment of anxiety and depression. An increase in time spent in open arm in EPM and increased struggling time in FST following long-term administration of olive oil indicated that olive oil has anxiolytic and antidepressant properties. Olive oil decreased brain 5-HT, 5-HIAA, and DA; however, DA metabolite homovalinic acid (HVA) were increased suggesting that it has neuroprotective effects. Olive oil reduced behavioral deficits via altering 5-HT and DA metabolism, hence could be used as a therapeutic agent for depression and anxiety. Chocano-Bedoya et al., (2013) examined whether long-term dietary patterns derived from a food-frequency questionnaire (FFQ) to predict the development of depression in middle-aged and older women. These investigators conducted a study on 50,605 participants (age range: 50-77 y) without depression at baseline (1996) who were followed until 2008. Long-term diet was assessed by using FFQs every 4 y since 1986. Prudent (high in vegetables) and Western (high in meats) patterns were identified by using a principal component analysis. Two definitions for clinical depression were used as follows: a strict definition that required both clinical diagnosis and use of antidepressants (3002 cases) and a broad definition that included women who reported either a clinical diagnosis or antidepressant use (7413 cases). After adjustment for age, BMI, and other potential confounders, no significant association was seen between the dietary patterns and depression risk. Under the broad definition, women with the highest scores for the Western pattern had 15% higher risk of depression than did women with the lowest scores, but after adjustment for psychological scores at baseline, results were insignificant. These results did not support association between dietary patterns from factor analysis and depression risk.

Milk Proteins. Vekovischeva et al., (2013) reported that milk proteins are the main components of feeding and have potential to change the mental condition. However, the effects of milk proteins after prolonged use remain poorly understood. These investigators compared the effects of two whey proteins (α-lactalbumin (α-lac) and native whey) with casein on social and individual behavior in mice. During a 30 d-long dietary intervention, male C57BL/6J mice had ad libitum access to diet containing 17% of one of three protein sources: α-lac, native whey or casein. Mice had voluntary access to a running wheel. Social behavior (group and resident-intruder activity) was tested at baseline and at the end of the intervention. Half of each dietary group was withdrawn from the diet and running wheel for 7 d, and social activity and individual behavior tests (open field, elevated-plus maze, light–dark box and forced swimming) were performed, to evaluate anxiety and depression. This study indicated that long-term ingestion of whey proteins may modulate behavior when compared with casein. Diet enriched with α-lac exhibited anxiolytic and antidepressive activities while the whey diet improved sociability. The differences between the diet groups were pronounced under the running wheel and the withdrawal of the experimental diet, suggesting the beneficial effects of the milk proteins in stressful situations. Diet-induced behavioral changes remained evident for a week after feeding suggesting that the proteins of the whey fraction have efficacy on the mental state of mice. Sihvola et al., (2013) examined the influence of consumption of a whey protein-in breakfast drink v. a carbohydrate drink v. control on subjective and physiological responses to mental workload in simulated work. Ten healthy subjects (seven women, median age 26 years, median BMI 23 kg/m(2) participated in this study. The subjects performed demanding work-like tasks after having a breakfast drink high in protein (HP) or high in carbohydrate (HC) or a control drink. Subjective states were assessed using the NASA Task Load Index (NASA-TLX), the Karolinska sleepiness scale (KSS) and the modified Profile of Mood States. Heart rate was recorded during task performance. The ratio of plasma tryptophan (Trp) to the sum of the other large neutral amino acids (LNAA) and salivary cortisol were also analyzed. The plasma Trp:LNAA ratio was 30% higher after the test drinks HP than after the control drink. The increase in heart rate was smaller after the HP and HC drinks when compared with the control drink during task performance. Subjective sleepiness was reduced more after the HC drink than after the control drink. There were no significant differences between the breakfast types in the NASA-TLX index, cortisol levels or task performance suggesting that whey protein or carbohydrates may improve coping with mental tasks in healthy subjects.

Robinson et al., (2013) reported that serotonergic medications can mitigate the negative affective biases in depression or anxiety, however its molecular mechanism of occurrence remains unknown. The negative affective biases may be driven by specific medial prefrontal-amygdala circuitry, hence these researchers investigated whether serotonin manipulation can alter affective processing within a dorsal medial prefrontal-amygdala circuit: the putative human homologue of the rodent prelimbic-amygdala circuit or 'aversive amplification' circuit. Pharmaco-fMRI design, subjects performed a forced-choice face identification task with word distractors in an fMRI scanner over two separate sessions. Subjects received dietary depletion of tryptophan on one session while on the other session they received a balanced placebo control diet. The dorsal medial prefrontal response was elevated in response to fearful relative to happy faces under depletion was accompanied by increase in positive dorsal medial prefrontal-amygdala functional connectivity suggesting that serotonin depletion engages a prefrontal-amygdala circuit during the processing of fearful relative to happy face stimuli. The same 'aversive amplification' circuit is also engaged during anxiety induced by shock anticipation. As such, serotonergic projections may inhibit engagement of the 'aversive amplification' circuit and dysfunction may contribute to the negative affective bias in mood and anxiety disorders providing explanation for the role of serotonin and serotonergic agents in the neurocircuitry of negative affective bias.

Exercise and Depression. Regular exercise has an antidepressant effect in human subjects. Animal studies have suggested that the antidepressant effect of exercise is attributable to an increase of brain 5-HT; however, the mechanism underlying the antidepressant action via exercise is unclear. In contrast, the effect of 5-HT on antidepressant activity has not been clarified because the therapeutic response to antidepressant drugs has a time lag in spite of the rapid increase of brain 5-HT. Lee et al., (2013) investigated the contribution of brain 5-HT to the antidepressant effect of exercise. Mice were fed a tryptophan-deficient diet and stressed using chronic unpredictable stress (CUS) for 4 weeks with or without the performance of either moderate or intense exercise on a treadmill 3 days per week. The onset of depression-like behavior was not attributable to reduction of 5-HT but to chronic stress. Regular exercise, whether moderate or intense, prevented depression-like behavior with an improvement of hippocampal cell proliferation without 5-HT recovery. The mice that exercised had increased hippocampal NE. Regular exercise prevented the impairment of short-term memory in a 5-HT-reduced state suggesting that: (1) chronic depletion of brain 5-HT may not contribute to the onset of depression-like behavior; (2) regular exercise, whether moderate or intense, prevents the onset of stress-induced depression-like behavior independent of brain 5-HT and is dependent on brain NE; and (3) regular exercise prevents tryptophan depletion-induced impairment of short-term memory.

Recently Imayama et al., (2013) investigated the adherence and changes in body measures and biomarkers of glucose metabolism and inflammation between antidepressant users and non-users in a 12-month controlled trial. These researchers assigned overweight or obese, postmenopausal women to: diet (10% weight loss goal, N=118); moderate-to-vigorous aerobic exercise (225 min/week, N=117); diet+exercise (N=117); and control (N=87). Women using antidepressants were classified as users (N=109). ANOVA and estimating equation were used to compare adherence (exercise, diet session attendance, and changes in percent calorie intake from fat, cardiopulmonary fitness, and pedometer steps) and changes in body measures (weight, waist and percent body fat) and serum biomarkers (glucose, insulin, homeostasis assessment-insulin resistance, and high-sensitivity C-reactive protein) between users and non-users. An interaction term (intervention×antidepressant use) tested effected modification. There were no differences in adherence except that diet session attendance was lower among users in the diet+exercise group. Changes in body measures and serum biomarkers did not differ by antidepressant use. Dietary weight loss and exercise improved body measures and biomarkers of glucose metabolism and inflammation independent of antidepressant use.

It is known that stress can have deleterious effects on health and academic performance. Stress-relieving activities include the non-medical use of prescription drugs (NMUPD). Betancourt et al., (2013) determined the associations between self-perceived academic load and stress, NMUPD (stimulants, depressants, and sleeping medication), and dietary pattern among college students. A questionnaire was used to evaluate academic load and stress, NMUPD, and dietary pattern were used on 275 first- and second-year students. In total, 27.6% reported NMUPD in the past 6 months, with higher use among students aged 21-30 years than in those aged 31-53 years. Those with high levels of stress had higher NMUPD than did those with low or moderate stress levels. Among those who reported NMUPD over 6 months, 74% reported that such use was effective as a coping strategy, and 35% reported that it helped them to improve academic performance. Although no significant association was noticed between NMUPD and dietary pattern, 57% of the participants reported that their appetites decreased when they engaged in NMUPD. Thus high level of stress was related to high NMUPD.

Obesity and Depression. Recently Trigueros et al., (2013) reported that overweight and obesity have a major impact on global health; its prevalence has increased in industrialized countries and diabetes and hypertension are the direct consequences. Pharmacotherapy provides reinforcement for obesity treatment, but should be an adjunctive support to diet, exercise, and lifestyle modification. At present, only Orlistat and Sibutramine have been approved by the FDA for long-term use, but Sibutramine was withdrawn by the European Medicines Agency. The development of functional foods for the prevention and/or treatment of obesity provides an opportunity for the food market and involve the knowledge of the mechanisms of appetite and energy expenditure as well as the metabolic sensation of satiety. Strategies for weight control management affect gut hormones as potential targets for the appetite regulation, stimulation of energy expenditure (thermogenesis), and modifications in the metabolic activity of the gut microbiota. Functional foods may also include fatty acids, phenolic compounds, soybean, plant sterols, dietary calcium and fiber. The present situation of the anti-obesity agents used in dietary therapy as well as some functional food ingredients with anti-obesity effects have been discussed in this report. Furthermore, Oberholzer et al., (2013) investigated the effect of Sibutramine on platelet ultrastructure and morphology in relation to known physiological effects of the compound. Six-week-old, female Spraque-Dawley rats were used in this study. The animals were placed on a high energy diet after which Sibutramine administration followed. Blood was drawn on the day of termination and platelet rich plasma was obtained to prepare plasma smears for analysis. Scanning electron microscopy was used to investigate the ultrastructure of the platelets. Platelets of the Sibutramine-treated animals showed smooth surface with limited pseudopodia as compared to control animals. Higher magnification of the platelets showed membrane tears and swelling, as seen in necrotic cells suggesting that Sibutramine alters the morphology of platelets to that of typical necrotic cells.

Butt et al., (2013) reported that spices have been an integral part of human diets. The bioactive components present in them are of significance owing to their therapeutic potential against various ailments. They prevent chronic ailment in addition to nutrition and included in the category of functional foods. Black pepper is an important healthy food owing to its antioxidant, antimicrobial potential and gastro-protective properties. Black pepper, with piperine as an active ingredient, has rich phytochemistry that includes volatile oil, oleoresins, and alkaloids. Recently cell-culture studies and animal modeling predicted the role of black pepper against number of diseases. The free-radical scavenging activity of black pepper might be helpful in chemoprevention and controlling progression of tumor growth. Additionally, the key alkaloid, piperine assist in cognitive brain functioning, boost nutrient's absorption and improve GIT functionality. The antioxidant, antimicrobial, anti-inflammatory, gastro-protective, and antidepressant activities of black pepper are now being investigated. Moreover, the synergistic interaction of black pepper with other drugs and nutrients is being explored.

Kaplan (2013) provided a review of seminal psychiatric research published in 2011 and 2012 and its clinical relevance for day-to-day practice. The review focused on conditions encountered by adolescent medicine physicians such as ADHD, autism, bipolar disorder, tic disorders, and MDD. Additionally, specific clinical situations for which psychiatric consultation must be obtained, as well as helpful resources and suggestions to mitigate the unavailability of appointments in a mental health office. In addition, Howland (2013) reported that compared to the general population, individuals with psychiatric illness, especially serious and chronic mood and psychotic disorders, are more likely to be overweight or obese, have higher rates of weight-related conditions, and have greater non-suicide mortality rates. Lorcaserin (Belviq (®)), Phentermine/Topiramate combination (Qsymia (®)), and

Bupropion/Naltrexone combinations are effective for the treatment of obesity, as an adjunct to a reduced-calorie diet and physical activity, although their absolute safety is yet to be established. Bariatric surgery is an effective approach for morbid obesity, but careful psychiatric assessment before and follow up after surgery is necessary. Behavioral lifestyle interventions to promote weight loss are effective and should be implemented along with or instead of drug therapies or surgery.

All guidelines for antihypertensive therapy recommend weight loss; anti-obesity drugs might be a helpful option. Siebenhofer et al., (2013) assessed the long-term effects of pharmacologically induced reduction in body weight with Orlistat, Sibutramine or Rimonabant on:- all cause mortality - cardiovascular morbidity - adverse events: - changes in systolic and/or diastolic BP - body weight reduction. Randomized controlled trials in adult hypertensive patients with a study duration of at least 24 weeks comparing pharmacologic interventions (Orlistat, Sibutramine, and Rimonabant) for weight loss with placebo. These researchers used the random effects method and investigated the cause of heterogeneity. The number of studies remained the same, with eight studies comparing Orlistat or Sibutramine to placebo. No study investigating Rimonabant for weight loss was identified. No study included mortality and cardiovascular morbidity as a pre-defined outcome. Incidence of GIT side effects was higher in Orlistat treated patients. Most frequent side effects of Sibutramine were xerostomia, constipation, and headache. Patients assigned to weight loss diets, Orlistat or Sibutramine reduced their body weight more effectively than patients in the usual care/placebo groups. BP reduction in patients treated with Orlistat was for systolic BP (SBP). In patients with elevated BP, Orlistat and Sibutramine reduced body weight to a similar extent. In the same trials, Orlistat reduced BP and Sibutramine increased BP. No trials investigating Rimonabant in people with elevated BP could be included. However long-term trials assessing the effect of Orlistat, Sibutramine and Rimonabant on mortality and morbidity are lacking.

Germ Cell Lines and Reproductive Robustness. Garcia et al., (2013) reported that animals can thrive on variable food resources as a result of autonomous processes and beneficial relationships with their gut microbes. Food intake elicits physiological changes, which are counteracted by transient systemic responses that maintain homeostasis in the organism. This integration of external information occurs through cellular sensory elements, such as nuclear receptors, which modulate gene expression in response to specific cues. Given the importance of germline stem cells (GSCs) for the development of the germline and the continuity of species, it is reasonable to assume that GSCs might be shielded from the negative influence of environmental perturbations. However, there are no mechanisms as yet available that protect GSCs from harmful dietary metabolites. Using Caenorhabditis elegans, these investigators reported that the somatic activity of the conserved nuclear receptor nhr-114/HNF4 protects GSC integrity from dietary metabolites. In the absence of nhr-114 and on certain bacterial diets, otherwise somatically normal animals accumulate germ cell division defects during development and become sterile. In nhr-114(-) animals, the induction of germline defects and sterility depend on bacterial metabolic status, with respect to tryptophan. This illustrates an animal-microbe interaction in which somatic nuclear receptor activity preserves the germline by buffering against dietary metabolites, through a somatic detoxifying response. These findings uncovered evolutionarily-conserved, soma-to-germline axis that maintains reproductive robustness on variable food resources.

Obesity and Psychiatric Medication. Central noradrenergic pathways are involved in feeding and cardiovascular control, physiological processes altered by obesity. Bello et al., (2013) determined how high-fat feeding and body weight gain alter the sensitivity to the feeding suppression and neural activation to a selective NE reuptake inhibitor, Nisoxetine. Acute administration of Nisoxetine resulted in a dose-dependent reduction in the 24 h refeeding response in male Sprague Dawley rats maintained on standard chow. In a similar fashion, Nisoxetine resulted in reductions in BP and increase in heart rate. The 3 mg/kg dose was subthreshold. In a separate experiment, 10 wk exposure to a high-fat diet (60% fat) resulted in weight gain and feeding suppression following administration of Nisoxetine (3 mg/kg) compared with animals fed a control ***diet*** (10% fat). Nisoxetine (3 mg/kg) induced neural activation, as measured by c-Fos immunohistochemistry, in the arcuate nucleus of the hypothalamus in animals exposed to the high-fat diet indicating that acute Nisoxetine can impact cardiovascular performance and that the feeding suppression to a low-dose Nisoxetine is enhanced as a result of high-fat ***diet*** and weight gain. Apter and Steingart (2013) reported that Psychiatric medications have many implications on weight and growth. Stimulant medications may produce appetite loss and thus affect growth. Second-generation antipsychotics which are widely used for psychosis and many other indications may cause weight gain and subsequent metabolic disease. Weight loss as seen in anorexia nervosa may interfere with the efficacy of antidepressants. Hainerová and Lebl (2013) reported that mutations in genes involved in energy balance regulation within the CNS lead to monogenic forms of obesities. Individuals with these mutations are characterized by early-onset obesity by endocrine abnormalities. Carriers of leptin gene mutations are able to normalize their body weight after daily s.c leptin administration. Pharmacotherapy targeting the specific-gene deficiencies has not been tested in other monogenic obesities. Mutations in the melanocortin 4 receptor gene (MC4R) represent the most common cause of human obesity. Several treatment options have been investigated in subjects with MC4R mutations. Few studies showed that an intensive life-style intervention induces similar weight reduction in MC4R mutation carriers in comparison to MC4R mutation noncarriers. However, long-term body weight maintenance is hardly achieved in MC4R mutation carriers. Sibutramine, Serotonin and NE reuptake inhibitor, in MC4R mutation carriers induced weight reduction and improved cardiometabolic health risks. This result was also found in homozygous MC4R mutation carrier. In vitro studies of melanocortin agonists activate mutated MC4R with impaired endogenous agonist functional response. An administration of intranasal adrenocorticotropic hormone was not effective in subjects with pro-opiomelanocortin gene mutations. Bariatric surgery has also been performed in few of MC4R mutation carriers. After gastric banding, lower body weight reduction and worse improvement of metabolic complications was found in MC4R mutation carriers versus noncarriers. However, preliminary results suggest that diversionary operations as gastric bypass represent a suitable method for MC4R mutation carriers as well. However, the management of monogenic obesities still remains a challenge.

Taurine. Toyoda and Iio (2013) reported that taurine is one of the most abundant amino acids in the CNS, and has various functions as a neuromodulator and antioxidant. Taurine is involved in depression; however, knowledge of its function in depression is limited. These investigators elucidated the effects of taurine on antidepressant-like behaviors in rats and depression-related signal transduction in the hippocampus. The rats fed a high taurine (HT: 45 mmol/kg taurine) diet for 4 weeks (HT4w) showed decreased immobility in the forced swim test (FS) compared to controls. Rats fed a low taurine (LT: 22.5 mmol/kg taurine) diet for 4 weeks or an HT diet for 2 weeks (HT2w) did not show difference in FS compared to controls. The expression of glutamic acid decarboxylase (GAD) 65 and GAD67 in the hippocampus was not affected by taurine supplementation. However, the phosphorylation of extracellular signal-regulated kinase1/2 (ERK1/2), protein kinase B (Akt), glycogen synthase kinase3 beta (GSK3β), and cAMP response element-binding protein (CREB) were increased in the hippocampus of HT4w and HT2w rats. Phosphorylated calcium/calmodulin-dependent protein kinase II (CaMKII) was increased in the hippocampus of HT4w rats only. No significant changes in these signaling molecules were observed in the hippocampus of rats fed an HT diet for 1 day suggesting that taurine supplementation has an antidepressant-like effect to change depression-related signal transduction in the hippocampus.

Tryptophan Conversion to Nicotinamide. Valproic acid (VPA) is a short-chained, branched fatty acid that is used in humans as an anticonvulsant and mood stabilizer, and increases the liver NAD concentration. In a study the effects of VPA on the conversion of tryptophan to nicotinamide was investigated. Shibata et al., (2013) fed rats diets containing various amounts of VPA for 14 d, 24-h urine samples were collected, and tryptophan and its catabolites were measured. The conversion of tryptophan to nicotinamide was increased by feeding a diet containing VPA. Of the intermediates formed during the conversion of tryptophan to nicotinamide, the tryptophan to 3-hydroxyanthranilic acid step was not affected by the administration of VPA, while such metabolites beyond quinolinic acid as nicotinamide and its catabolites were increased. This increase was dependent on the intake of VPA.

Lithium and Ascorbate. Lithium (Li) is a trace element that is essential in the human diet due to its importance for health and proper functioning of an organism. However, the biological activity of this metal in crop plants, which are the primary dietary sources of Li, is still poorly understood. Kalinowska et al., (2013) performed a study to analyze two Li chemical forms on the growth and the L-ascorbic acid content in the Li accumulation and translocation in butterhead lettuce (Lactuca sativa L. var. capitata) cv. Justyna. The plants were grown in a nutrient solution enriched with Li in the form of LiCl or LiOH at the following concentrations: 0, 2.5, 20, 50 or 100 mg Li dm(-3). The results indicated that the presence of Li(+) ions in the root environment reduced the yield of edible parts of the lettuce if the Li concentration in a nutrient solution had reached 20 mg Li dm(-3). However, a yield reduction was found to be significant only for LiOH. In plants exposed to 50 mg Li dm(-3), both shoot and root fresh weights (FW) decreased, regardless of the supplied Li chemical form. On the other hand, under the lowest LiOH dose, increase in the root FW was noted, suggesting beneficial effects of Li on the growth of lettuce plants. However, Li concentrations and forms did not affect the L-ascorbic acid content in the lettuce leaves. Regardless of which Li form was used, Li accumulated mainly in the root. An exception was the higher concentration of Li in the shoots than in the roots of plants supplied with 100 mg Li dm(-3) in LiCl, and there were same Li concentrations in both organs of plants supplied with 100 mg Li dm(-3) in LiOH. The effectiveness of Li translocation from roots to shoots rose with increasing Li concentrations in the growth medium, suggesting a translocation of this metal throughout the plant and that Li toxicity in lettuce plants is related to a high accumulation of this element in the root and shoot, causing a reduction in the yield, in the presence either of LiCl or LiOH, but not affecting the L-ascorbic acid accumulation in the leaves.

Chronic Social Stress and Fluoxetine on Meal Pattern. Both chronic stress and antidepressant drugs have been associated with changes in body weight. Kumar et al., (2013) investigated the mechanisms by which stress and antidepressants interact to affect meal patterns. A group of mice was subjected to the chronic social defeat stress model of major depression followed by fluoxetine treatment and analyzed for food intake using metabolic cages. Chronic social defeat stress increased food intake by increasing meal size, an effect that was reversed by fluoxetine treatment. In an attempt to gain mechanistic insight into changes in meal patterning induced by stress and fluoxetine, fasting serum samples were collected every 4h hour over a 24-h period, and acyl-ghrelin, leptin, and corticosterone were estimated. Chronic stress induced a peak in acyl-ghrelin levels prior to the onset of the dark phase, which was shifted in mice treated with fluoxetine indicating that stress increases food intake by decreasing satiation, and that fluoxetine can reverse stress-induced changes in meal patterns.

Aromatic Amino Acids and Obesity. Recently, Cappola et al., (2013) described an association of branched-chain amino acids (BCAA) and aromatic amino acids (AAA) with obesity and insulin resistance. These researchers investigated the impact of BCAA on behavioral functions. Supplementation of either a high-sucrose or a high-fat diet with BCAA induced anxiety-like behavior in rats compared with control groups fed on unsupplemented diets. These behavioral changes were associated with decrease in the concentration of tryptophan (Trp) in brain tissues and serotonin but no difference in serotonin synaptic function. The anxiety-like behaviors and decreased Trp in the brain of BCAA-fed rats were reversed by supplementation of Trp but not by fluoxetine, suggesting that the behavioral changes are independent of the serotonergic pathway of Trp metabolism. Instead, BCAA supplementation lowered the brain Trp-derived metabolite, kynurenic acid, which was normalized by Trp indicating that high-energy diets with BCAA causes neurobehavioral impairment. The elevated levels of BCAA in obesity suggest a potential mechanism for explaining the association of obesity and mood disorders.

Opioid antagonists and Obesity. Clapper et al., (2013) studied the effect of antagonism of opioid systems (e.g., with Naltrexone) as an anti-obesity strategy, and is particularly effective when co-administered with dual inhibitors of dopamine and NE reuptake (e.g., Bupropion). Previously, these investigators demonstrated that amylin enhances the food intake lowering and weight loss effects of neurohormonal (e.g., leptin, cholecystokinin, melanocortins) and small molecule (e.g., Phentermine, Sibutramine) agents. They characterized the interaction of amylin with Naltrexone/Bupropion on energy balance. Wild-type and amylin knockout mice were responsive to the food intake lowering effects of either Naltrexone (1mg/kg, s.c) or Bupropion (50mg/kg, s.c) suggesting that they act independently of amylinergic systems and interact additively when given in combination with amylin. To test this, diet-induced obese rats were treated (for 11 days) with vehicle, rat amylin (50 μg/kg/d, infused s.c), Naltrexone/Bupropion (1 and 20mg/kg, respectively by twice daily s.c injection) or their combination. Amylin+Naltrexone/Bupropion combination therapy exerted additive effects to reduce cumulative food intake, body weight, and fat mass. In a separate study, the effects of amylin and Naltrexone/Bupropion administered at the same doses for 14 days were compared to a pair-fed group. Although the combination and pair-fed groups lost a similar amount of body weight, rats treated with the combination lost 68% more fat and maintained their lean mass supporting combined amylin agonism with opioid and catecholaminergic signaling systems for the treatment of obesity. In conclusion, diet comprosing of vitamins, minerals, amino acids, and metabolites augment antidepressant action, improve symptoms in anxiety disorders, depression, neurodegenerative diseases, brain injury, ADHD, and schizophrenia, and attenuate the side effects of other medications. Hence it is significant to detect and correct vitamin and mineral deficiencies for recovery. Generally low in adverse effects when taken in therapeutic doses, nutrients can be combined for more benefits as illustrated in Figure 9.

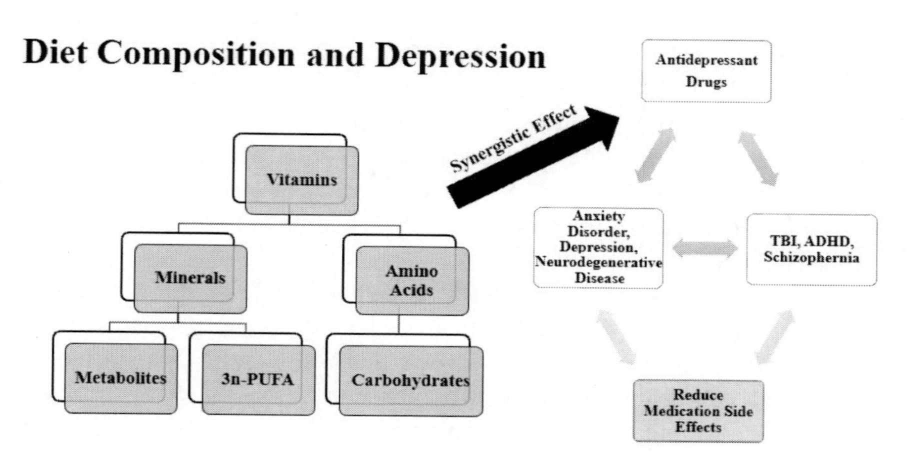

Figure 9. A diagram illustrating that vitamins, minerals, amino acids, and metabolites augment antidepressant action, improve symptoms in anxiety disorders, depression, neurodegenerative diseases, brain injury, ADHD, and schizophrenia, and attenuate medication side effects. Detection and correction of vitamin and mineral deficiencies is essential for recovery. Generally low in adverse effects when taken in therapeutic doses, nutrients can be combined for greater benefits. Further studies are needed to validate these treatments (Akhondzadeh et al., 2013).

Hypericum for Weight Reduction. Garcia-de la Cruz et al., (2013) conducted a study to assess the anti-obesity effect of Hypericum silenoides Juss and Hypericum philonotis Cham. & Schlecht in male Wistar rats fed with a cafeteria diet. Adult male Wistar rats with an initial body weight of 290-320 g were used in this trial. The rats were fed with a cafeteria diet for 77 days. Hypericum species were administered orally at a dose of 10, 30 or 100 mg/kg of body weight daily for 35 days. Body weight, food intake, anorexic effect and serum glucose, lipid profile, alanine transaminase (ALT), aspartate transaminase (AST) and atherogenic index (AI), were estimated. Inhibitory lipase activity assay and forced swimming test were also carried out. Oral administration of H. silenoides and H. philonotis extracts resulted in a significant decrease in body weight and serum glucose levels in obese male Wistar rats. Treatment with H. silenoides showed anorexic and antidepressant effects and also decreased total cholesterol, triglycerides and high-density lipoprotein-cholesterol, while low-density lipoprotein-cholesterol, AI, AST and ALT were not changed. The dichloromethane extract of H. silenoides (half maximal inhibitory concentration) and hexane extract of H. philonotis showed lipase inhibitory activity. Thus H. silenoides and H. philonotis extracts showed anti-obesity activity in cafeteria-diet-fed rats providing evidence for the use of the Hypericum genus for weight reduction.

Falvinoid Antioxidants. Flavonoids are plant phenolic metabolites that are widely distributed in the human diet. These antioxidants have received significant attention because of their neuroprotective, cardioprotective, and chemopreventive actions. While a major focus has been on the flavonoids' antioxidant properties, many of the health benefits of flavonoids and their in vivo metabolites are due to their modulatory actions in cells through direct interactions with proteins, and not due to their antioxidant function. Flavonoids are present in the circulation at very low concentrations, insufficient to exert effective antioxidant effects. The enzyme paraoxonase 1 (PON1) is associated with high-density lipoprotein (HDL), and is responsible for many of HDLs' antiatherogenic properties. Atrahimovich et al., (2013) demonstrated that the flavonoid, Glabridin binds to rePON1 and affects the enzyme's 3D structure. This interaction protects the enzyme from inhibition by an atherogenic component of the human carotid plaque. The structure-activity relationships of 12 flavonoids from different subclasses with rePON1 using Trp-fluorescence quenching, modeling calculations and Cu(2+)-induced low-density lipoprotein (LDL) oxidation was investigated. The 'protein-binding' mechanism is involved by which flavonoids exert their beneficial effect. Flavonoids' capacity to interact with the enzyme's rePON1 hydrophobic groove determines their pro/antioxidant behavior.

Curcumin. The root extract, curcumin (diferuloylmethane), is a constituent of the ancient herbal medicine, Jiawei-Xiaoyaosan that has been used for dyspepsia, stress, and mood disorders. Curcumin possesses biological actions that result in changes in oxidative stress, inflammation, and cell-death pathways. Curcumin has been studied for its therapeutic applications in cancer, aging, endocrine, immunological, gastrointestinal, and cardiac diseases because of its safety profile. In addition, data in animal models and in humans have been collected in stroke, AD, and PD and its efficacy in stress and mood disorders. Kulkarni et al., (2008) reported that curcimin exerts its antidepressant action by augmenting brain regional serotonergic and dopaminergic neurotransmission. Recently Witkin and Li (2013) have also reported beneficial effects of curicumin in several neurodegenerative diseases. Current understanding of the biological basis for antidepressant-relevant biochemical and behavioral changes shows convergence with some mechanisms known for standard antidepressants. In addition, the mechanisms of the antidepressant-like action of curcumin also coincides with those of other diseases. Although curcumin is a primary ingredient in anti-aging pills, cosmetic creams, eye treatments, and diet products, it presents a significant challenge for disease treatment and prevention and in overcoming its low oral bioavailability. Although multiple approaches to this problem are being examined, a solution to the bioavailability issue will be needed to ensure appropriate curcumin delivery employing emerging nanotechnological approaches.

References

Apter, A; Steingart, L. (2013) Interaction between weight and medications in psychological illnesses of children, *World Rev Nutr Diet.* 106, 174-180.

Atrahimovich, D; Vaya, J; Khatib, S. (2013) The effects and mechanism of flavonoid-rePON1 interactions. Structure-activity relationship study., *Bioorg Med Chem.* 21, 3348-3355.

Bello, N.T; Walters, A.L; Verpeut, J.L; Cunha, P.P. (2013) High-fat diet-induced alterations in the feeding suppression of low-dose nisoxetine, a selective norepinephrine reuptake inhibitor., *J Obes.* 2013, 457047.

Betancourt, J; Ríos, J.L; Pagán, I; Fabián, C; González, A.M; Cruz, S.Y; González, M.J; Rivera, W.T; Palacios, C. (2013) Non-medical use of prescription drugs and its association with socio-demographic characteristics, dietary pattern, and perceived academic load and stress in college students in Puerto Rico., *P R Health Sci J.* 32, 89-94.

Brownley, K.A; Girdler, S.S; Stout, A.L; McLeod, M.N. (2013) Chromium supplementation for menstrual cycle-related mood symptoms., *J Diet Suppl.* 10, 345-356.

Butt, M.S; Pasha, I; Sultan, M.T; Randhawa, M.A; Saeed, F; Ahmed, W. (2013) Black pepper and health claims: a comprehensive treatise., *Crit Rev Food Sci Nutr.* 53, 875-886.

Coppola, A; Wenner, B.R; Ilkayeva, O; Stevens, R.D; Maggioni, M; Slotkin, T.A; Levin, E.D; and Newgard, C.B. (2013) Branched-chain amino acids alter neurobehavioral function in rats. Am J Physiol Endocrinol Metab. 304, E405–E413.

Fashner, J; Gitu, A.C. (2013) Common gastrointestinal symptoms: irritable bowel syndrome. *FP Essent.* 413: 16-23.

Flemmer A. (2013) [Mood and food: eating for a good mood]. *Kinderkrankenschwester.* 32, 53-54.

Ford, A.C; Moayyedi, P. (2013) Dyspepsia., *Curr Opin Gastroenterol*. 29, 662-668.

García-de la Cruz, L; Galvan-Goiz, Y; Caballero-Caballero, S; Zamudio, S; Alfaro, A; Navarrete, A. (2013) Hypericum silenoides Juss. and Hypericum philonotis Cham. & Schlecht. extracts: in-vivo hypolipidaemic and weight-reducing effects in obese rats., *J Pharm Pharmacol.* 65, 591-603.

Garcia-de-la Cruz, L; Galvan-Goiz, Y; Caballero-Caballero, S. (2013) Hypericum silenoids Jus and Hypercum philonotis Cham. & Schlecht. Extracts: in-vivo hypolipidemic and weight-reducing effects in obese rats. J Pharm Pharmacol. 65, 591-603.

Hainerová, I.A; Lebl, J. (2013) Treatment options for children with monogenic forms of obesity., *World Rev Nutr Diet.* 106, 105-112.

Hoirisch-Clapauch, S; Mezzasalma, M.A; Nardi, A.E. (2013) Pivotal role of tissue plasminogen activator in the mechanism of action of electroconvulsive therapy. *J Psychopharmacol.* Oct 9.

Imayama, I; Alfano, C.M; Mason, C; Wang, C; Duggan, C; Campbell, K.L; Kong, A; Foster-Schubert, K.E; Blackburn, G.L; Wang, C.Y; McTiernan, A. (2013) Weight and metabolic effects of dietary weight loss and exercise interventions in postmenopausal antidepressant medication users and non-users: a randomized controlled trial., *Prev Med.* 57, 525-532.

Kalinowska, M; Hawrylak-Nowak, B; Szymańska, M. (2013) The influence of two lithium forms on the growth, L-ascorbic acid content and lithium accumulation in lettuce plants., *Biol Trace Elem Res.* 152, 251-257.

Kaplan, G. (2013) What is new in adolescent psychiatry? Literature review and clinical implications., *Adolesc Med State Art Rev.* 24, 29-42.

Kulkarni, S.K; Bhutani, M.K; Bishnoi, M. (2008) Antidepressant activity of curcumin: involvement of serotonin and dopamine system. *Psychopharmacology (Berl).* 201, 435-442.

Kumar, J; Chuang, J.C; Na, E.S; Kuperman, A; Gillman, A.G; Mukherjee, S; Zigman, J.M; McClung, C.A; Lutter, M. (2013) Differential effects of chronic social stress and fluoxetine on meal patterns in mice., *Appetite.* 64; 81-88.

Laporta, J; Peters, T.L; Weaver, S.R; Merriman, K.E; Hernandez, LL. (2013) Feeding 5-hydroxy-l-tryptophan during the transition from pregnancy to lactation increases calcium mobilization from bone in rats., *Domest Anim Endocrinol.* 44, 176-184.

Lee, H; Ohno, M; Ohta, S; Mikami, T. (2013) Regular moderate or intense exercise prevents depression-like behavior without change of hippocampal tryptophan content in chronically tryptophan-deficient and stressed mice., *PLoS One*. 8(7), e66996.

Lehto, S.M; Ruusunen, A; Tolmunen, T; Voutilainen, S; Tuomainen, T.P; Kauhanen, J. (2013) Dietary zinc intake and the risk of depression in middle-aged men: a 20-year prospective follow-up study., *J Affect Disord*. 150, 682-685.

Liu, W; Zhai, X; Li, H; Ji, L (2014) Depression-like behaviors in mice subjected to co-treatment of high-fat diet and corticosterone are ameliorated by AICAR and exercise., *J Affect Disord*. 156,171-177.

Lucas, M; Chocano-Bedoya, P; Shulze, M.B; Mirzaei, F; O'Reilly, E.J; Okereke, O.I; Hu, F.B; Willett, W.C; Ascherio, A. (2014) Inflammatory dietary pattern and risk of depression among women., Brain Behav Immun. 36, 46-53.

Mezuk, B; Johnson-Lawrence, V; Lee, H; Rafferty, J.A; Abdou, C.M; Uzogara, E.E; Jackson, J.S. (2013) Is ignorance bliss? Depression, antidepressants, and the diagnosis of prediabetes and type 2 diabetes., *Health Psychol*. 32, 254-263.

Młyniec, K; Budziszewska, B; Reczyński, W; Doboszewska, U; Pilc, A; Nowak, G. (2013) Zinc deficiency alters responsiveness to antidepressant drugs in mice., *Pharmacol Rep*. 65, 579-592.

Nascimento E, Guzman-Quevedo O, Delacourt N, da Silva Aragão R, Perez-Garcia G, de Souza SL, Manhães-de-Castro R, Bolaños-Jiménez F,Kaeffer B. Long-lasting effect of perinatal exposure to L-tryptophan on circadian clock of primary cell lines established from male offspring born from mothers fed on dietary protein restriction. PLoS One. 2013;8(2):e56231.

Oberholzer, H.M; Van Der Schoor, C; Pretorius, E. (2013) The effect of sibutramine on platelet morphology of Spraque-Dawley rats fed a high energy diet., *Microsc Res Tech*. 76, 653-657.

Pałucha-Poniewiera, A; Brański, P; Wierońska, J.M; Stachowicz, K; Sławińska, A; Pilc, A.(2013) The antidepressant-like action of mGlu5 receptor antagonist, MTEP, in the tail suspension test in mice is serotonin dependent., *Psychopharmacology (Berl)*. Aug 20.

Persons, J.E; Robinson, J.G; Ammann, E.M; Coryell, W.H; Espeland, M.A; Harris, W.S; Manson, J.E; Fiedorowicz, J.G. (2013) Omega-3 fatty acid biomarkers and subsequent depressive symptoms., *Int J Geriatr Psychiatry*. Dec 11.

Perveen, T; Hashmi, B.M; Haider, S; Tabassum, S; Saleem, S; Siddiqui, M.A. (2013) Role of monoaminergic system in the etiology of olive oil induced antidepressant and anxiolytic effects in rats., I*SRN Pharmaco*l. 2013, 615685.

Robinson OJ, Overstreet C, Allen PS, Letkiewicz A, Vytal K, Pine DS, Grillon C. The role of serotonin in the neurocircuitry of negative affective bias: serotonergic modulation of the dorsal medial prefrontal-amygdala 'aversive amplification' circuit. Neuroimage. 2013 Sep;78: 217-223.

Shibata, K; Kondo, R; Sano, M; Fukuwatari, T. (2013) Increased conversion of tryptophan to nicotinamide in rats by dietary valproate. Biosci Biotechnol Biochem. 77, 295-300.

Siebenhofer, A; Jeitler, K; Horvath, K; Berghold, A; Siering, U; Semlitsch, T. (2013) Long-term effects of weight-reducing drugs in hypertensive patients., *Cochrane Database Syst Rev*. 3, CD007654.

Sihvola, N; Korpela, R; Henelius, A; Holm, A; Huotilainen, M; Müller, K; Poussa, T; Pettersson, K; Turpeinen, A; Peuhkuri, K. (2013) Breakfast high in whey protein or carbohydrates improves coping with workload in healthy subjects., *Br J Nutr.*110, 1712-1721.

Skarupski, K.A; Tangney, C.C; Li, H; Evans, D.A; Morris, M.C. (2013) Mediterranean diet and depressive symptoms among older adults over time., *J Nutr Health Aging.* 17, 441-445.

Toyoda, A; Iio, W. (2013) Antidepressant-like effect of chronic taurine administration and its hippocampal signal transduction in rats., *Adv Exp Med Biol.* 775, 29-43.

Trigueros, L; Peña, S; Ugidos, A.V; Sayas-Barberá, E; Pérez-Álvarez, J.A; Sendra, E. (2013) Food ingredients as anti-obesity agents: a review., *Crit Rev Food Sci Nutr.* 53, 929-942.

Vekovischeva, O.Y; Peuhkuri, K; Bäckström, P; Sihvola, N; Pilvi, T; Korpela, R. (2013) The effects of native whey and α-lactalbumin on the social and individual behaviour of C57BL/6J mice., *Br J Nutr.* 110, 1336-1346.

Witkin, J.M; Li, X. (2013) Curcumin, an active constiuent of the ancient medicinal herb Curcuma longa L.: some uses and the establishment and biological basis of medical efficacy. CNS Neurol Disord Drug Targets. 12, 487-497.

Yu, Z.M; Parker, L; Dummer, T.J. (2013) Depressive symptoms, diet quality, physical activity, and body composition among populations in Nova Scotia, Canada: Report from the Atlantic Partnership for Tomorrow's Health., *Prev Med.* Dec 29.

Chapter 7

Disease-Specific Depression and Diet (Recent Update)

Abstract

Depression is involved in several chronic diseases including dietary imbalance, developmental disorders, and postnatal malnutrition. In this chapter a brief description of malnutrition and cortical spreading depression, dietary risks of depression, late-life depression, and depression associated with obesity, metabolic syndrome, and coronary artery diseases is described and its possible prevention and/or treatment with dietary interventions including fruits and vegetables, Mediterrenean diet, curcumin, and intake of moderate tea/coffee. The basic molecular mechanism of Charnoly body formation involved in the etiopathogenesis of depression as a consequences of compromised hippocampal mitochondrial bioenergetics and its prevention by antioxidants is also discussed.

Keywords Major depressive disorders (MDD), Hippocampus, Charnoly body (CB), multidrug-resistant (MDR) Malignancies

Almost all biological creatures suffer from depression depending on the physicochemical experiences and challenges they experience in their life. Depression is characterized by hopelessness, frustration, negative thoughts, and worthlessness. The types of diet consumed can modulate our mood. Various social, physical, mental, economical, psychological, biochemical, physiological, and pharmacological factors can also influence our mood which is reflected as either depression or anxiety. It has been hypothesized that brain region-specific serotonergic neurotransmission is impaired in depression and can be alleviated by consuming tryptophan-rich diet as tryptophan is the precursor of serotonin (5-HT). In general drugs developed to alleviate depression have been designed to enhance brain region-specific serotonergic neurotransmission, which is significantly compromised in depression due to reduced availability of its precursor, tryptophan or 5-hydrotryptophan (5-HTP). Both tryptophan as well as 5-HTP enhance the serotonin synthesis in the CNS and alleviate depression. However major depressive disorders (MDDs) are refractory to such non-pharmacological therapeutic interventions.

Although serotonergic drugs are effective to a certain extent in alleviating cardinal symptoms of depression, these are associated with serious side effects. For instance, antidepressants have low margin of safety as well as therapeutic index. These drugs require a sufficiently high levels in the brain to be effective. It may take as many as 2-4 weeks to have therapeutic benefits. Another serious drawback is that these drugs cannot be discontinued abruptly as it may adversely impact the biological system. Increased incidences of suicides have been noticed in MDD patients who were on antidepressants and suddenly stopped taking medications including SSRIs. A person with suicidal tendency is a severe case of depression according to Beck depression Scale. Although drug addiction is the most serious cause of depression, chronic illnesses such as cancers, rheumatoid arthritis, chronic infections, post-traumatic stress disorders, war wounded and rape victims, early childhood abuse, post-surgical patients, post-partum women, astronauts, divorced couples, death of beloved ones, hypothyroid patients, chronic progressive neurodegenerative disorders such as PD, AD, drug addiction, schizophrenia and many others chronic illnesses are associated with depression, which may have significant impact on human performance and productivity. In addition to food, there is now growing realization that genes can play a significant role in regulating mood. Recent evidence suggests the involvement of genes in regulating serotonergic neurotransmission in depression. Since several factors involved in depression are difficult to regulate, dietary manipulation is the most effective, simple, economical non-pharmacological approach to alleviate depression particularly in obesity. In general diets rich in tryptophan has been shown to produce anti-depressant effect. Although several foods are rich in serotonin; as such serotonin does not cross the blood brain barrier. Hence we need to consume tryptophan-rich diets because it can cross the blood brain barrier and converted to 5-HT in the presence of rate limiting enzyme tryptophan hydroxylase and 5-HTP decarboxylase, and vitamin B_6. Tryptophan is a neutral amino acid, naturally less abundant in proteins, and essential as it cannot be synthesized by the body. Hence has to be supplemented exogenously through specific dietary selections as discussed earlier.

Vitamin B_6 is chemically called as pyridoxine. Pyridoxine is water soluble and requires its consumption on a daily basis. Pyridoxine (Vitamin B_6) exists in other metabolically-active forms, called as vitamers; such as pyridoxine, pyridoxamine phosphate, pyridoxal, pyridoxal phosphate, and a metabolically-incative form pyridoxic acid which is excreted through urine and feces. Pyridoxal phosphate is the most metabolically-active form of vitamin B_6 and acts as a cofactor for various decarboxylation steps in the body. Pyridoxine is converted to pyridoxal by enzyme called pyridoxine oxidase, and pyridoxal is converted to pyridoxal phosphate (PLP) by enzyme, pyridoxal kinase. We developed the improved procedure to estimate various pyridoxine vitamers from the biological samples and CSF for the clinical diagnosis and prognosis of pyridoxine-deficiency-induced seizures in children (Sharma and Dakshinamurti, 1992). Recent studies have shown that the gene encoding pyridoxal kinase are mutated in patients with PD and other progressive neurodegenerative disorders associated with depression.

Usually healthy diets are rich in tryptophan. These diets must be consumed on a regular basis. For instance milk, bread, soy bean, nuts, spinach, papaya, pumpkin, pineapple, orange, Tofu, cheese, meat, eggs, fish are rich sources of tryptophan in addition to omega-3 fatty acids, vitamin B_6, Vitamin B_1, and vitamin B_{12}, Vitamin D and Viamin E, required for mood alleviation and healthy life. Whereas diets rich in caffeine, cigarette smoking, drugs of abuse, alcohol consumption, aspartame, diet Pepsi Coca Cola (containing simple carbohydrates and saturated fats like pizza, humbergers, and French fries) are the poor source of tryptophan and can have deleterious impact on sleep, sex, food intake, digestive system, cardiovascular system and CNS to cause depression. Diets that are rich in simple carbohydrates and saturated fats should be avoided to prevent depression. Usually obese persons are accompanied with MDDs. Their preference to consume simple carbohydrates and fat-rich diet is a futile attempt to enhance brain region-specific serotonergic neurotransmission as carbohydrate-rich diet induces insulin secretion from the pancreas and insulin. Tryptophan is neutral and essential amino acid and have to be consumed from the dietary sources as it is not synthesized in the body. Moreover, it is less abundant, hence it is important to consume diets rich in tryptophan to meet daily requirements of serotonin in the CNS for a healthy life. Increased consumption of carbohydrate and fat-rich diet by depressed obese person is to increase the brain regional availability of tryptophan. Release of insulin by consuming carbohydrate rich diet makes it possible for tryptophan to enter CNS as insulin acts as a carrier for the tryptophan to enhance its availability in the CNS. Hence it will be advisable to recommend tryptophan-rich diet to an obese person suffering from MDD rather than diet rich in simple carbohydrates and saturated fats to enhance brain regional tryptophan levels to alleviate depression. The presence of vitamin B_6 is also equally important because in the absence of coenzyme, pyridoxal phosphate, the enzyme 5-HTP decarboxylase cannot synthesize 5-HT (Dakshinamurti et al., 1990). In addition to serotonin, various other neurotransmitters including GABA, NE, and dopamine may be involved in depression. However drugs targeted to these neurotransmitters and their receptor subtypes, proved less effective in alleviating typical symptoms of depression. Hence serotonergic mechanism of depression has dominated to explain as well as alleviate depressive disorders. The main advantage of the nonpharmacological approach is to alleviate depression through dietary manipulation of CNS serotonergic neurotransmission and seems more physiological without any adverse effects as this treatment is free from addiction and deleterious adverse effects associated with the chronic use of antidepressants.

Boutayeb and Boutayeb (2005) reported that currently non communicable diseases are the biggest cause of death worldwide. Beside mortality, these diseases also cause morbidity and disability. Their increased prevalence is associated to multi-morbidity. Because they need costly prolonged treatment and care, these diseases have social and economical consequences that affect individuals, households, and the whole society. They raise the equity problem between and within countries. These researchers provided a systematic review on multimorbidy of non-communicable diseases and health equity in WHO Eastern Mediterranean countries by reviewing Medline/PubMed, EMBASE and other sources. Of the 26 contributions selected, twelve dealt with comorbidity of depression and mental disorders with other chronic diseases. Another 11 publications were related to multimorbidity of diabetes, cardiovascular diseases (CVDs), hypertension, metabolic syndrome, and obesity. Female gender, low income, low level of education, old age, and unemployed/retired were the primary victims of multimorbidity. Geographically, no contribution was issued from North African countries. In eastern Mediterranean countries the multidimensional transition is increasing in multimorbidity of depression and mental diseases, cardiovascular diseases, diabetes, cancer and respiratory diseases with the highest burden among the least disadvantaged individuals. It has been recommended that health ministries in WHO Eastern Mediterranean countries should pay attention to the association between equity and multimorbidity and develop cost effective strategies based on early diagnosis, healthy diet, physical activity, and refraining from smoking and alcohol. Diet modifies key biological factors associated with the development of depression; however, associations between diet quality and depression are not fully understood. Quirk et al., (2013) evaluated evidence regarding the association between diet quality and depression. Twenty-five studies from nine countries met eligibility criteria. Best-evidence analyses found limited evidence to support an association between traditional diets (Mediterranean or Norwegian diets) and depression and a conflicting evidence for associations between (i) a traditional Japanese diet and depression, (ii) a "healthy" diet and depression, (iii) a Western diet and depression, and (iv) individuals with depression and the likelihood of eating a less healthy diet. This was the first study to synthesize and analyze evidence regarding diet quality, dietary patterns and depression.

There are cognitive strategies in targeted depression, anxiety, sleep, vascular risk factors, diet, and exercise. Preventable risk factors are smoking, addiction, poor diet and lack of exercise as illustrated in Figure 10.

Cognitive Strategies in Targeted Depression

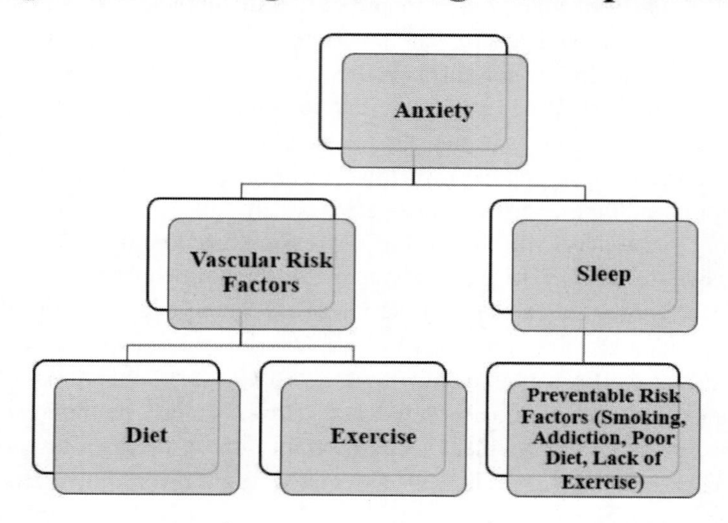

Figure 10. A diagram illustrating cognitive strategies in targeted depression, anxiety, sleep, vascular risk factors, diet, and exercise. Preventable risk factors such as smoking, addiction, poor diet and lack of exercise.

Dietary Imbalance and Developmental Disorders. It is known that developmental disorders (DDs) are the leading cause of disability in developed countries and also in the US. Ibrahim and El-Sayed (2013) highlighted the role of dietary imbalances in the incidence of DD to determine which dietary supplements can aid in the treatment of the DD. DDs are a group of conditions that result from abnormal CNS development and cause impaired function. They can begin at any time from prenatal to 22 years of age and the disability presents throughout life time. Down syndrome, autism, neural tube defects, schizophrenia, cretinism, and ADHD are the most common DDs. Their occurrence may be attributable to the lack of certain dietary nutrients. Particularly, essential vitamins, minerals, and ω-3 fatty acids are deficient in the general population and in patients suffering from mental disorders. Usually, most of these disorders treated with prescription drugs cause undesirable side effects. Therefore, psychiatrists recommend complementary nutritional remedies. Daily supplements of nutrients, such as that contain amino acids, reduce symptoms, because they are converted into neurotransmitters that alleviate depression and other mental disorders.

Postnatal Malnutrition. Postnatal depression is a condition that affects women and the development of their infants. There is a lack of evidence for treatment and prevention strategies that are safe for mothers and infants. Certain dietary deficiencies in a pregnant or postnatal woman's diet may cause postnatal depression. By correcting these deficiencies postnatal depression can be prevented. Specific examples of dietary supplements aimed at preventing postnatal depression include: omega-3 fatty acids, iron, folate, s-adenosyl-L-methionine, cobalamin, pyridoxine, riboflavin, vitamin D, and calcium. To assess the benefits of dietary supplements for preventing postnatal depression either in the antenatal period, postnatal period, or both, the investigators searched the Cochrane Pregnancy and Childbirth Group's Trials Register. Randomized controlled trials, involved women who were pregnant or who had given birth in the previous six weeks, who were not depressed or taking antidepressants. The trials could use as intervention any dietary supplementation alone or in combination with another treatment compared with other preventive treatment, or placebo, or standard clinical care. Miller et al., (2013) assessed two controlled trials. One trial compared oral 100 μg selenium yeast tablets with placebo, taken from the first trimester until birth. Eighty-three women were randomized to each arm of the trial. Sixty-one women completed the selenium group, 44 of whom completed an Edinburgh Postnatal Depression Scale (EPDS). In the placebo group, 64 women completed the trial, 41 of whom completed an EPDS. Selenium had an effect on EPDS scores but did not reach statistical significance. There was a high risk of attrition bias due to a large proportion of women withdrawing from the study or not completing an EPDS. The other trial compared DHA and EPA with placebo. The trial randomized 126 women at risk of postpartum depression to three group: 42 were allocated to EPA, 42 to DHA, and 42 to placebo. Three women in the EPA group, four in the DHA group, and one woman in the placebo group were lost to follow-up. Women who were found to have MDD, bipolar disorder, substance abuse or dependence, suicidal ideation or schizophrenia at recruitment were excluded from the study. The women who discontinued the intervention (five in the EPA group, four in the DHA group and seven in the placebo group) were included in the intention-to-treat analysis, while those who were lost to follow-up were not. Women received supplements or placebo from recruitment at a gestational age of 12 to 20 weeks until their final review visit six to eight weeks postpartum. The outcome measure was the Beck Depression Inventory (BDI) score at the fifth visit (six to eight weeks postpartum). No benefit was found for EPA or DHA-rich fish oil supplementation in preventing postpartum depression. No benefit was found in the secondary outcomes of the presence of MDD at six to eight weeks postpartum, the number of women who commenced antidepressants, maternal estimated blood loss at delivery or admission of neonates to the neonatal intensive care unit indicating that there is insufficient evidence that selenium, DHA or EPA can prevent postnatal depression. However there is currently no evidence to recommend any other dietary supplement for the prevention of postnatal depression. Early maternal exposure to a high-fat diet (HFD) may also influence the brain development of progeny and affect physiology and behavior. Giriko et al. (2013) investigated the somatic, physical, sensory-motor and neurobehavioral development of the offspring of dams fed an HFD (52% calories from fat, mainly saturated) and the offspring of dams fed a control diet (CD - 14.7% fat) during lactation from the 1st to the 21st postnatal day (P) in rats. Maternal body weights were evaluated during lactation. In the progeny, somatic (body weight, head and lengths axes) and physical (ear unfolding, auditory conduit opening, eruption of the incisors and eye opening) development of the reflex responses (palm grasp, righting, vibrissa placing, cliff avoidance, negative geotaxis, auditory startle response and free-fall righting) were determined during suckling. Depressive and aggressive behaviors were tested with the forced swimming test (FST) and the "foot-shock" test on days 60 and 110, respectively. The open field test was used to assess motor function. Compared to controls, the HFD-pups exhibited decreases in body weight (P7-P21) and body length (P4-P18), but by days P71 and P95, these pups were overweight. All indicators of physical maturation and the consolidation of the reflexes, vibrissa placing, auditory startle responses, free-fall righting and negative geotaxis, were delayed in HFD-progeny. The pups from HFD dam rats also exhibited reduced swimming and climbing times in the FST and increased aggressive behavior without any change in locomotion, suggesting developmental and neurobehavioral changes in the rat offspring of dams fed the HFD during lactation and disruption of physical and sensory-motor maturation, increased susceptibility to depression, and aggressive behavior. Although there is no evidence to suggest that changes in iron stores are consequence of aging; iron deficiency anemia is prevalent in older age, particularly after the age of 80 and has undesirable health outcomes including increased susceptibility to falling and depression. Serum ferritin concentrations also decline. Chronic inflammation is a common condition in older people, making the measurement of iron status difficult, and elevated circulating hepcidin is responsible for changes in iron metabolism that result in systemic iron depletion. Other contributory factors are poor diet and medications, such as aspirin. There are concerns about possible adverse effects of iron supplements, either in relation to pro-inflammatory effects in the gut or inappropriate tissue iron deposition. Brain iron levels are increased with age-related degenerative diseases, but it remains unknown if this is the cause or a consequence of the disease, and genetic factors are likely to play a role. In order to maintain body iron within the normal range a personalized approach is needed, taking into account factors that may affect iron metabolism and the strategies for preventing iron deficiency or overload (Fairweather-Tait et al., 2013).

Malnutrition and Cortical Spreading Depression (CSD). Malnutrition early in life can disrupt neurotransmitter systems in the brain, affecting electrophysiological activity. The opioid receptor antagonist Naloxone can affect the EEG and behavior in animals and humans, and patients on drug-abuse treatment use it as a therapy. This work in the rat determined whether malnutrition early in life modulates the action of naloxone on CSD. Guedes et al., (2013) induced malnutrition by feeding the dams during the gestation and lactation with a low-protein diet (8% protein). The male pups received a single daily s.c injection of Naloxone (10 mg/kg/day) from the 7th to the 28th postnatal day, and were (30-40 days of life) subjected to a 4-hours CSD recording session at two points on the parietal cortical surface. Compared to well-nourished rats receiving a 23% protein diet, malnourished animals displayed lower body weights and higher CSD velocities of propagation, confirming the facilitating effect of malnutrition on CSD. Naloxone reduced in well-nourished rats the CSD propagation velocity, as compared to saline-injected controls. In contrast, the effect of naloxone was less intense in the malnourished condition, and the CSD velocity difference between malnourished-naloxone and malnourished-saline groups were not significant, suggesting involvement of opioid-based mechanisms in excitability-related neural processes, which influence CSD propagation, and that early malnutrition attenuates the impairing action of Naloxone on CSD. Furthermore, da Silva Germano et al., (2013) evaluated the effects of hypercaloric diet in different phases of life on CSD in adult rats. Newborn Wistar rats were suckled by dams fed a high-lipid (cafeteria) hypercaloric diet during the lactation period. After suckling, part of the pups remained in the high-lipid diet until the end of the experiment in adulthood, and the other part received the control (lab chow) diet. A third group received the hypercaloric diet only at adulthood. When the animals reached 90-93 days of life, CSD was recorded. CSD propagation velocities and CSD amplitudes were reduced in the groups L and FL, but not in the group Ad, in comparison with a control group (C), fed the lab chow diet during the entire life. CSD velocity changes observed in adulthood were associated with the hypercaloric dietary treatment during brain development, providing evidence in favor of permanent or long-lasting electrophysiological effects due to deleterious effects of nutritioinal stress during brain growth spurt.

Diet and Risk of Depression. Sanhueza et al., (2013) reviewed the association between dietary variables and the risk of depression. These investigators searched fifteen databases. Only longitudinal studies for which outcomes were unipolar depression and/or depressive symptoms in adults were included. Participants were in the age range 18-97 years and the study sample size was in the range 526-27111. Follow-up ranged from 2 to 13 years. The diversity of dietary variables and nonlinear associations precluded formal meta-analysis and so a narrative analysis was undertaken. Variables inversely associated with depression risk were the consumption of nutrients such as folate, omega-3 fatty acids, and monounsaturated fatty acids; foods such as olive oil and fish; and a diet rich in fruits, vegetables, nuts, and legumes. Some of these associations varied by sex and some showed a nonlinear association.

Socioeconomic Status. It has been noticed that among the 78 million obese Americans, *l*ow-socioeconomic-status (SES) Latinos are misrepresented. Drieling et al., (2013) performed a study which provides guidance for obesity-reduction strategies by evaluating food security, educational community resource utilization, education level, depression, sex, and length of US residence as predictors of diet and physical activity. This study used baseline data for a weight-loss trial among lower-SES obese (BMI 30 to 55) Latino immigrants enrolled at a community health clinic. Physical activity was measured using 7-day pedometer recording. Dietary intake was measured using a food frequency questionnaire including; education community resource use (nutrition and physical activity classes), education level, US residence (years), food security, and depressive symptoms. Data were analyzed using multivariate-adjusted linear regression models. More than one third of participants were sedentary (<5,000 steps/day), and 41% had low fruit and vegetable intake (<5 servings/day). The educational resource use, male sex, less education, fewer depressive symptoms, and shorter US residence time were associated with more physical activity. Educational resource use was positively associated with fruit and vegetable intake. Male sex was associated with more sweet-beverage and fast-food intake. Fewer depressive symptoms were associated with lower sweet-beverage intake. Thus, obesity-reduction strategies among low-SES Latino immigrants might emphasize educational resource use and interventions for psychosocial and sociodemographic characteristics. Jacka et al., (2013) conducted a large prospective Norwegian Mother and Child Cohort Study by recruiting pregnant women between 1999 and 2008. Data were collected during pregnancy and when children were 6 months and 1.5, 3, and 5 years of age. Latent growth curve models were used to determine linear development in children's internalizing and externalizing problems from 1.5 to 5 years of age as a function of diet quality during pregnancy and at 1.5 and 3 years. Diet quality was evaluated by dietary pattern extraction and characterized as "healthy" or "unhealthy." The sample comprised

23,020 women and their children. Adjustments were made for sex of the child, maternal depression, maternal and paternal age, maternal educational attainment, household income, maternal smoking before and during pregnancy, mothers' parental locus of control, and marital status. Higher intakes of unhealthy foods during pregnancy predicted externalizing problems among children. Children with an unhealthy diet postnatally had higher levels of both internalizing and externalizing problems. Children with a low level of postnatal healthy diet also had higher incidence of both internalizing and externalizing problems. Early nutritional exposures were related to the risk for behavioral and emotional problems. Generally children who were overweight or obese were at increased risk for depression and development of unhealthy weight control behaviors (UWCBs), including using diet pills, purging, or fasting. Armstrong et al., (2013) performed a study on 106 children/adolescents 8-17 years of age. BMI, Depression Inventory-Short Form, and questionnaires assessing perception of overweight and UWCBs were used in this study. Depression was hypothesized to mediate the relationship between perception of overweight and UWCBs. This study indicated that depressive symptoms mediate the relationship between youth perception of overweight and UWCBs accounting for youth BMI z-score. The model explained 24% of the variance in UWCBs. This study presented a potential mechanism by which youth perception of overweight may influence UWCBs. Miyaki et al., (2013) examined the associations of socio-economic status (SES) with dietary intake of folate and health outcomes in Japanese workers. This cohort consisted of 2266 workers. SES was assessed by a self-administered questionnaire. Intakes of nutrients were assessed with a validated, brief and self-administered diet history questionnaire (BDHQ). The degree of depressive symptoms was estimated by the validated K6 scale. Multiple linear regression and stratified analysis were used to evaluate the associations of intake with the confounding factors. Path analysis was conducted to describe the impacts of intake on health outcomes. Education levels and household incomes were associated with intake of folate and depression scales. After adjusting for age, sex and total energy intake, years of education affected the folate intake. The structural equation model revealed that the indirect effect of folate intake was significant in the pathway of education level to depression scale. Thus both education and income were associated with depression; thus increase in folate intake may alleviate the harms of social disparities on mental health. Furthermore, Moran et al., (2013) compared the effect of different diet compositions on anthropometric, reproductive, metabolic, and psychological outcomes in PCOS. A literature search was conducted using Australasian Medical Index, CINAHL, EMBASE, Medline, PsycInfo, and EBM reviews. Inclusion criteria were women with PCOS not taking anti-obesity medications and weight-loss or maintenance diets comparing different dietary compositions. Studies were assessed for risk of bias. A total of 4,154 articles were retrieved and six articles from five studies met the selection criteria, with 137 women included. There were subtle differences between diets, with greater weight loss for a monounsaturated fat-enriched diet; improved menstrual regularity for a low-glycemic index diet; increased free androgen index for a high-carbohydrate diet; reductions in insulin resistance, fibrinogen, total, and high-density lipoprotein cholesterol for a low-carbohydrate or low-glycemic index diet; improved quality of life for a low-glycemic index diet; and improved depression and self-esteem for a high-protein diet. Weight loss improved PCOS regardless of dietary composition, suggesting that weight loss should be targeted in all overweight women with PCOS through reducing caloric intake and healthy food choices irrespective of diet composition.

Imigrant Women and Depression. It has been reported that immigrant women in Canada have a higher prevalence of postpartum depression symptomatology than Canadian-born women. There exists a need to synthesize information on the contextual factors and social determinants of health that influence immigrant women's reception of and behavior in accessing existing mental health services. The research question was: what are the ethno-culturally defined patterns of help-seeking behaviors and decision-making and other predictive factors for therapeutic mental health care access and outcomes with respect to postpartum depression for immigrant women in Canada? Higginbottom, et al., (2013) incorporated a systematic review using narrative synthesis of reports (peer- and non-peer reviewed) of empirical research and aims to provide stakeholders with perspectives on postpartum mental health care services as experienced by immigrant women. To reach this goal they used integrated knowledge translation, thus partnering with key stakeholders throughout the planning, implementation and dissemination stages to ensure topic relevancy and impact on future practice and policy. The search and selection strategies established systematic review methodologies as outlined by the Centre for Reviews and Dissemination and also incorporated guidelines for selection and appraisal of gray literature. Two search phases (a database and a gray literature phase) identified literature for screening and final selection based on an inclusion/exclusion checklist. Quality appraisal was performed using the tools produced by the Centre for Evidence Based Management. The narrative synthesis was informed by Popay et al. (2006) framework using identified tools for each of its four elements. The integrated knowledge translation plan ensured key messages were delivered in an audience-specific manner to optimize their impact on policy and practice change throughout health service, public health, immigration and community sectors. The narrative synthesis methodology facilitated understandings and acknowledgement of the broader influences of theoretical and contextual variables, such as race, gender, socio-economic status, pre-migration history and geographical location. This review aimed to have a substantive and sustainable impact on health outcomes, practice, programs and/or policy in the context of postpartum mental health of immigrant women.

Late-Life Depression. Peltzer and Phaswana-Mafuya (2013) conducted a national population-based study with a sample of 3,840 individuals aged 50 years or above in South Africa. The questionnaire included socio-demographic characteristics, health variables, anthropometric and BP measurements as well as questions on depression symptoms in the past 12 months. Regression analysis was performed to assess the association of socio-demographic factors, health variables, and depression. The prevalence of symptom-based depression was 4.0%. In multivariable analysis, functional disability, lack of quality of life, and chronic conditions (*angina, asthma, arthritis, and nocturnal sleep problems*) were associated with depression, suggesting that it is a public health problem requiring interventions to reduce occurrence. Factors associated with depression, including functional disability, poor quality of life, and chronic condition could be used to guide interventions. The identification of protective and risk factors can help in developing public health care policies to improve quality of life among older adults.

Life Style Factors. It is known that diet, exercise, and sleep play a significant role in the development, progression and treatment of MDD. Lopresti et al. (2013) summarized animal- and human-based studies on the relationship between these three lifestyle factors and MDD, and their influence on depression: namely *neurotransmitter processes, immuno-inflammatory pathways, HPA axis disturbances, oxidative stress and antioxidant defence systems,* *neuroprogression, and mitochondrial disfunction.* Their studies highlighted that emphasis in clinical studies on the influence of diet, sleep, and exercise on MDD and their effect on physiological processes will improve our understanding and treatment of MDD. Mental health interventions, taking into account the bidirectional relationship between these lifestyle factors may also enhance the efficacy of interventions associated with MDD.

Fruits and Vegetables Intake. McMartin et al. (2013) examined the association between fruit and vegetable intake (FVI) and mental health disorders. This study used data from the Canadian Community Health Survey (CCHS), repeated with five waves between 2000 until 2009 (n=296,121 aged 12 years or older). FVI was assessed based on frequency of consumption. The primary outcome was a major depressive episode over the previous 12 months. Regression models adjusted for age, gender, household income, education, physical activity, chronic illness, and smoking. In the first wave, greater FVI was associated with lower odds of depression. Relative to those with the lowest FVI, those with the greatest FVI also had lower odds of suffering from distress. Poor mental health status and previous diagnosis of a mood disorder and anxiety disorder also demonstrated inverse associations with FVI, suggesting importance of a healthy diet in the prevention of depression and anxiety.

Mediterrean Diet. The Mediterranean lifestyle has been a habit for people in Western civilizations living around the Mediterranean sea who worked hard and survived with few seasonal foods. Chedraui and Pérez-López (2013) reported that interactions between genetic (genome) and environmental factors (epigenome) operate during entire lifespan. The aging is associated with cellular and functional alterations that induce cellular dysfunction. Epigenetic mechanisms of aging are modifiable by appropriate preventive action mediated by sirtuins, caloric restriction, dietary components, adipose tissue-related inflammatory reactions, and physical activity. Adherence to the Mediterranean diet was associated with longevity and reduced risk of developing chronic diseases, including cancer, metabolic syndrome, depression, cardiovascular, and neurodegenerative diseases. Some dietary components, such as olive oil, antioxidants, omega-3 and -6 polyunsaturated fatty acids, polyphenols and flavonoids, provide anti-aging effects. Physical activity also displayed a positive effect, producing caloric consumption and regulation of adipose and pancreatic function. The strength of some food patterns may be a way of recommending for food and health policies. These authors discussed various ways of improving health during mid-life, focusing on certain groups of functional foods and healthy habits which may reduce or prevent age-related chronic diseases. Psaltopoulou et al., (2013) examined the association between adherence to a Mediterranean diet and risk of stroke, depression, cognitive impairment, and PD. Publications from PubMed were those providing effect estimates of relative risk (RR) for the association between Mediterranean diet and the aforementioned outcomes. Increased adherence to Mediterranean diet was associated with reduced risk for stroke, depression, and cognitive impairment. Moderate adherence was associated with reduced risk for depression and cognitive impairment, whereas the protective trend concerning stroke was marginal. Subgroup analyses highlighted the protective actions of high adherence in terms of reduced risk for ischemic stroke, mild cognitive impairment, dementia, particularly AD. The protective effects of Mediterranean diet in stroke prevention was more significant among males. The protective effects of high adherence seemed independent of age, whereas the favorable actions of moderate adherence faded away with more advanced age, suggesting that adherence to a Mediterranean diet may contribute to the prevention of brain diseases; this may be of special value given the aging of Western societies. Given the reported health benefits of a Mediterranean diet (MedDiet) and delay in cognitive decline, a study determined the level of adherence to a MedDiet using 11-point scale and relationships with cognitive function and psychological well-being. Crichton et al., (2013) analyzed data from 1183 adults, aged 40-65. Food frequency questionnaires were used to calculate mean intakes in a MedDiet and foods consumed in an Australian diet. Outcome measures included self-reported cognitive failures, memory, anxiety, stress, self-esteem, general health and physical function. The majority of Australians (71.7%) had a medium adherence to a MedDiet pattern. Overall MedDiet adherence was not related to cognitive function. However, intakes of plant foods in the MedDiet were positively associated with physical function and general health, and negatively associated with anxiety, depression, and perceived stress. A significant proportion of the diet in the Australian sample came from foods not consumed in a MedDiet. This was the major limitation when attempting to compare MedDiet adherence in different populations. Moreover global standardization of serving sizes and food groups are required for proper comparison. Sanchez-Villegas et al. (2013) compared in a randomized trial the effects of two Mediterranean diets versus a low-fat diet on depression risk after 3 years of intervention. This was a multicenter, primary prevention trial of cardiovascular disease based on community-dwelling men aged 55 to 80 years and women aged 60 to 80 years at high risk of cardiovascular disease attending primary care centers. Primary analyses were performed on an intention-to-treat basis. Cox regression models were used to assess the relationship between the nutritional intervention and the incidence of depression. 224 new cases of depression were identified during follow-up. There was an inverse association with depression for participants consuming Mediterranean diet supplemented with nuts compared with those assigned to the control group, although this was not significant. However, when the analysis was restricted to participants with DM2, the effect of the intervention with the Mediterranean diet supplemented with nuts reached significance suggesting that a Mediterranean diet supplemented with nuts could exert a beneficial effect on the risk of depression among DM2 patients.

Persons et al., (2013) determined the relationship between the omega-3 fatty acid of RBC membranes, in particular DHA and EPA, and baseline and new-onset depressive symptoms in post-menopausal women to characterize the association between dietary omega-3 fatty acid intake and depressive symptomatology. Study participants included 7086 members of the Women's Health Initiative Memory Study (aged 63-81 years) who had an assessment of RBC omega-3 fatty acid concentrations at the baseline screening visit. Depressive symptoms at baseline and follow-up were characterized using the Burnam eight-item scale for depressive disorders and inferred by antidepressant medication use. In multivariable-adjusted models, primary exposure, RBC DHA + EPA, was not related to depressive symptoms at baseline or follow-up, nor were RBC total omega-3, DHA, or EPA. However, dietary intake of omega-3 was positively associated with depressive symptoms, although this did not persist at follow-up, suggesting that there exists no relationship between RBC omega-3 levels and depressive symptoms, and associations between dietary omega-3 and depressive symptoms are variable. Furthermore, biomarkers of omega-3 status were not related to risk of depression in post-menopausal women. Rienks et al., (2013) performed a study on Participants (aged 50-55 years) who completed a food frequency questionnaire. Depressive symptoms were measured in 2001 and 2004 using the validated 10-item Centre for Epidemiologic Studies Depression scale. Multiple logistic regression was used for cross-sectional analysis (8369 women) and longitudinal analysis (7588) to assess the associations between dietary patterns and prevalence of depressive symptoms, and then for longitudinal analysis (6060) on their associations with the incidence of depressive symptoms in 2004, while adjusting for sociodemographic and lifestyle factors. Six dietary patterns were identified from factor analysis: cooked vegetables, fruit, Mediterranean style, meat and processed meat, dairy, and high fat and sugar. Consumption of the Mediterranean-style diet had association with lower prevalence and lower incidence of depressive symptoms. None of the associations found for other dietary patterns were significant after adjustment for confounders. A dose-response relationship was found when women were grouped according to Mediterranean-style diet, supporting that this dietary pattern by mid-aged women may have a protective influence against the onset of depressive symptoms and have a potential role in the prevention and management of depression.

Mediterranean diet and Cognition. Previous studies reported beneficial effects of the Mediterranean diet (MedDiet) on cognitive function, but results were inconsistent. Martinez-Marinez-Lapiscina et al., (2013) assessed the effect on cognition using MedDiets in comparison with a low-fat control diet. 522 participants were assessed at high vascular risk (44.6% men, age 74.6 ± 5.7 years at cognitive evaluation) enrolled in a multicentre, randomized, primary prevention trial (PREDIMED), after a nutritional intervention comparing two MedDiets (supplemented with either extra-virgin olive oil (EVOO) or mixed nuts) versus a low-fat control diet. Global cognitive performance was examined by Mini-Mental State Examination (MMSE) and Clock Drawing Test (CDT) after 6.5 years of nutritional intervention. After adjustment for sex, age, education, Apolipoprotein E, family history of cognitive impairment/dementia, smoking, physical activity, BMI, hypertension, dyslipidemia, diabetes, alcohol and total energy intake, participants on MedDiet+EVOO showed higher mean MMSE and CDT scores with significant differences. The adjusted means of MMSE and CDT scores were also higher for participants allocated to the MedDiet+Nuts. These results did not differ after controlling for depression suggesting that an intervention with MedDiets enhanced with either EVOO or nuts improved cognition compared with a low-fat diet.

Cognitive impairment is common in heart failure patients. Poor dietary habits are associated with reduced neurocognitive function in other medical populations, including diabetes and AD. Alosko (2013) examined whether dietary habits help moderate the relationship between heart failure severity and cognitive function. A total of 152 persons with heart failure completed neuropsychological testing and a fitness assessment. Dietary habits were assessed using the Conversation-Diet questionnaire, a nutrition measure in primary care settings. Better dietary habits attenuated the adverse impact of heart failure severity on frontal functioning. Follow-up analyses revealed consumption of foods high in sodium was associated with reduced cognitive function suggesting that dietary habits can moderate the association between heart failure and performance on tests of attention and executive function.

Katsiardanis et al., (2013) investigated the association of dietary habits with cognitive function among elders (>65 years). Sociodemographic, dietary information, serum measurements, and Mini-Mental State Examination (MMSE) assessments were performed for 237 elderly men and 320 women. All models were adjusted for age, education, social activity, smoking, depression symptomatology (using the Geriatric Depression Scale), MedDietScore (range 0-55), and metabolic syndrome. About 49.8% men and 66.6% women had MMSE scores <24. Adherence to the Mediterranean diet was moderate. Indicative cognitive impairment (MMSE score <24) was positively associated with age and low education in women and with depressive symptoms, low education status, and low social activity in men. Adherence to the Mediterranean diet was positively associated with MMSE score in men, but inversely associated in women. The intake of pulses, nuts, and seeds was associated with lower likelihood of having MMSE score<24 in men. Only the Mediterranean dietary pattern showed a significant association with MMSE score for cognitive impairment (i.e., protective in men, but not in women), while individual food groups or nutrients did not reach significance. These findings supported the role of diet in the prevention of mental disorders, and state a hypothesis for a sex-diet interaction on cognitive function among elders.

Anxiety and depression contribute to morbidity in elderly and may be associated with diet. Hodge et al. (2013) investigated the association between diet and psychological distress as a biomarker for depression. Dietary patterns were defined by factor analysis or the Mediterranean Diet Score (MDS); depression and anxiety were assessed 12 years later. A total of 8,660 healthy men and women and aged 50-69 years from the Melbourne Collaborative Cohort Study were included. At baseline (1990-1994), diet (food frequency questionnaire), education, Socio-Economic Indices for Areas (SEIFA) - Index of Relative Socio-economic Disadvantage, medication use, social engagement, physical activity, smoking status, alcohol use, and health conditions were assessed; at follow-up (2003-2007), psychological distress was assessed using the Kessler Psychological Distress Scale (K10). Logistic regression was used to identify associations between diet and a K10 score ≥20, indicative of psychological distress. The MDS was inversely associated with psychological distress, with the odds ratio in the top-scoring group relative to the lowest scoring group being 0.72. Stronger adherence to a traditional Australian-style eating pattern was also associated with a lower K10 score, with the odds ratio for having a K10 score indicative of psychological distress for the top 20% of adherence to this pattern relative to the lowest being 0.61 indicating that a Mediterranean-style diet was associated with less psychological distress, through provision of a healthy nutrient profile. The Australian dietary pattern, which included foods high in fat and sugar content along with whole foods, also showed a weak inverse association. Adherence to this pattern may reflect a feeling of belonging to the community associated with less psychological distress.

Methyl donor deficiencies and chronic stress cause depression but their interaction has not been investigated. Javelot et al., (2013) performed a study in which, methyl donor deficient diet and chronic stress condition consisted respectively of a B_2, B_9, B_{12}, and choline-free diet and a chronic mild stress. Rats were assigned to six groups with three "diet" conditions (free-feeding, pair-fed and methyl donor deficient diet) and two "stress" conditions (no-stress and stress) and were evaluated in the open-field, the elevated plus-maze and the forced swimming test. After the behavioral evaluation, corticosterone and homocysteine plasma levels were measured and dopamine, DOPAC, serotonin, 5HIAA were determined in brain areas. Rats given a methyl donor deficient diet for 11 weeks inducing elevated plasma homocysteine levels were compared to pair-fed and free-feeding rats with or without unpredictable chronic mild stress. Regardless of stress environmental conditions, the methyl donor deficient diet decreased plasma corticosterone levels and caused disinhibition in the elevated plus-maze condition. However, stress augmented the effects of the deficient regimen on rearing in the open-field and climbing in the forced swim test. The dietary changes involved in behavior and plasma corticosterone could be caused by homocysteine-induced decreases in dopamine and 5-HT metabolites in selective brain regions and could be noted regardless of stress-conditions, methyl donor deficient diet decreased DOPAC/dopamine and 5HIAA/serotonin ratios in striatum and hypothalamus and 5HIAA/serotonin ratio in the sensorimotor cortex. These data are relevant to the neuropsychiatric disorders associated with folate deficiency and homocysteinemia.

Rosenberg et al., (2013) compared behavioral outcomes (physical activity, sedentary behavior, smoking cessation, diet) between the intervention and usual care conditions which was a randomized trial among 214 adults with depression and poorly controlled diabetes and/or coronary heart disease that promoted health behavior change and pharmacotherapy to improve health. Behavioral outcomes were measured with the International Physical Activity Questionnaire (physical activity, sitting time) and the Summary of Diabetes Self-Care Activities Measure (smoking, diet, exercise). Regression models among completers (N=185) were conducted for age, education, smoking status and depression. The participants had more days/week following a healthy eating plan and more days of participation in 30 min of physical activity compared to usual care. Intervention participants were more likely to meet physical activity guidelines compared to usual care. Diet and activity improved for those on intervention, while there were no differences in some aspects of diet (fruit and vegetable and high-fat food intake), smoking status and sitting time between conditions in the TEAMcare trial.

Food allergy is associated with psychological distress in both child and parent. It is unknown whether parental distress is present prior to clinical diagnosis or whether experiences at clinic can reduce any distress. Knibb and Semper (2013) assessed anxiety and depression in parents and the impact of suspected food allergy on the families before and after a visit to an allergy clinic. 124 parents visiting an allergy clinic for the first time to have their child assessed for food allergy completed a study-specific questionnaire and the Hospital Anxiety and Depression Scale; 50 parents completed these 4-6 wk later in their own home. Most parents (86.4%) reported suspected food allergy had an impact on their family life; 76% had made changes to their child's diet. 32.5% of parents had mild-to-severe anxiety before their clinic visit; 17.5% had mild-to-moderate depression. Post-clinic, 40% had mild-to-severe anxiety; 13.1% had mild-to-moderate depression. There were no differences in anxiety or depression scores before and after the clinic visit indicating that anxiety and depression are present in a small proportion of parents prior to diagnosis of food allergy in their child and this did not reduce in the short term after the clinic visit.

A study was performed to investigate food consumption, nutrient intakes and serum metabolic biomarkers in depressive, anxiety and alcohol abuse disorders in comparison with the remaining from a population-based nationwide sample. Rintamaki et al., (2013) conducted this study based on the Health 2000 Survey data of which 5504 subjects aged 30 and over 3009 women and 2495 men. Depressive disorder, anxiety disorders, and alcohol addiction were diagnosed using the Composite International Diagnostic Interview (M-CIDI). The consumption of food and beverage, and nutrient intakes were measured with a food frequency questionnaire, and biomarkers of depression were determined in blood samples. No similar differences with both genders were found in the intakes of energy, dietary fibre or macronutrients or in biomarkers in depressive or anxiety disorders. Women suffering from depressive disorder consumed more soft drinks and those suffering from anxiety disorders consumed more oils, polyunsaturated fatty acids and less potatoes than the remaining participants. Men suffering from depressive disorder consumed less sweets and chocolate and those with anxiety disorder consumed more tea compared with the remaining participants. In alcohol addiction, the intake of carbohydrate was lower in both genders indicating a difference in the usual diet between individuals with alcohol addiction and the remaining participants. No consistent difference in both genders between those with depressive or anxiety disorders and the remaining was observed.

Dietary Manipulation of Dairy Milk Fat. Rico and Harvatine (2013) reported that milk fat depression (MFD) caused by ruminal biohydrogenation occurs in dairy cattle. Nine cows were used to analyze recovery from diet-induced MFD. A high-fiber, low-oil diet was fed during the control and recovery periods, and a low-fiber, high-oil (LFHO) diet was fed during the induction period. Milk yield was not affected by the treatment. Milk fat percentage and yield decreased during induction and were lower by d 3 and 5, respectively. Milk fat concentration increased when cows were fed the recovery diet and were not different from control on d 19 and 15, respectively. Yield of fatty acids (FA) decreased during the induction period and was lower than that of controls by d 5. A biphasic response was seen for milk fat Trans isomers, where trans-11 C18:1 and cis-9, trans-11 conjugated linoleic acid (CLA) were elevated initially and trans-10 C18:1 and trans-10, cis-12 CLA increased during the induction period. A similar biphasic response was seen during recovery from MFD, with trans-10 C18:1 and trans-10, cis-12 decreasing initially and trans-11 C18:1 and cis-9, trans-11 CLA increasing slightly during the second phase. Recovery from diet-induced MFD occurred with a short lag when dietary fiber and oil concentrations are corrected. This time course identified factors causing MFD and set expectations during recovery from MFD. Altenhofer et al., (2013) performed a study on 95 cows which were fed soy bean oil and rapeseed oil as a nutritional supplement to improve the nutritional quality of milk. These studies suggested that feeding of oil supplements has significant impact on milk fat composition and on human health, by decreasing fats with a negative effect (saturated fatty acid and cholesterol) while increasing others with positive (monounsaturated fatty acid, PUFA, and conjugated linolenic acid) effects. Boerman et al., (2014) evaluated the effect of a blend of synthetic antioxidants on the yield of milk and its components and fatty acid composition in cows fed a diet to cause milk fat depression (MFD). These investigators hypothesized that synthetic antioxidant to diets with a high rumen unsaturated fatty acid load (RUFAL) would decrease the severity of MFD. Sixteen lactating cows with two 21-d periods, were fed a corn silage and grass silage-diet containing 15% distillers grains. The diet contained 34% neutral detergent fiber, 18% crude protein, 26% starch, and 4.3% total fatty acids (dry matter basis). Cows were fed the diet without supplementation (control; CON) or supplemented with 0.02% (dry matter basis) of a synthetic antioxidant (AOX). Milk samples were collected in the beginning of the study for baseline values and at the end of each period (d 20-21) and analyzed for milk components and fatty acid composition. Dry matter intake and milk yield were unaffected by treatment. No effect of treatment on yields of fat, protein, lactose, 3.5% fat-corrected milk, energy-corrected milk, feed efficiency, body weight, or body condition score was observed. Milk fat and yield were both reduced by the high RUFAL diets. A tendency for AOX to increase the concentration of milk fat and decrease the concentration of milk protein was noticed. Yields of de novo and preformed fatty acids were not affected by treatment, although a trend for a slight increase in the yield of 16-carbon fatty acid for AOX compared with CON was detected. Treatment had minor effects on milk fatty acids, except for linoleic acid, which were over 90% higher for AOX compared with CON, indicating that milk fat concentration and yield are reduced by a high RUFAL diet containing 15% distillers grains; however, AOX did not overcome the MFD induced by this diet.

It is known that removing His from a postruminal AA infusion decreases milk protein and increases milk fat content. Feather meal is an inexpensive protein source, high in rumen undegradable protein but low in His. Stahel et al., (2013) investigated dietary feather meal for creating a His deficiency or imbalance to alter milk composition. Four dietary treatments were fed for 4 wk each to 8 multiparous mid-lactation cows in a replicated 4 × 4 Latin square design. A standard-protein control diet (SP-C) was formulated to provide 3,100 g/d of metabolizable protein (MP). Feather meal was added to the control diet either to replace the MP isonitrogenously (SP-FM) or to increase the MP supply to 3,484 g/d (HP-FM). As an isonitrogenous control for HP-FM, a high-protein diet (HP-C) was formulated with His-adequate protein sources to provide the same MP content as HP-FM. Dry matter intake tended to decrease when feather meal was fed. The flows of digestible His, Met, and Lys, and plasma concentrations of these AA were reduced on both feather meal diets. The flows of total digestible essential AA were not different between HP-FM and SP-C. The DMI depression on HP-FM prevented an imbalance of excess AA over His, and created a deficiency of His, Met, and Lys compared with SP-C. Milk production decreased on the 2 feather meal treatments, partly explained by a tendency for DMI to decrease. Milk yield was lowest on SP-FM at 30.3 kg/d and highest on HP-C at 37.9 kg/d. Milk fat yield was not affected by diet but protein and lactose yields were both lower with feather meal. Protein yields were 860 and 998 g/d, whereas lactose yields were 1,384 and 1,561 g/d for SP-FM and HP-FM, respectively resulting in a higher fat content and lower protein on FM diets. The ratio of solids-not-fat:fat in milk was lowest on SP-FM at 2.11 compared with 2.56 on SP-C. Adding feather meal to the diet by replacing MP was more effective at lowering the solids-not-fat:fat ratio than increasing the MP content with an imbalanced protein source. Conjugated linoleic acids (CLA), and the trans-10,cis-12 (t10,c12-CLA) isomer are potent modulators of milk fat synthesis in dairy cows. Studies in mice revealed that t10,c12-CLA was responsible for hepatic lipodystrophy and decreased adipose tissue with changes in the fatty acid distribution. Kramer et al., (2013) investigated the fatty acid distribution of lipids in body tissues compared to their distribution in milk fat in early lactating cows in response to CLA treatment. Effects in mammary gland were analyzed at gene expression level. Twenty-five heifers were fed a diet supplemented with (CLA groups) or without (CON groups) a rumen-protected CLA supplement that provided 6 g/d of c9,t11- and t10,c12-CLA. Five groups of randomly assigned cows were analyzed according to experimental design based on feeding and time of slaughter. Cows in the first group received no CLA supplement and were slaughtered one day postpartum (CON). Milk samples were taken from the remaining cows in CON and CLA groups at 42 (period 1) and 105 (period 2) days in milk (DIM). Tissue samples from liver, retroperitoneal fat, mammary gland and M. longissimus (13th rib) were obtained and analyzed for fatty acid distribution. Genes involved in lipid metabolism of the mammary gland were analyzed using microarray. Both supplemented CLA isomers increased in milk fat. Furthermore, fatty acids increased at the expense of de novo-synthesized fatty acids. Total and single trans-octadecenoic acids also increased. Fatty acid distribution of the mammary gland showed similar changes to those in milk fat, due to residual milk but without affecting gene expression. Liver fatty acids were not altered except for trans-octadecenoic acids, which were increased. Adipose tissue and M. longissimus were marginally affected by CLA, suggesting that CLA leads to alterations in milk fat depression but only marginally affected tissue lipids. Gene expression of the mammary gland was not influenced by CLA supplementation. Metzler-Zebeli et al., (2013) investigated the effect of increasing barley grain on the microbial composition and LPS concentrations in the rumen and colon of goats. Effects were compared with respect to the responses of ruminal and colonic pH and short-chain fatty acid (SCFA) generation. Growing goats were fed diets containing 0, 30, or 60% coarsely ground barley grain for 6 weeks. Ruminal ciliate protozoa were counted with Bürker counting chamber, and qPCR was used to compare bacterial populations. Increasing dietary grain level increased ruminal numbers of entodiniomorphids. With the 60% grain diet, there was a reduction in ruminal abundance of the genus Prevotella and Fibrobacter succinogenes, whereas the ruminal abundance of Lactobacillus spp. increased compared to the 0 and 30% grain diets. In the colon, abundance of the genus Prevotella and F. succinogenes increased in goats fed the 60% grain diet compared to those fed the other diets. Colonic abundance of Clostridium cluster I was related to the presence of grain in the diet. Ruminal LPS concentration decreased in response to the 60% grain diet, whereas its colonic concentration increased in response to the same diet. These results provided insight on the adaptive response of rumen protozoa and rumen and bacterial populations to increasing dietary levels of grain in goats. Although luminal pH affects microbial populations, fermentable substrate flow to the caprine hindgut may have played a role for colonic bacterial populations.

During diet-induced milk fat depression (MFD), the short and medium-chain fatty acids (SMCFA), synthesized in the mammary gland, are reduced to a much greater extent than the long-chain fatty acids (LCFA) that originate from the circulation. Vyas et al., (2013) hypothesized that increased availability of SMCFA might rescue conjugated linoleic acid (CLA)-induced MFD in lactating dairy cows. To test this hypothesis, 4 rumen-fistulated lactating cows (128 ± 23 d in milk) were used in a 4 × 4 Latin square design with 3-wk experimental periods. Treatments were applied during the last 2 wk and included 3× daily infusion of a total of (1) 230 g/d of LCFA (blend of 59% cocoa butter, 36% olive oil, and 5% palm oil); (2) 420 g/d of butterfat (BF); (3) 230 g/d of LCFA with 27 g/d of CLA (LC-CLA), containing 10 g/d of trans-10,cis-12 CLA; and (4) 420 g/d of butterfat with 27 g/d of CLA (BF-CLA). Butterfat provided 50% of C16 (115 g/d) and similar amounts of C18 FA as found in LCFA, such that the difference between the BF and LCFA treatments was 190 g/d of SMCFA. No treatment effects were observed for DMI or milk yield. Milk fat content was reduced by 41 and 32%, whereas milk fat yield was reduced by 41 and 38% with LC-CLA and BF-CLA, respectively, compared with their respective controls. Abomasal infusion of CLA reduced de novo synthesized fatty acid (DNFA; SMCFA and 50% C16:0) concentration, whereas DNFA tended to be greater with BF infusion. An interaction was observed between SMCFA and CLA as the increased availability of SMCFA reduced stearoyl-CoA-desaturase-1 gene expression, whereas it reduced lipoprotein lipase (LPL), 1-acylglycerol-3-phosphate O-acyltransferase 6 (AGPAT-6), sterol regulatory element-binding protein cleavage-activating protein (SCAP), and peroxisome proliferator-activated receptor γ (PPAR-γ) gene expression in the presence of CLA. The mRNA expression of genes involved in fatty acid synthesis [acetyl-coenzyme A carboxylase α (ACACA) and fatty acid synthase (FASN)], fatty acid uptake (LPL), and triglyceride synthesis [AGPAT-6 and diacylglycerol O-acyltransferase 1 (DGAT-1)] along with protein abundance of the ACC and FASN were reduced with CLA. However, the increased availability of SMCFA had no significant effect on lipogenic gene expression except for LPL, whose expression was increased with BF infusion. The nutritional manipulation by increasing the intestinal availability of SMCFA was not sufficient to rescue CLA-induced MFD.

Bichi et al., (2013) demonstrated that addition of marine algae (MA) to the diet of dairy ruminants is an effective strategy to enhance the milk content of some bioactive lipids, but it has also been associated with milk fat depression. Little is known, however, about the persistency of the response to dietary MA in sheep. Based on previous experiments with dairy ewes fed sunflower oil plus MA, it was hypothesized that the response might be mediated by time-dependent adaptations of the rumen microbiota, which could be evaluated indirectly through milk fatty acid (FA) profiles. Animal performance and milk FA composition in response to MA in the diet were studied using 36 ewes distributed in 6 lots and allocated to 2 treatments (3 lots/treatment) consisting of a total mixed ration supplemented with 25 g of sunflower oil (SO)/kg of dry matter plus 0 (SO; control diet) or 8 g of MA/kg of dry matter (SOMA diet). Diet supplementation with MA did not affect milk yield but did decrease milk fat content. Differences in the latter were detected from d 18 onward and reached -17% at the end of the experiment (i.e., on d 54). Compared with the control diet, the SOMA diet caused a reduction in milk 18:0 and its desaturation product (cis-9 18:1) that lasted for the whole experimental period. This decrease, together with the progressive increase in some fat synthesis inhibitors, especially trans-10 18:1, was related to the persistency of milk fat depression in lactating ewes fed MA. Additionally, inclusion of MA in the diet enhanced the milk content of trans-11 18:1, cis-9,trans-11 18:2, and C20-22 n-3 polyunsaturated FA, mainly 22:6 n-3, suggesting that the ruminal microbiota did not adapt to the dietary supply of very long chain n-3 PUFAs.

Feeding unsaturated oils to lactating cows impair ruminal biohydrogenation (BH) of unsaturated fatty acids (USFA) and increase ruminal outflow of BH intermediates such as trans-10, cis-12 CLA that are considered to be potent inhibitors of milk fat synthesis. Supplementing lactating cow's rations containing plant origin oils with monensin and/or vitamin E may minimise the formation of trans-10 isomers in the rumen, thereby preventing milk fat depression. Khodamoradi et al., (2013) evaluated the effects of monensin and vitamin E in the diets of lactating cows containing whole cottonseed, as the main source of FA on feed intake, milk production and composition, milk fatty acid profile, efficiency of nitrogen (N) utilization, efficiency of net energy (NE) and nutrients digestibilities. Four multiparous lactating dairy cows were assigned to a 4 × 4 Latin square design. Each experimental period lasted 21 days with a 14 days of treatment adaptation and a 7 days of data collection. The control diet was a total mixed ration (TMR) consisted of 430 g/kg forage and 570 g/kg of a concentrate mixture on dry matter (DM) basis. Cows were assigned to one of the four dietary treatments including control diet (C), control diet supplemented with 150 mg of vitamin E/kg of DM (E), control diet supplemented with 24 mg of monensin/kg of DM (M) and control diet supplemented with 150 mg of vitamin E and 24 mg of monensin/kg of DM (EM). Dry matter intake (DMI) ranged from 19.1 to 19.5 kg/d and was similar among the dietary treatments. Dietary vitamin E or monensin had no effect on milk production, milk fat, protein and lactose concentrations, efficiency of utilization of nitrogen and net energy for lactation (NEL). Digestibility of DM, organic matter (OM), crude protein (CP) and ether extract (EE) was not affected. Digestibility of neutral detergent fibre (NDF) was higher in cows fed with the M and EM diets in relation to those fed the C and E diets.

Feeding the M diet decreased milk fat concentration of C16:0, the milk fat concentration of C18:2n-6 FA tended to be increased. Dietary supplementation with vitamin E or monensin had no effect on milk fat concentrations of saturated, unsaturated, monounsaturated, polyunsaturated, short chain and long chain FA, but decreased milk fat concentration of medium chain fatty acids (MCFA), suggesting that vitamin E and/or monensin did not improve milk fat content or minimize the formation of trans-10 FA isomers in the rumen when cottonseed was included in the diet as the main source of fatty acids.

CLA Supplementation and Milk Fat Depression. Trans-10, cis-12 conjugated linoleic acid (CLA) causes milk fat depression in dairy cows, but CLA effects on glucose metabolism are not clear. Hotger et al., (2013) investigated endogenous glucose production (eGP) and glucose oxidation (GOx), as well as hepatic genes involved in glucose production in cows supplemented either with 50 g of rumen-protected CLA (9% trans-10,cis-12 and 10% cis-9,trans-11; CLA; n=10) or 50 g of control fat (24% C18:2; Ctrl; n=10) from wk 2 before parturition to wk 9 of lactation. Animal performance data were recorded and blood metabolites and hormones were taken weekly from 2 wk before to 12 wk after parturition. During wk 3 and 9 after parturition, glucose tolerance tests were performed and eGP and GOx were measured by [U-(13)C] glucose infusion. Liver biopsies were taken at the same time to measure total fat and glycogen concentrations and gene expression of pyruvate carboxylase, cytosolic phosphoenolpyruvate carboxykinase, glucose-6-phosphatase, and carnitine palmitoyl-transferase 1. Conjugated linoleic acid feeding reduced milk fat, but increased lactose output; milk yield was higher starting 5 wk after parturition in CLA-fed cows than in Ctrl-fed cows. Energy balance was more negative during CLA supplementation, and plasma concentrations of glucose were higher immediately after calving in CLA-fed cows. Conjugated linoleic acid supplementation did not affect insulin release during glucose tolerance tests, but reduced eGP in wk 3, and eGP and GOx increased with time after parturition. Hepatic gene expression of cytosolic phosphoenolpyruvate carboxykinase tended to be lower in CLA-fed cows than in Ctrl-fed cows. In spite of lower eGP in CLA-fed cows, lactose output and plasma glucose concentrations were greater in CLA-fed cows than in Ctrl-fed cows, suggesting a CLA-related glucose sparing effect due to lower glucose utilization for milk fat synthesis and because of an efficient whole-body energy utilization in CLA-fed cows.

Tea and Coffee Consumption. Tea and coffee, after water, are the most commonly consumed beverages and are the sources of caffeine and antioxidant polyphenols in the American diet. Bhatti et al., (2013) assessed the effects of chronic tea and/or coffee consumption. Green tea, was associated with reduced risks for stroke, diabetes and depression, and improved levels of glucose, cholesterol, abdominal obesity and BP. Habitual coffee consumption was associated with reduced mortality, both for all-cause and cardiovascular deaths. In addition, coffee intake was associated with increased risks of heart failure, stroke, diabetes mellitus and some cancers. However, coffee was associated with neutral to reduced risks for both atrial and ventricular arrhythmias. Caffeine at high doses increased anxiety, insomnia, calcium loss and risk of fractures. Hence coffee and tea can be recommended as health-promoting additions to an adult diet. However adequate dietary calcium intake may be important for tea and coffee drinkers.

Fructose and Metabolic Syndrome. Lustig (2010) reported that the Atkins Diet is usually low in carbohydrate and high in fat, whereas the Japanese diet is high in carbohydrate and low in fat. Yet both promote weight loss. A common feature of both diets is that they eliminate the monosaccharide fructose. Sucrose and high fructose corn syrup consist of glucose and fructose. Glucose when polymerized forms starch, which has a high glycemic index, generates an insulin response, and is not very sweet. Fructose is found in fruit, does not generate an insulin response, and is very sweet. Fructose consumption has increased globally, paralleling the obesity and chronic metabolic disease pandemic. Sugar (fructose-containing mixtures) is a source of "empty calories," no different from any other empty calorie. However, fructose is unlike glucose. In the hypercaloric glycogen-replete state, intermediary metabolites from fructose metabolism overwhelm hepatic mitochondrial capacity, which promotes de novo lipogenesis and leads to hepatic insulin resistance, which drives chronic metabolic disease. Fructose also facilitates ROS formation, which leads to cellular dysfunction and aging, and promotes changes in the brain's reward system, which drives excessive consumption. Thus, fructose can exert detrimental health effects in ways that mimic those of ethanol. The only distinction is that because fructose is not metabolized in the CNS, it does not exert neuronal depression experienced by those taking ethanol. Hence fructose may be thought of as "alcohol without the buzz."

Flavonoids. Neurodegenerative, neurological and psychiatric diseases are a group of pathologies with social and economic burden. Since brain disorders continue to be pathological conditions for which surgery cannot be frequently used, treatments are based on drugs that alleviate the symptoms. Despite all efforts in finding more efficient therapeutic agents, the requirement for neuroprotective drugs which can cross the blood-brain barrier (BBB) has been a challenge. Flavonoids are known by their antioxidant activities thus preventing oxidative stress, which is believe to be one of the causes of disorders affecting the CNS. They can also modulate both enzymes and receptors activities, and regarded as multi-target biotherapeutics or drugs. Grosso et al. (2013) emphasized the benefits of flavonoids in the diet for the treatment of AD, PD, epilepsy, depression, and schizophrenia. The antioxidant effect of flavonoids and their effects not related with antioxidant activity have been reviewed. Flavonoids have positive impacts on human health. These are a family of phenolic compounds, are widely present in our diet and exist in traditional Chinese medicines, in which they act as the major active functional ingredients. Xu (2013) analyzed different subclasses of flavonoids for their protective roles in promoting the expression of synaptic proteins, synaptotagmin, and post-synaptic density protein-95 in cultured rat cortical neurons. Among the 65 flavonoids, (-)-catechin, luteolin, and isorhamnetin induce the expression of synaptic proteins. Similar results were revealed in the flavonoid-treated hippocampal neurons. The identification of these synapse-promoting flavonoids could be useful in discovering potential drugs, or food supplements, for treating various neurodegenerative diseases, including AD and depression.

Talbinah. Talbinah is a barley syrup cooked with milk and sweetened by honey. The Prophet Mohammad recommended it when sad events happen for soothing hearts and relieving sadness. Badrasawi et al., (2013) performed 3-week clinical trial to determine the effect of Talbinah on mood and depression among elderly people. A sample of 30 depressed elderly subjects (21 men and 9 women) was selected from the long term care facility. Three interview-based validated scales (Geriatric Depression Scale, Depression Anxiety Stress Scales, and Profile of Mood States) were used to determine mood, depression, stress, and anxiety. The nutritional value of Talbinah was examined using proximate food analysis, mineral and differential amino acid analysis. The results indicated that Talbinah is a high carbohydrate food with high tryptophan: branch chain amino acids ratio (1:2). There was a significant decrease in depression, stress, and mood disturbances scores suggesting that Talbinah reduces depression and enhances mood. Hence ingestion of foods such as Talbinah may provide a mental health benefit to elderly people.

Folate Deficiency. Folate deficiency has been linked to neurodegenerative and stress-related diseases such as stroke, dementia, and depression. The role of the neurotrophins nerve growth factor (NGF) and neurotrophin-3 (NT-3) in stress-related disorders and neurodegeneration has gained attention in recent years. Uracil misincorporation is involved in the neuropsychiatric dysfunction induced by experimental folate deprivation. Eckart et al., (2013) conducted a study in a 2×2 design, aged mice lacking uracil-DNA N-glycosylase (Ung(-/-)) versus wild-type (Ung(+/+)) controls subjected to a folate-deficient diet versus a regular diet for three months. Folate deficiency led to decreased NGF protein levels in the frontal cortex and amygdala. In the hippocampus, NGF levels were increased in UNG (-/-) mice on the normal diet, but not under folate deficiency, while in UNG (+/+) mice, folate deprivation did not affect hippocampal NGF content. NT-3 protein was neither affected by genotype nor by folate deficiency, suggesting that folate deficiency affects NGF levels in the frontal cortex, amygdala, and hippocampus. The decrease in NGF in the hippocampus in response to folate deficiency in Ung(-/-) mice may contribute to enhanced anxiety and depression-like behavior as well as to hippocampal neurodegeneration.

Tomato-Rich Diet. Lycopene in tomatoes is the most powerful antioxidant amongst the carotenoids. Niu et al., (2013) investigated the relationship between different vegetables, including tomatoes/tomato products (a major source of lycopene), and depressive symptoms in a community-based elderly population. These researchers analyzed 986 community-dwelling elderly Japanese aged 70 years and older. Dietary intake of tomato was assessed using a self-administered diet-history questionnaire, and depressive symptoms were evaluated using the 30-item Geriatric Depression Scale with 2 cut-off points: 11 (mild and severe) and 14 (severe) or use of anti-depressive agents. The prevalence of mild and severe depressive symptoms was 34.9% and 20.2%, respectively. After adjustments for potentially confounding factors, the odd ratios of having mild and severe depressive symptoms by increasing levels of tomatoes/tomato products were 1.00, 0.54, and 0.48. Similar relationship was noticed in the case of severe depressive symptoms, without any significant relationship with intake of other kinds of vegetables and depressive symptoms suggesting that a tomato-rich diet is related to lower prevalence of depressive symptoms and that it may have a beneficial effect on the prevention of depressive symptoms. Further studies are required to confirm these findings.

Bone Broth. The preparation and consumption of bone broth is recommended to patients as part of the gut and psychology syndrome (GAPS) diet for autism, ADHD, dyslexia, dyspraxia, depression and schizophrenia as part of the diet. However, bones are known to sequester the heavy metal lead, contamination with which is widespread throughout the environment. Such lead can be mobilized from the bones. Monro (2013) hypothesized that bone broth might carry a risk of being contaminated with lead. A study of lead concentrations in three different types of chicken broth showed that such broths contain significantly high levels of lead as compared to water with which the broth was made. In particular, broth made from skin and cartilage taken off the bone and chicken-bone broth had significantly high lead concentrations. In view of the dangers of lead intake to the human body, it was recommended that physicians must consider the risk of lead contamination when advising patients bone broth diets.

Hippocampal and PFC Atrophy in Depression. Ota and Duman (2013) reported atrophy of neurons and structural alterations of limbic brain regions, including the prefrontal cortex (PFC) and hippocampus, in brain imaging and postmortem studies of depressed patients. Their findings suggested that prolonged negative stress can induce changes comparable to those seen in MDD, through dendritic retraction and decreased spine density in PFC and hippocampal CA3 pyramidal neurons. Interestingly, environmental and pharmacological manipulations, including antidepressant medication, exercise, and diet, could block or even reverse many of the molecular changes induced by stress, providing a clear link between these factors and susceptibility to MDD. In this report, the authors discussed the environmental and pharmacological factors, as well as the contribution of genetic polymorphisms in the regulation of neuronal morphology and plasticity in MDD and preclinical stress models. Particularly, the pro-depressive changes induced by stress and the reversal of these changes by antidepressants, exercise, and diet.

Overeating and Deep Brain Stimulation. Hedonic overconsumption contributing to obesity involves abnormal activation within the mesolimbic dopamine system. Dysregulation of dopamine signaling in the nucleus accumbens shell (NAS) has been implicated in reward-seeking behaviors, such as binge eating, which contributes to treatment resistance in obesity (Wise, 2012). Direct modulation of the NAS with deep brain stimulation (DBS), a surgical procedure under investigation in humans for the treatment of MDD, obsessive-compulsive disorder, and addiction, may also be effective in ameliorating binge eating. Halpern et al., (2013) examined the ability of DBS of the NAS to block this behavior in mice. *c-Fos* immunoreactivity was estimated as a marker of DBS-mediated neuronal activation. NAS DBS reduced binge eating and increased *c-Fos* in this region. DBS of the dorsal striatum had no influence on this behavior, demonstrating anatomical specificity for this effect. The dopamine D_2 receptor antagonist, Raclopride, attenuated the action of DBS, whereas the D_1 receptor antagonist, SCH-23390, was ineffective, suggesting that dopamine signaling involving D_2 receptors underlies the effect of NAS DBS. To determine the translational relevance to the obese state, chronic NAS DBS was also examined in diet-induced obese mice and was found to reduce caloric intake and induce weight loss suggesting the involvement of the mesolimbic dopaminergic pathways in the hedonic mechanisms contributing to overeating and obesity, and the ability of NAS DBS to modulate this system.

NASA Space Travel and Pomegranate Diet. NASA plans for extended space travel, and space radiation can have negative impact on cognitive skills as well as physical and mental health. With long-term space travel, astronauts may be exposed to increased radiation levels. An antioxidant-enriched diet may offer protection against the cellular effects of radiation and may provide neuroprotection from the deleterious effects of radiation-induced cognitive and behavioral skills. Dulcich and Hartman (2013) performed a study on ninety-six C57BL/6 mice (48 pomegranate fed and 48 control) irradiated with proton radiation (2 Gy), and two-month postradiation behaviors were assessed using behavioral tests to measure cognitive and motor functions. Proton irradiation induced depression-like behaviors in the tail suspension test, but this effect was ameliorated by the pomegranate diet. Males, in general, displayed worse coordination and balance than females on the rotarod task, and the pomegranate diet ameliorated this effect. Pomegranates may protect the brain (*and therefore behavior*) from the deleterious effects of radiation by a number of mechanisms. Particles can strike DNA, causing damage and apoptosis, also strike water molecules, generating ROS that cause inflammation, vascular damage, and suppressed neurogenesis. Pomegranate's neuroprotective, antioxidant, anti-inflammatory, and provascular (via NOS) activation may protect against these deleterious effects.

Gluten-Free Diet and Depression. van Hees et al., 2013 investigated whether long-term adherence to a gluten-free diet is related to depression in 2265 coeliac disease (CD) patients.

Diet adherence was compared based on depressive symptoms. The life-time prevalence rate of depressive symptoms was 39.0%, of whom 11.9% suffered from depressive symptoms. Adherence to gluten-free diet was strict in 50.2% of patients, sufficient in 46.3%, and insufficient in 3.6%. Insufficient adherence was not associated with depressive symptoms. Keeping a gluten-free diet for longer than five years was associated with lower OR of depressive symptoms compared to being on a diet for less than two years suggesting that lifetime depressive symptoms may be present in one third of the CD patients who adhere to gluten-free diet. Long-term adherence to the gluten-free diet may reduce the risk of depressive symptoms.

Fish Intake and Depression. Psychological distress is becoming significant public health priority in both high- and low-income countries. Psychological distress, defined as symptoms of depression and anxiety, is an important public health issue in developing countries. However little is known about the extent to which adverse dietary factors are associated with psychological distress in South Asians. Evidence that depressive symptoms are inversely related to n-3 (ω-3) fatty acids is growing among US adults. Fish is a rich source of poly unsaturated fatty acids (PUFAs). PUFAs play an important role in the normal function of neuronal cells, neurotransmission, and membrane synthesis. Several reports indicate an association between a deficiency of PUFA and depression. Bhattacharryya et al., (2013) compared the associations of diet and psychological distress in men and women in Goa, India. Cross-sectional study of consecutive attendees in nine urban and rural general practices in 2004-2005. All participants completed an FFQ on their dietary intake in a typical week. Psychological distress was measured using the Kessler Psychological Distress Scale (K10), a WHO-validated screening instrument. Consecutive attendees (n 1512; 601 men and 911 women) aged 30 to 75 years participated. Moderate and high scores of psychological distress were detected in more women than men. Those who ate one or more portions of fish weekly had half the prevalence of distress in both sexes and this was independent of age, marital status, education, income, religion and living alone, suggesting that psychological distress can be reduced with fish intake. Further work is required to establish a temporal relationship. Rutkowska et al., (2013) conducted a study to examine the effects of diet supplemented with fish oil, which is rich in n-3 PUFAs and n-3 PUFAs enriched phospholipids ("super lecithin") obtained from eggs on anhedonic-like response and body weight in the rat chronic mild stress (CMS) model of depression. Neither fish oil nor n-3 PUFAs enriched egg yolk phospholipids reversed disturbances caused by CMS, such as anhedonic-like state or reduction of body weight gain. Beydoun et al., (2013) assessed whether self-reported depressive symptoms were inversely associated with n-3 fatty acid intakes by using a cross-sectional study in 1746 adults (aged 30-65 y). The 20-item Center for Epidemiologic Studies-Depression Scale (CES-D) was used, with a CES-D score ≥16 suggestive of elevated depressive symptoms (EDS). By using the mean of two 24-h dietary recalls, n-3 highly unsaturated fatty acids (HUFAs; ≥20 carbons), n-3 polyunsaturated fatty acids (PUFAs; ≥18 carbons), and plausible ratios with n-6 (ω6) fatty acids were estimated. EDS prevalence was 18.1% among men and 25.6% among women. In women, the uppermost tertile (tertile 3) of n-3 PUFAs was associated with reduced odds of EDS by 49%, with a sex differential. The n-3 PUFA: n-6: PUFA ratio was inversely related to EDS among women. A similar pattern was noted for n-3 HUFA: n-6 HUFA among women. For CES-D subscales, n-3 PUFA was inversely related to somatic complaints, whereas positive affect was directly related to n-3 HUFA (% of energy; total population and among women), n-3 HUFA: n-6 HUFA (women), and n-3 HUFA: n-6 PUFA (total population and among women). Among women, higher intakes of n-3 fatty acids [absolute (n-3) relative to n-6 fatty acids (n-3: n-6)] were associated with lower risk of depressive symptoms, specifically in somatic complaints (mainly n-3 PUFAs) and positive affect (mainly n-3 HUFAs).

Relatively little is known about the dietary intake and nutritional status of community-based individuals with eating disorders. Allen et al., (2013) collected data to from the Western Australian Pregnancy Cohort (Raine) Study that followed participants from birth to young adulthood to (i) describe the dietary intake of population-based adolescents with an eating disorder and (ii) examine associations between eating disorder symptoms, fatty acid intake and depression in adolescents with and without eating disorder. These researchers utilized self-report data from the 17-year Raine Study assessment. Participants comprised 429 female adolescents who completed comprehensive questionnaire measures on dietary intake, eating disorder symptoms and depressive symptoms. Adolescents with an eating disorder reported lower intake of total fat, saturated fat, omega-6 fatty acid, starch, vitamin A and vitamin E compared to adolescents without eating disorder. Adolescents with an eating disorder and pronounced depressive symptoms also reported lower intake of polyunsaturated fat and omega-3 and omega-6 fatty acid than adolescents with an eating disorder but no marked depression. Omega-3 and omega-6 fatty acid correlated negatively with eating disorder symptoms and with depressive symptoms. A relationship was noticed between low omega-3 and omega-6 fatty acid intake and depressive symptoms in adolescents with eating disorders. Persons et al., (2013) determined the relationship between the omega-3 fatty acid content of red RBCs, in particular DHA and EPA, and baseline and new-onset depressive symptoms in post-menopausal women. These investigators characterized the association between dietary omega-3 fatty acid intake and depressive symptomatology in 7086 subjects of the Women's Health Initiative Memory Study (aged 63-81 years) who had an assessment of RBC omega-3 fatty acid at the baseline screening visit. Depressive symptoms at baseline and follow-up were characterized using the Burnam eight-item scale for depressive disorders and inferred by antidepressant medication use. Primary exposure and RBC DHA + EPA, were not related to depressive symptoms at baseline or follow-up, nor were RBC total omega-3, DHA, or EPA. In contrast, dietary intake of omega-3 was positively associated with depressive symptoms at baseline for dietary, although this did not persist at follow-up. No relationship between RBC omega-3 levels and subsequent depressive symptoms was evident, and associations between dietary omega-3 and depressive symptoms were variable. Biomarkers of omega-3 status did not appear to be related to risk of depression in post-menopausal women.

Low levels of DHA have been linked to a number of mental illnesses such as memory loss, depression and schizophrenia. While DHA is beneficial in improving memory and cognition, the influence of dietary fats on the neurotransmitters and receptors in cognitive function remains unknown. Yu et al., (2013) investigated serotonin receptor (5-HT(1A) and 5-HT2A), cannabinoid receptor (CB1) and GABA(A)) receptor binding densities in the brain of male rats fed a high-saturated-fat (HF) diet, as well as the effect of DHA on HF diet. Alterations of these receptors in the post-mortem rat brain were detected by [(3)H]-WAY-100635, [(3) H]-ketanserin, [(3)H]-CP-55,940 and [(3)H]-muscimol binding autoradiography, respectively. In the hippocampus, the 5-HT(1A), CB1 and GABA(A) receptor binding densities increased in response to an HF diet, while in the hypothalamus, 5-HT(1A) and CB1 binding densities increased in HF-fed rats. DHA prevented the HF-induced increase of receptors binding density in the hippocampus and hypothalamus. Furthermore, DHA attenuated 5-HT2A receptor binding density in the caudate putamen, anterior cingulate cortex and medial mammillary nucleus, which was increased in HF group, indicating that an HF diet increased 5-$HT_{(1A)}$, 5-HT_{2A}, CB_1 and $GABA_{(A)}$ receptor binding densities in the brain regions involved in cognitive function and that dietary DHA can attenuate such alterations. These findings provided insight into the mechanism by which DHA ameliorates reduced cognitive function associated with an HF diet. It is now known that the brain DHA, 22:6n-3 accumulates during brain development and is essential for normal neurological function. Chen and Su (2013) evaluated whether brain development was the critical period in which DHA deficiency leads to dysregulation of the HPA axis in response to stress later in life. These investigators exposed rats to an n-3 fatty acid-deficient diet or the same diet supplemented with fish oil as an n-3 fatty acid-adequate diet either throughout the preweaning period from embryo to weaning at 3 weeks old or during the postweaning period from 3 to 10 weeks old. Exposure to the n-3 fatty acid-deficient diet during the preweaning period resulted in decrease in hypothalamic DHA levels and a reduced male offspring body weight. DHA deficiency during the preweaning period increased and restraint stress-induced changes in colon temperature and serum corticosterone levels, caused increase in GABA(A) antagonist-induced heart rate changes and enhanced depressive-like behavior in the forced swimming test and anxiety-like behavior in the plus-maze test in later life. These effects were not seen in male rats fed the n-3 fatty acid-deficient diet during the postweaning period suggesting that brain development is the critical period in which DHA deficiency leads to excessive HPA responses to stress and elevated behavioral indices of depression and anxiety in adulthood. These effects of hypothalamic DHA deficiency during brain development may involve a $GABA_{(A)}$ receptor-mediated mechanism.

PUFA & Cytokines in Depression. It is known that proinflammatory cytokines play a significant role in depression-like behavior and apoptosis in the limbic system after myocardial infarction (MI). Gilbert et al., (2013) reported that a PUFA n-3 diet or the combination of Lactobacillus helveticus R0052 and Bifidobacterium longum R0175 probiotics, when given before the ischemic period, reduce circulating proinflammatory cytokines as well as apoptosis in the limbic system. These investigators determined if the same nutritional interventions maintain their beneficial effects when initiated after the onset of the reperfusion period and attenuate depression-like behavior observed after MI. MI was induced by the occlusion of the left anterior descending coronary artery for 40 min in rats. After the onset of reperfusion, animals were fed with a high-or low-PUFA n-3 diet, combined or not with one billion live bacteria of L. helveticus and B. longum. At 3 d post-MI, caspase-3 enzymatic activities and terminal 2'-deoxyuridine, 5'-triphosphate (dUTP) nick-end labelling (TUNEL)-positive cells were decreased in the CA1, dentate gyrus (DG) and amygdala with the high-PUFA n-3 diet, as compared to the three other diets. Probiotics attenuated caspase-3 activity and TUNEL-positive cells in the DG and the medial amygdala. At 2 weeks post-MI, depression-like behavior was observed in the low-PUFA n-3 diet without probiotics-group, and this behavior was attenuated with the high-PUFA n-3 diet or/and probiotics indicating that a high-PUFA n-3 diet or the administration of probiotics, after the onset of reperfusion, are beneficial to attenuate apoptosis in the limbic system and post-MI depression in the rat.

Fish and PUFA consumption are thought to play a role in mental health; however, many studies do not consider multiple sources of PUFA. Jacka et al., (2013) analyzed data from 935 women aged 20–93 years. A validated and comprehensive dietary questionnaire ascertained the consumption of n-3 and n-6 PUFA. Another assessed fish and energy intake and provided data for a dietary quality score. The General Health Questionnaire-12 (GHQ-12) measured psychological symptoms and a clinical interview (Structured Clinical Interview for DSM-IV-TR Research Version, Non-patient edition) assessed depressive and anxiety disorders. Median dietary intakes of long-chain n-3 fatty acids (310 mg/d) were below dietary target levels. The only PUFA related to depressive and anxiety disorders was DHA. There was a non-linear relationship between DHA intake and depression; those in the second tertile of DHA intake were nearly 70% less likely to report a depressive disorder compared to those in the first tertile. The relationship of DHA to anxiety disorders was linear; for those in the highest tertile of DHA intake, the odds for anxiety disorders were reduced by nearly 50% after adjustments, including adjustment for diet quality scores, compared to the lowest tertile. Those who ate fish less than once per week had higher GHQ-12 scores, and this relationship was obvious in smokers, suggesting that the relationship between DHA and depressive disorders may be non-linear. As discussed above neuroinflammation is present in the majority of acute and chronic neurological disorders. Excess or chronic inflammation in the brain exacerbate neuronal damage and loss. Identifying modulators of neuroinflammation is an active area of study since it may lead to novel therapies. n-3 PUFA are anti-inflammatory in non-neural tissues; their role in neuroinflammation is less explored. Orr et al., (2013) studied the relationship between n-3 PUFA and neuroinflammation in animal models of brain injury and aging. Protective effects of n-3 PUFA in models of sickness behavior, stroke, aging, depression, PD, diabetes, and cytokine- and irradiation-induced cognitive impairments were observed. However, studies that test the direct effects of n-3 PUFA in neuroinflammation in vivo are still lacking. Future research in this area is needed to determine if n-3 PUFA target neuroinflammatory pathways. Hence, n-3 PUFA bioactive metabolites may provide novel therapeutic targets for neurological disorders with a neuroinflammatory component.

Telomer Length & PUFA. Telomere length is regulated by the enzyme telomerase, and is linked to exposure to proinflammatory cytokines and oxidative stress. Shorter telomere length has been associated with poor health behaviors, age-related diseases, and early mortality. Supplementation of n-3 PUFA lowered the concentration of serum proinflammatory cytokines. Kiecolt-Glaser et al., (2013) assessed whether n-3 PUFA also affects leukocyte telomere length, telomerase, and oxidative stress. In addition to testing for group differences, changes in the n-6: n-3 PUFA ratio were assessed to account for individual differences in adherence, absorption, and metabolism. The four-month trial included 106 healthy sedentary overweight middle-aged and older adults who received (1) 2.5g/day n-3 PUFAs, (2) 1.25g/day n-3 PUFAs, or (3) placebo capsules. Supplementation lowered oxidative stress as measured by F2-isoprostanes. The estimated geometric mean log-F2-isoprostanes were 15% lower in the two supplemented groups compared to placebo. Although group differences for telomerase and telomere length were insignificant, changes in the n-6: n-3 PUFA plasma ratios helped clarify the influence of intervention: telomere length increased with decreasing n-6: n-3 ratios suggesting that lower n-6: n-3 PUFA ratios can impact cell aging. The triad of inflammation, oxidative stress, and immune cell aging represents pre-disease mechanisms that may be ameliorated through nutritional interventions. This research increased our understanding of the impact of the n-6: n-3 PUFA balance. NIH State of the Science Conference panel concluded that insufficient evidence is available to recommend the use of any primary prevention therapy for AD or cognitive decline with age. Despite the insufficient evidence, therapies with varying levels of evidence for safety and efficacy are taken by the public and discussed in the media. One example is the long-chain n-

3 (omega-3) PUFA (n-3 LC-PUFA), DHA and EPA, found in some fish and dietary supplements.

Palm Oil and depression. Choi et al., (2013) hypothesized that supplementing diets with palm oil would promote adipocyte differentiation in adipose tissue of feedlot steers, and that soybean oil supplementation would depress adipocyte differentiation. Twenty-eight Angus steers were assigned to 3 groups of 9 or 10 steers and fed a basal diet without additional fat (control), with 3% palm oil (rich in palmitic acid), or with 3% soybean oil (rich in PUFA), for 10 wk, top-dressed daily. Palm oil had no effect on ADG, food intake, or G:F, whereas soybean oil depressed ADG, food intake, and G:F. Marbling scores tended to be increased in palm oil-fed steers than in soybean oil-fed steers. Subcutaneous (SC) adipocyte mean volume was greater in palm oil-fed steers than in soybean-supplemented cattle. Similarly, glucose and acetate incorporation into total lipids was greater in sc adipose tissue of palm oil-fed steers cells, respectively) than adipose tissue of soybean oil-fed steers in cells, respectively). Glucose-6-phosphate dehydrogenase and NADP-malate dehydrogenase activities were greater in sc adipose tissue of palm oil-fed steers than in adipose tissue of control steers. Palm oil did not increase palmitic acid or decrease oleic acid in sc adipose tissue or LM, but decreased myristoleic, palmitoleic, and cis-vaccenic acid in adipose tissue, indicating a depression in stearoyl-coenzyme a desaturase activity. Soybean oil increased the proportion of α-linolenic acid in adipose tissue and muscle and increased linoleic acid and 18:1trans-10 in muscle, indicating that palm oil promotes lipid synthesis in adipose tissue without decreasing feed efficiency or increasing the palmitic acid content of beef.

Diet, Depression, and Sexual Abuse. Bonomi et al., (2013) examined the relationship between physical/sexual and non-physical dating violence victimization from age 13 to 19 and health in late adolescence/early adulthood. The sample comprised 585 subjects completed an online survey to assess: 1) current health (depression, disordered eating, binge drinking, smoking, and frequent sexual behavior); and 2) dating violence victimization from age 13 to 19 (assessed using questions covering physical, sexual, and non-physical abuse, including technology-related abuse involving stalking/harassment via text messaging and email). Multivariable models compared health indicators in never-exposed subjects to those exposed to physical/sexual or non-physical dating violence only. The multivariable models were adjusted for age and other non-dating abuse victimization (bullying; punched, kicked, choked by a parent/guardian; touched in a sexual place, forced to touch someone sexually). Compared to non-exposed females, females with physical/sexual dating violence victimization were at increased risk of smoking; depressive symptoms; eating disorders (using diet aids; vomiting to lose weight); and frequent sexual behavior (5+ intercourse and oral sex partners); having anal sex). Compared to non-exposed females, females with non-physical dating violence were at increased risk of smoking, depressive symptoms (down/hopeless); lost interest, eating disorders (fasting; vomiting), having 5+ intercourse partners, and having anal sex. For males, no health differences were observed for those experiencing physical/sexual dating violence compared to those who did not. Compared to non-exposed males, males with non-physical dating violence were at increased risk of smoking and abnormal eating (fasting, using diet aids, vomiting). For females, more pronounced adverse health was observed for those exposed to physical/sexual versus non-physical dating violence. For both females and males, non-physical dating violence victimization contributed to poor health. Obese patients rarely achieve long-term weight loss with only lifestyle interventions.

Carbohydrate-Rich Diet and Depression. Depression is associated with a high-carbohydrate diet, lack of interest in proper oral hygiene, and xerostomia with the use of antidepressants. Patients often consult their dentists as a result of changes affecting the hard dental substance and the soft-tissues. Lambrecht et al., (2013) identified adverse drug interactions between the antidepressants and medications to provide practicing dentists an overview of the scientific literature. These investigators performed a literature search using PubMed, Cochrane and the specific search items. The review (1984-2009) focused on medicines used in dental practice (*vasoconstrictors, non-opioid analgesics, non-steroidal anti-inflammatory drugs, antibiotics, antifungals and benzodiazepines*). There are various drug interactions between antidepressants and medicines used in dentistry. When two or more drugs are co-administered, a drug interaction must be anticipated though many of these interactions are potential problems, but do not seem to be real clinical issues, suggesting that the drug interaction can be minimized by careful history-taking, skillful dose adjustment, and safe administration of the therapeutic agent. The odds for experiencing depressive symptoms in diabetic patients are twice more than nondiabetic persons, and depression is an independent predictor for the onset of diabetes. Recently Haghighatdoost and Azadbakht (2013) reviewed the data on the treatment of depression in diabetic patients and reported that there is association between diabetes and depression. However, depression remains unrecognized and untreated in two-thirds of diabetic patients, which may lead to incrased diabetes complications. A strategy for managing depression among diabetic patients is the use of diet to improve both health problems. Because of similar pathophysiology for chronic diseases and depression, similar dietary recommendations could be useful. However, few studies have been conducted among diabetic patients. Regarding the complications of diabetes such as renal diseases and coronary heart diseases, the proper macronutrients should be clarified in depressed diabetic patients. Recent studies are investigating the association of overall dietary patterns and depression. Studies of single nutrients on depression produced inconsistent results, and failed to consider the complex interactions between nutrients. Lai et al., (2013) performed a study to review recent literature and conduct meta-analyses addressing the association between dietary patterns and depression. Six electronic databases were searched up to August 2013 that examined the association of diet and depression among adults. The healthy diet pattern was associated with a reduced odds of depression. No significant association was observed between the Western diet and depression; however, the studies were very limited for a precise estimate of this effect, suggesting that high intakes of fruit, vegetables, fish, and whole grains may be associated with a reduced depression risk.

Sucrose is not present in the internal milieu as such, so it is unlikely that it may have a direct influence on cognitive functions, behavior, and knowledge. However, during the digestive process, disaccharides are released into monosaccharides, in the case of sucrose into glucose and fructose, which reach the liver via the portal vein. Finally, they go into bloodstream in the form of glucose as very low-density lipoproteins (VLDL). Brain needs a constant supply of glucose from the bloodstream. Adult brain requires about 140 g of glucose per day, which represents up to a 50% of total carbohydrates consumed daily in the diet. The intake of a food or beverage enriched with sucrose has been associated with improved mental alertness, memory, reaction time, attention and ability to solve mathematical problems, as well as a reduction in fatigue, both in healthy individuals and patients with AD. An adequate nutrition of brain contributes to structural and functional integrity of neurons. In major mental illnesses such as schizophrenia, depression and AD, and nutritional deficiencies at cellular level are involved. At present, several studies highlight the need to improve understanding of the molecular mechanisms involved in the deterioration of cognitive performance and mechanisms through which, the nutritive components of the diet, particularly the sucrose, may modify such functions (Navarro and Llamas 2013).

Metabolic Disorders and Depression. The biological mechanisms that link the development of depression to metabolic disorders such as obesity and diabetes remain obscure. Dopamine and plasticity-related signaling in mesolimbic reward circuitry is implicated in the pathophysiology and etiology of depression. Sharma and Fulton (2013) determined the impact of a high-fat diet (HFD) on depressive-like behavior and biochemical alterations in brain reward circuitry to understand the neural processes that contribute to depression in the diet-induced obesity (DIO). Adult male C57Bl6 mice were placed on a HFD or ingredient-matched, low-fat diet for 12 weeks. At the end of the diet regimen, anxiety and depressive-like behavior, corticosterone levels and biochemical changes were assessed in the midbrain and limbic brain regions. Nucleus accumbens (NAc), dorsolateral striatum (DLS) and ventral tegmental area were subjected to SDS-PAGE and immunoblotting using antibodies against D1A receptor, D2 receptor, and brain-derived neurotrophic factor (BDNF), phospho-DARPP-32(thr75), phospho-CREB and ΔFosB. HFD mice showed decreases in open arm time and center time activity in elevated plus maze and open field tasks, respectively, and increased immobility (behavioral despair) in the forced swim test. Corticosterone levels following acute restraint stress were elevated in HFD mice. These mice had higher D2R, BDNF and ΔFosB, but reduced D1R, protein expression in the NAc. The expression of BDNF in both the NAc and DLS and phospho-CREB in the DLS was positively correlated with behavioral despair suggesting that chronic consumption of high-fat food and obesity induce plasticity-related changes in reward circuitry that are associated with a depressive-like phenotype. As increases in striatal BDNF and CREB activity are implicated in depressive behavior and reward, and that these signaling molecules may mediate the effects of high-fat feeding and DIO to promote negative emotional states and depressive-like symptoms.

High Fat Diet and Mitochondrial Function. It is known that high-fat diet (HFD) can cause peripheral and neuronal insulin resistance, and brain mitochondrial dysfunction. Although the dipeptidyl peptidase-4 inhibitor, Vildagliptin, is known to improve peripheral insulin sensitivity, its effects on neuronal insulin resistance and brain mitochondrial dysfunction caused by a HFD are unknown. Pipatpiboon et al., (2013) tested the hypothesis that Vildagliptin prevents neuronal insulin resistance, brain mitochondrial dysfunction, and learning and memory deficit caused by HFD. Male rats were divided into two groups to receive either a HFD or normal diet (ND) for 12 weeks, after which rats were fed with either Vildagliptin (3 mg/kg/day) or vehicle for 21 days. The cognitive function was tested by the Morris Water Maze prior to brain removal for studying neuronal insulin receptor (IR) and brain mitochondrial function. In HFD rats, neuronal insulin resistance and brain mitochondrial dysfunction were demonstrated, with impaired learning and memory. Vildagliptin prevented neuronal insulin resistance by restoring insulin-induced long-term depression and neuronal IR phosphorylation, IRS-1 phosphorylation and Akt/PKB-ser phosphorylation. It also improved brain mitochondrial dysfunction and cognitive function. Vildagliptin restored neuronal IR function, increased glucagon-like-peptide 1 levels and prevented brain mitochondrial dysfunction, thus attenuating the impaired cognitive function caused by HFD.

Depression-induced Neuronal Atrophy. Atrophy of neurons and gross structural alterations of limbic brain regions, including the prefrontal cortex (PFC) and hippocampus, have been reported in brain imaging and postmortem studies of depressed patients. Prolonged negative stress can induce changes comparable to those seen in MDD, through dendritic retraction and decreased spine density in PFC and hippocampal CA3 pyramidal neurons. Environmental and pharmacological manipulations, including antidepressant medication, exercise, and diet, can reverse molecular changes induced by stress, providing a clear link between these factors and susceptibility to MDD. Ota and Duman (2013) discussed the environmental and pharmacological factors, as well as the contribution of genetic polymorphisms in the regulation of neuronal morphology and plasticity in MDD and preclinical stress models. In particular, these investigators highlighted the pro-depressive changes incurred by stress and the reversal of these changes by antidepressants, exercise, and diet.

Hippocampal Charnoly Body (CB) Formation in Depression. Atrophy in the hippocampus is one of the most significant neuroanatomical findings in depressed patients, and current therapies for depression tend to enhance hippocampal neurogenesis. Charnoly body is a pleomorphic, multilemmaller, electron dense membraneous structure of degenerated mitochondria that is formed as a consequence of chronic nutritional and/or environmental-induced oxidative and nitrative stresss due to free radical overproduction in a highly vulnerable cell. Charnoly body formation in the zinc containing hippocampal and olfactory lobe neurons occurs due to metallothionein-3 (MT-3) deficiency in AD (Sharma et al., 2013a, Sharma et al., 2013b, Sharma and Ebadi 2014a, Sharma and Ebadi 2014b). Hippocampal atrophy is noticed in AD patients. CB formation in the vulnerable neurons of the hippocampus is implicated in depression. Hippocampal CB formation triggers depressive symptoms. Nutritional rehabilitation and Omega-3 fatty acids (PUFA) including EPA and DHA inhibit CB formation and augment hippocampal mitochondrial regeneration to enhance neurogenesis promoting antidepressant action. MT3 inhibits CB formation to prevent hippocampal damage in the AD patients where MT3 levels are significantly reduced as a function of cognitive impairment. Accumulation of CBs at the junction of axon hillock as well as at the synaptic terminal may inhibit axoplasmic flow of ions, neurotransmitters, and mitochondria in various neurodegenerative disorders including AD, PD and drug addiction patients suffering from severe depression and memory loss. Thus CB formation in the aging brain is responsible for impaired brain regional neurotransmission involved in neurocybernatics. MTs inhibit CB formation by serving as free radical scavengers and prevent senile dementia by boosting the mitochondrial bioenergetics. In general MTs transgenic (MT_{trans}) mice are lean and agile, whereas MTs double knock (MT_{dko}) mice are obese and lethargic as noticed among depressed persons. Hence drugs or antioxidants should be targeted to inhibit CB formation in the hippocampus to prevent progressive neurodegeneration in MDDs. Delayed motor learning in postnatal undernourished developing rats occurs due to CB formation. Nutritional and Zinc supplementation inhibits CB formation by augmenting mitochondrial regeneration. Exogenous administration of the mithochndrial ubiquinone (NADH) oxidoreductase (complex-1) inhibitor, 1-methyl, 4-phenyl, 1,2,3,6-tetrahydropyridine (MPTP) (10 mg/kg, i.p) for 7 days caused severe immobilization in MT_{dko} mice, whereas MT_{trans} mice could still walk with their stiff legs and erect tail, indicating the neuroprotective role of MTs in PD and depression. These findings also suggest that MTs preserve mitochondrial bioenergetics by serving as free radical scavengers, involved in CB pathogenesis (Sharma and Ebadi, 2014). The mammalian CNS is especially dependent on the omega-3 (n-3) fatty acid, DHA for normal signaling and function, and n-3 fatty acid deficiencies are contributing factors in increasing the prevalence of MDD. However, the reasons for which omega-3 fatty acids and mood are interlinked remain unknown. Recently, Kang and Gleason (2013) discovered that the fat-1 transgenic mouse has high levels of DHA in the brain because it can convert n-6 to n-3 fatty acids, exhibits increased hippocampal neurogenesis suggesting a mechanism by which omega-3 could influence depression and mood. Hence n-3 fatty acids, and DHA, may prevent and treat depression by virtue of their effects on the hippocampal neurogenesis. Because DHA can be obtained through the diet, increasing DHA intake in depressed patients or those at risk for depression may be one way of managing the depression and providing aid to those who have not been able to achieve remission via pharmacological interventions.

Sedentary Behavior and Depression. Evidence suggests sitting time is associated with a range of health issues in adults, yet the relationship between sedentary behavior and health indicators in young people is less clear. Age-related increases in sedentary behavior are well-documented; the behavioral patterns of adolescent girls are of particular concern. More than one third of adolescent girls' sedentary behavior time is accumulated through use of recreational screen-based behaviors. Costigan et al., (2013) investigated the association between recreational screen-based sedentary behavior and the physical, behavioral, and psychosocial health indicators for adolescent girls. In adition, these researchers searched studies that had adjusted sedentary behavior indicators for physical activity. A structured electronic search of all publication years (through December 2011) was conducted to identify studies in: CINAHL, Communications and Mass Media Complete, ERIC, MEDLINE with Full Text, PsycINFO, and SPORTDiscus with Full Text. Included publications were observational and interventional studies involving adolescent girls (12-18 years) that examined associations between screen-based, sedentary behavior and health indicators (physical, psychosocial, and/or behavioral). 33 Studies evaluated health indicators of screen-based sedentary behaviors among adolescent girls. Strong evidence for a positive association between screen-based sedentary behavior and weight status was observed. A positive association was observed between screen-time and sleep problems, musculoskeletal pain and depression. Negative associations were identified between screen time and physical activity/fitness, screen time and psychological well-being, and screen time and social support. The relationship between screen-based sedentary behavior and diet quality was inconclusive. Less than half of the studies adjusted sedentary behavior indicators for physical activity suggested that screen-based sedentary behavior is associated with deleterious health consequences, but additional longitudinal studies are needed to better understand the health impacts. In addition, screen-time guidelines for youth should be updated according to rapid technological advances.

Obesity and Depression. According to WHO, in 2010 there are over 1 billion overweight adults worldwide with 400 million adults who are obese. Obese people may present with gastroesophageal reflux, non-alcoholic fatty liver, and gallstones. Obesity is a major risk factor for diabetes, cardiovascular disease, musculoskeletal disorders, obstructive sleep apnea, and cancers (prostate, colorectal, endometrial, and breast). Fock and Khoo (2013) emphasized that the main cause of obesity is an imbalance between calories consumed and calories expended, although, genetics and diseases such as hypothyroidism, Cushing's disease, depression, and use of medications such as antidepressants and anticonvulsants are responsible for fat accumulation in the body. The primary treatment for obesity is dieting, physical exercise, and cognitive behavioral therapy. Calorie-restriction strategies are one of the most common dietary plans. Low-calorie diet refers to a diet with a total dietary intake of 800-1500 calories, while very low-calorie diet has <800 calories daily. These dietary regimes need to be balanced in macronutrients, vitamins, and minerals. In general, 50% of the dietary calories should come from carbohydrates, 10% from proteins, and 30% from fats, of which 10% of total fat consist of saturated fats. After reaching the desired body weight, the amount of dietary calories may be increased gradually to maintain a balance between calories consumed and calories expended. Regular physical exercise enhances the efficiency of diet through increase in the satiating efficiency of a fixed meal, and is useful for maintaining diet-induced weight loss. By calorie restriction and exercise, weight loss of 5-8.5 kg is observed 6 months after intervention. After 48 months, a mean of 3-6 kg could be maintained, indicating that obesity is preventable and treatable. Dieting and physical exercise can produce weight loss that can be maintained. Infact obesity increases the odds of developing depression. Depressed mood not only impairs motivation, quality of life and overall functioning but also increases the risks of other complications. Abdominal obesity is a significant predictor of depression and anxiety risk than overall adipose mass. Metabolic abnormalities from central obesity that lead to metabolic disease may also be responsible for the increased incidence of depression in obesity. Hryhorczuk et al. (2013) reported that a higher mass of dysfunctional adipose tissue is associated with metabolic disturbances that are either directly or indirectly implicated in the control of emotions and mood. To better comprehend the development of depression in obesity, these researchers addressed the link between adiposity, diet, negative emotional states, and the evidence that alterations in glucocorticoids, adipose-derived hormones, insulin, and inflammatory signaling, characteristic of central obesity may be involved.

Morgan et al., (2013) evaluated whether gaps in public and professional beliefs remain by comparing beliefs of the public and health professionals on the helpfulness of interventions and likely prognosis for six mental health problems: depression, depression with suicidal thoughts, early schizophrenia, chronic schizophrenia, social phobia, and post-traumatic stress disorder. Mental health literacy surveys based around persons with a mental disorder were carried out in a representative sample of the public (n=6019) in 2011 and samples of general practitioners, psychiatrists, and psychologists (n=1536) in 2012. Respondents were asked to rate the helpfulness of interventions and the likely outcome with or without appropriate professional treatment. There were many differences in treatment beliefs. Medium-sized differences tended to be consistent and related to the greater belief by the public in the helpfulness of close family or friends, a counsellor, vitamins and minerals, a special diet or avoiding certain foods, and having an occasional alcohol drink to relax. In contrast, professionals showed a greater belief in psychotherapy and cognitive behavior therapy for depression and anxiety, and antipsychotics for schizophrenia. Findings on prognosis showed small differences in beliefs. Nutritional risk screening is done to identify individuals at risk of malnourishment. Ramage-Morin and Garriguet (2013) presented the assessment of nutritional risk based on a national sample representative of householders aged 65 or older. Data from the Canadian Community Health Survey-Healthy Aging were used to estimate the prevalence of nutritional risk. Factors associated with nutritional risk were examined with restricted and full logistic models. The distribution of responses on the SCREEN II-AB nutritional risk instrument was reported. 34% of Canadians aged 65 or older were at nutritional risk. Women were more likely than men to be at risk. Among people with depression, 62% were at nutritional risk, compared with 33% without depression. Level of disability, poor oral health, and medication were associated with nutritional risk, as were living alone, low social support, infrequent social participation, and not driving on a regular basis. Lower income and education were also associated with nutritional risk, indicating that nutritional risk is common among seniors living in private households in Canada.

Metabolic Signals and Obesity. Central obesity and related metabolic changes correlate positively with depression. Excessive intake of foods high in saturated fat promotes weight gain, visceral fat accumulation and increased risk of depressed mood. Endocrine changes associated with abdominal obesity include HPA dysregulation and altered plasma levels of cortisol, leptin, adiponectin, resistin and insulin, implicated in the control of emotion and mood. Obesity-induced impairments in brain glucocorticoids (GCs), leptin and insulin receptor signaling link hypercortisolemia and leptin and insulin resistance to depression. Central fat accumulation also enhances the release of inflammatory cytokines (e.g., TNF-α, IL-1β) and signals (C-reactive protein) that may enhance neuroinflammatory responses and depressive behavior. Increased entry of saturated free fatty acids into the brain may also propagate neuroinflammation, leptin/insulin resistance and, eventually, depression. Increased vulnerability to external stressors, negative emotional states and adverse cognitive style (e.g., poor self-image) associated with overweight and obesity may augment consumption of energy-dense "comfort" foods to fuel a vicious circle of central obesity, metabolic dysfunction, and depression.

Sullivan et al., (2013) evaluated the use of endoscopic aspiration therapy for obesity. Aspiration therapy involves endoscopic placement of a gastrostomy tube (A-Tube) and the AspireAssist siphon assembly to aspirate gastric contents 20 minutes after meal consumption. These investigators performed a pilot study of 18 obese subjects who were assigned (2:1) to groups that underwent aspiration therapy for 1 year plus lifestyle therapy (n = 11; mean BMI, 42.6 ± 1.4 kg/m (2)) or lifestyle therapy only (n = 7; mean BMI, 43.4 ± 2.0 kg/m (2)). Lifestyle intervention comprised a 15-session diet and behavioral education program. Ten of the 11 subjects who underwent aspiration therapy and 4 of the 7 subjects who underwent lifestyle therapy completed the first year of the study. After 1 year, subjects in the aspiration therapy group lost 18.6% ± 2.3% of their body weight (49.0% ± 7.7% of excess weight loss [EWL]) and those in the lifestyle therapy group lost 5.9% ± 5.0%. Seven of the 10 subjects in the aspiration therapy group completed an additional year of therapy and maintained a 20.1% ± 3.5% body weight loss. There were no adverse effects of aspiration therapy on eating behavior and no evidence of compensation for aspirated calories with increased food intake. No episodes of binge eating in the aspiration therapy group or serious adverse effects were reported suggesting that, aspiration therapy may be a safe and effective long-term weight loss therapy for obesity. In addition, adolescence is a transitional life phase that is associated with heightened risk for two major health conditions - obesity and mental health problems. Given the comorbidity of obesity and depression, an aspect that warrants further exploration is the association between obesogenic risk and obesity in the expression of depressive symptoms. Haore et al., (2013) conducted a systematic review to evaluate the relationships between obesogenic risk factors (physical activity, sedentary behavior, diet and weight status) and depression in adolescents. Relationships were found between lack of physical exercise, heightened sedentary behavior, poor diet quality, obesity or overweight and depression in adolescence. These investigators emphasized that the finding that obesogenic risk factors are associated with poor adolescent mental health should be interpreted with caution as data are generated from non-representative samples with less than optimal study design and methodology.

Childhood Obesity. Dolinsky et al., (2013) reported that with the rising prevalence of childhood obesity, pediatricians are called upon to treat overweight children. The primary treatment options are behavioral lifestyle modification, pharmacotherapy, and surgery. The primary childhood obesity treatment is lifestyle modification and has been shown to be effective in improving the severity of overweight and obesity. Several guidelines discuss appropriate methods for lifestyle modification in overweight and obese children. These authors summarized three recent guidelines/recommendations and described a child obesity treatment program in the US. Finally, evidence for pharmacologic and surgical treatment options has been discussed, which can be valuable treatment options for select patients. Furthermore, Heal et al., (2013) reported that obesity is an important causative factor in morbidity, disability and premature death. Increasing levels of obesity will impose enormous health, financial and social burdens on worldwide society unless effective interventions are implemented. For many obese individuals, diet and behavioral modification need to be supplemented by pharmacotherapy. Preclinical research has increased understanding of the complex nature of the hypothalamic regulation of food intake and has generated new molecular targets for the development of drugs for obesity treatment. Some approaches, for example, fixed-dose drug combinations, have demonstrated an ability to deliver levels of efficacy that are not achievable with the current antiobesity drug therapies. The regulatory and marketing landscape for development, registration and commercialization of novel centrally acting drugs for the treatment of obesity and related metabolic disorders has changed significantly. Now greater emphasis is placed on tolerability and safety, as well as efficacy. The therapeutic approaches to tackle obesity that are in late-stage clinical development and drugs in late-stage development for the treatment of obesity and future directions have been discussed in this report.

Silenoides, Obesity and Depression. A study was carried out to assess the anti-obesity effect of Hypericum silenoides Juss and Hypericum philonotis Cham. & Schlecht in male Wistar rats fed with a cafeteria diet. García-de la Cruz et al., (2013) used adult male rats with an initial body weight of 290-320 g in a trial. The rats were fed with a cafeteria diet for 77 days. Hypericum species were administered orally at a dose of 10, 30 or 100 mg/kg of body weight daily for 35 days. Body weight, food intake, anorexic effect and serum glucose, lipid profile, alanine transaminase (ALT), aspartate transaminase (AST) and atherogenic index (AI), were assessed. Additionally, inhibitory lipase activity assay and forced swimming test were also carried out. H. silenoides and H. philonotis extracts decreased body weight and serum glucose levels in obese male rats. Treatment with aqueous extract of H. silenoides exhibited anorexic and antidepressant effects and also decreased total cholesterol, triglycerides and high-density lipoprotein-cholesterol, while low-density lipoprotein-cholesterol, AI, AST and ALT were not affected. The dichloromethane extract of H. silenoides and hexane extract of H. philonotis demonstrated the most potent lipase inhibitory activity. Some H. silenoides and H. philonotis extracts showed a significant anti-obesity activity in cafeteria-diet-fed rats as well.

Inherited Metabolic Disease. Eminoglu et al., (2013) performed a study to investigate the quality of life (QoL) of patients with inherited metabolic diseases (IMD) who were treated with restrictive diet. A total of 68 patients (35 boys, 33 girls) with IMD (organic acidemia

[OA], n = 14; disorder of carbohydrate metabolism [CMD], n = 33; and disorder of amino acid metabolism [AMD], n = 21) and their parents were inteviewed. Both parents completed a QoL Scale for Metabolic Diseases-Parent Form, a KINDL parent questionnaire, and a depression form. All patients aged ≥4 years completed a questionnaire themselves, including the KINDL-Kid and KINDL-Kiddo self-reports. The interviews were carried out with patients and their parents in a clinical setting. The patients with bad diet compliance had lower scores for school labeling and perception of disease on both the parent and child questionnaire forms. The patients were divided into three groups (OA, CMD, and AMD) for further analysis. Differences were seen between groups with regard to scores of physical function and school performance according to QoL Scale for Metabolic Diseases-Parent Form. According to parent perceptions, the CMD patients had better QoL with regard to emotional wellbeing. As negative effects of the disease increased, the QoL of IMD patients and their parents decreased in emotional, physical, and cognitive function. Application of expanded newborn scanning programs, early diagnosis, regular follow up, and family education will reduce the effects of the disease and improve the QoL of both families and children.

Energy Balance and Obesity. Gonnissen et al., (2013) reported the effect of energy- and food-reward homeostasis for maintaining energy balance and its disruption may lead to metabolic disorders, including obesity and diabetes. Circadian alignment, quality sleep and sleep architecture in relation to energy-and food-reward homeostasis are crucial. A reduced sleep duration, quality sleep and REM sleep affect substrate oxidation, leptin and ghrelin concentrations, sleeping metabolic rate, appetite, food reward, HPA-axis activity, and gut-peptide concentrations, enhancing a positive energy balance. Circadian dysregulation affects sleep architecture and the glucose-insulin metabolism, substrate oxidation, homeostasis model assessment of insulin resistance (HOMA-IR) index, leptin concentrations and HPA-axis activity. Mood disorders such as depression; reduced dopaminergic neuronal signaling shows decreased food reward. A good sleep hygiene, together with circadian alignment of food intake, a regular meal frequency, and particular attention for protein intake or diets, contributes in curing sleep abnormalities and overweight/obesity features by preventing overeating; normalizing substrate oxidation, stress, insulin and glucose metabolism including HOMA-IR index, and leptin, GLP-1 concentrations, lipid metabolism, appetite, energy expenditure and substrate oxidation; and normalizing food reward. Synchrony between circadian rhythm and metabolic processes including meal patterns plays an important role in the regulation of energy balance and body-weight control. Additive effects of circadian alignment including meal patterns, sleep restoration, and protein diets in the treatment of overweight and obesity have been suggested.

Milk Proteins as Antidepressants. Milk proteins are the main components of everyday feeding and demonstrate a potential to change the mental condition. However, the effects of milk proteins after prolonged use remain poorly understood. Vekovischeva et al., (2013) compared the effects of two whey proteins (α-lactalbumin (α-lac) and native whey) with casein on social and individual behavior in mice. Maze, light–dark box and forced swimming) were performed, to evaluate anxiety and depression-like status. The long-term ingestion of whey proteins may modulate behavior when compared with casein. Diet enriched with α-lac exhibited anxiolytic and antidepressive activities During a 30 d dietary intervention, male C57BL/6J mice had ad libitum access to an experimental diet containing 17% (w/w) of one of three protein sources: α-lac, native whey or casein. Mice had voluntary access to a running wheel. Social behavior (group and resident-intruder activity) was tested at baseline and at the end of the intervention. Half of each dietary group was then withdrawn from the diet and running wheel for 7 d, and social activity and individual behavior tests (open field, elevated-plus while the whey diet improved sociability). The differences between the dietary groups were significant under the running wheel and the withdrawal of the experimental diet, suggesting that the beneficial effects of the milk proteins are evident in stressful situations. Diet-induced behavioral changes remained visible for a week after feeding, suggesting that the proteins of the milk whey fraction have significant efficacy on the mental state.

Chronic emotional stress is associated with increased cortisol release and metabolic disorders. However, few studies have evaluated the influence of chronic stress on calcium oxalate (CaOx) stone disease and its recurrence. Arzoz-Fabregas et al., (2013) enrolled 128 patients over a period of 20 months. All patients were CaOx stone formers with a recent stone episode (<3 months); 31 were first-time stone formers (FS) and 33 recurrent stone formers (RS). Dimensions of chronic stress were evaluated with self-reported validated questionnaires measuring stressful life events, perceived stress, anxiety, depression, burnout and satisfaction with life. An ad hoc self-reporting questionnaire was designed to evaluate stress-related specifically to stone episodes. Blood and urine samples were collected to determine cortisol levels and urinary composition. In addition, epidemiological data, socioeconomic information, diet and incidences of metabolic syndrome (MetS) were reported. No significant differences were observed in the scores of cases and controls on any of the questionnaires dealing with stress. The number and the intensity of perceived stressful life events were higher in RS than in FS, but there were no differences between the two groups in other parameters of stress. RS had higher glucose, uric acid, blood cortisol, and urine calcium levels than FS. RS also had lower economic levels and more frequent incidences of MS than FS. Although no differences were observed in cases and controls among any dimension of chronic stress, the number and intensity of stressful life events were higher in RS than in FS. These differences correlated with variations in blood and urinary levels and with metabolic disorders, indicating an association between chronic stress and risk of recurrent CaOx stone formation.

Eating Disorders and Depression. Wojsciak (2013) performed a study to assess the influence of food-restricted diets (anorexia models) on iron management and activity of rats. They divided 48 rats into 6 groups: 1 control (K) and 5 testing groups (K/2, GI, GII, GIII, GIV). K was fed ad libitum. K/2 received half the portion of the diet of K. The other groups received 100 % of the diet eaten by K, but with different models of food restriction: GI-1 day on, 1 day starvation; GII-2 days on, 2 days starvation; GIII-3 days on, 3 days starvation; and GIV-4 days on, 4 days starvation. As a result, all testing groups ate half of the diet consumed by the control group. The concentrations of iron in selected tissues, ferritin, and selected iron management parameters in blood were examined, as well as the animals' activities associated with food craving. The animal anorexia models had a significant influence on the blood concentrations of hemoglobin), hematocrit, RBC, iron levels in liver, kidney, and heart, the serum ferritin concentration and the rats activity; with no influence on the other parameters. In general, the negative effects of starvation models on iron management parameters and activity of animals were observed. However, these effects were dependent on the model of anorexia more than on the quantity of food intake. The negative effect of food deprivation on iron deficiency and rat activities were observed in all groups; however, the maximum effect was noticed in those animals which were subjected to chronic starvation. Acute deprivations caused the reduction of activity in the rats, however, chronic starvation caused an increase in the activity of the first phase of the experiment, followed by a decline in the subsequent phase suggesting that stress and frustration as well as depression may be caused by insufficient food intake, and as a result, by iron deficiency in a diet similar to human anorexia. In addition, treatment resistance is a common frustration in eating disorders. Attempts to identify the features of this resistance and subsequently develop novel treatments have had modest effects. Halmi (2013) reviewed that examined treatment resistant features expressed in core eating disorder psychopathology, comorbidities and biological features. The core eating disorder psychopathology of anorexia nervosa via vulnerable neurobiological features and conditioned learning to deal with life events. Thus it is reinforcing and ego syntonic resulting in resistance to treatment. The severity of core features such as preoccupations with body image, weight, eating and exercising predicts greater resistance to treatment. Bulimia nervosa patients are less resistant to treatment with treatment failure related to greater body image concerns, impulsivity, depression, diet restriction and poor social adjustment. For those with binge eating disorder overweight in childhood and high emotional eating predicts treatment resistance, suggesting that a diagnosis of an anxiety disorder and perfectionism may confer treatment resistance in anorexia nervosa a substance use disorder or personality disorder with impulse control problems may produce resistance to treatment in bulimia nervosa. Traits such as perfectionism, cognitive inflexibility and negative affect with genetic influences may also affect treatment resistance. Pharmacotherapy and novel therapies have been developed to address treatment resistance. Atypical antipsychotic drugs have shown some effect in treatment resistant anorexia nervosa and Topiramate and SSRIs are helpful for the treatment of resistant binge eating disorder patients. There are insufficient trials to evaluate the novel psychotherapies which are primarily based on the psychopathological features of the eating disorders, suggesting that treatment resistance in eating disorders is generally predicted by the severity of the core eating disorder psychopathology which develops from an interaction between environmental risk factors with genetic traits and a vulnerable neurobiology. Future investigations of the biological features and neurocircuitry of the eating disorders psychopathology and behaviors may provide information for more successful treatment interventions. Ferreira et al., (2013) performed a study to assess how an individual perceives himself within his group having physical appearance as a reference, the Social Comparison through Physical Appearance Scale (SCPAS). This scale measures by assessing the social ranking based on physical appearance, and not the tendency to make comparisons of the general physical appearance or specific body parts. Its psychometric characteristics are investigated in a sample of 828 female participants from normal population. These findings showed good consistency coefficients and test-retest reliability. The two parts of the SCPAS were associated to social comparison and shame measures, to anxiety, depression and stress indicators, and to eating disorders symptomatology. The scale discriminates between a clinical sample of 91 patients with an eating disorder and a non-clinical sample of 102 participants. Social comparison through physical appearance with peers and models partially mediates the effect of the dissatisfaction with weight on disordered eating and drive for thinness.

Toothware and Depression. A multidisciplinary healthcare approach is required in the management of tooth wear patients with underlying mental health disorders. Ahmed (2013) reviewed the main psychological and mental conditions that are manifested in the form of tooth wear. These conditions include depression, eating disorders, and alcohol and drug use disorders. These researchers reviewed the comorbidity of these conditions and the relevance of other medical conditions and lifestyle factors, such as gastroesophageal reflux disorder, smoking, and diet, in the expression of tooth wear. Dentists and Dental Care Professionals can have an important role in identifying mental disorders through the observed tooth wear. They can also monitor patients' response and compliance to medical treatment through the monitoring of tooth wear.

Heart Failure and Depression. Despite the increasing prevalence of heart failure with preserved left ventricular function, there are no specific treatments because the mechanism of impaired relaxation is inadequately understood. Evidence indicates that cardiac relaxation may depend on nitric oxide (NO), generated by NOS requiring the co-factor tetrahydrobiopterin (BH (4)). Recently, Jeong et al. (2013) reported that hypertension-induced diastolic dysfunction was accompanied by cardiac BH (4) depletion, NOS uncoupling, a depression in myofilament cross-bridge kinetics, and S-glutathionylation of myosin binding protein C (MyBP-C). These investigators hypothesized that the mechanism by which BH(4) ameliorates diastolic dysfunction is by preventing glutathionylation of MyBP-C and thus reversing changes of myofilament properties that occur during diastolic dysfunction. Deoxycorticosterone acetate (DOCA)-salt mouse model was used, which represents mild hypertension, myocardial oxidative stress, and diastolic dysfunction. Mice were divided into two groups that received control diet and two groups that received BH(4) supplement for 7days after developing diastolic dysfunction at post-operative day 11 and were assessed by echocardiography. Left ventricular papillary detergent-extracted fiber bundles were isolated for the determination of force and ATPase activity. Sarcomeric protein glutathionylation was assessed by immunoblotting. DOCA-salt mice exhibited diastolic dysfunction that was reversed after BH(4) treatment. Diastolic sarcomere length and relengthening were also restored to control by BH(4) treatment. pCa(50) for tension increased in DOCA-salt compared to sham but reverted to sham levels after BH(4) treatment. Maximum ATPase rate and tension cost (ΔATPase/ΔTension) decreased in DOCA-salt compared to sham, but increased after BH(4) treatment. Cardiac MyBP-C glutathionylation increased in DOCA-salt compared to sham, but decreased with BH(4) treatment. MyBP-C glutathionylation correlated with the presence of diastolic dysfunction suggesting that by depressing S-glutathionylation of MyBP-C; BH(4) ameliorates diastolic dysfunction by reversing a decrease in cross-bridge turnover kinetics. These data provided evidence for modulation of cardiac relaxation by post-translational modification of myofilament proteins.

Inflammatory Diet and Depression. Inflammation is considered as a mechanism leading to depression, but the association between inflammatory dietary pattern and depression risk is unknown. Lucas et al., (2014) identified a dietary pattern that was related to plasma levels of inflammatory biomarkers (C-reactive protein, IL-6, TNF-α receptor 2), and conducted a prospective analysis of the relationship of this pattern and depression risk among participants in the Nurses' Health Study. A total of 43,685 women (aged 50-77) without depression at baseline (1996) were followed up until 2008. Dietary information was obtained from food frequency questionnaires completed between 1984 through 2002 and computed as cumulative average of dietary intakes with a 2-year latency applied. They used a strict definition of depression that required both self-reported physician-diagnosed depression and use of antidepressants, and a broader definition that included women who reported either clinical diagnosis or antidepressant use. During the 12-year follow-up, 2594 cases of depression were documented and 6446 using the broader definition. After adjustment for BMI and other potential confounders, relative risks comparing extreme quintiles of the inflammatory dietary pattern were 1.41 for the strict definition and 1.29 for the broader definition of depression. The inflammatory dietary pattern was associated with a higher depression risk suggesting that chronic inflammation may underlie the association between diet and depression.

Vitamin D Deficiency and Depression. Epidemiological evidence suggests that low levels of vitamin D may predispose people to depression and cognitive impairment. While rodent studies demonstrated that prenatal vitamin D deficiency is associated with altered brain development, there is a lack of research examining adult vitamin D (AVD) deficiency. Groves et al., (2013) examined the impact of AVD deficiency on behavior and brain function in the mouse. Ten-week old male C57BL/6J and BALB/c mice were fed a control or vitamin D deficient diet for 10 weeks prior to, and during behavioral testing. A broad range of behavioral domains, excitatory and inhibitory neurotransmission in brain tissue, and, in separate groups of mice, locomotor response to d-Amphetamine and MK-801 was tested. AVD deficiency resulted in hyperlocomotion in a novel open field and reduced GAD65/67 levels in brain tissue. AVD-deficient mice had altered behavior on the elevated plus maze, altered responses to heat, sound and shock, decreased glutamate and glutamine, and increased GABA and glycine. By contrast C57BL/6J mice had no further behavioral changes but elevations in serine, homovanillic acid (HVA) and 5-HIAA. Although the behavioral phenotype of AVD did not seem to model a specific disorder, the overall reduction in GAD65/67 levels associated with AVD deficiency may be relevant to a number of neuropsychiatric conditions. This study demonstrated an association between AVD deficiency and changes in behavior and brain neurochemistry in the mouse. Vitamin D deficiency when the serum 25-hydroxyvitamin D (25-OHD(3)) concentration was < 20 ng/mL, has joined vitamin A deficiency as nutrition-responsive medical conditions. Glade (2013) reported that adequate vitamin D status is linked to decreased risks of cancers of the esophagus, stomach, colon, rectum, gallbladder, pancreas, lung, breast, uterus, ovary, prostate, urinary bladder, kidney, skin, thyroid, and hematopoietic system (e.g., Hodgkin's lymphoma, non-Hodgkin's lymphoma, multiple myeloma); bacterial infections; rheumatoid arthritis; Crohn's disease; periodontal disease; multiple sclerosis; asthma; type 2 diabetes; cardiovascular disease; stroke; peripheral artery disease; hypertension; chronic kidney disease; muscle weakness; cognitive impairment; AD; clinical depression; and premature death. On the other hand, inadequate vitamin D status during pregnancy may be associated with increased risk for the development of type 1 diabetes in the offspring. Despite the heavy reliance on serum 25-OHD(3) concentration for the diagnosis of vitamin D status, local tissue vitamin D intoxication may be present in individuals with much lower serum 25-OHD(3) concentrations. An individual's serum 25-OHD (3) concentration may appear to be "low" independent of sunlight exposure or vitamin D intake. Serum 25-OHD (3) concentration is poorly responsive to increases in vitamin D intake, and the prolonged routine consumption of maga doses of vitamin D may interfere with the regulation of phosphate homeostasis by fibroblast growth factor-23 (FGF23) and the Klotho gene product that is detrimental to health. In view of these observations, curbing excessive enthusiasm for increasing vitamin D intake recommendations may be regulated.

Minor Dietary Inadequacy and Depression. Minor dietary inadequacies, which are responsible for a decline in an enzyme's efficiency, could influence mood states. When diet does not provide an optimal intake of micronutrients, supplementation may benefit mood. Long and Benton (2013) evaluated the data base and studies were included if they considered aspects of stress, mild psychiatric symptoms, or mood in the general population; randomized and placebo-controlled; to evaluate the influence of multivitamin/mineral supplements for at least 28 days. Supplementation reduced the levels of stress. Fatigue and confusion were also reduced suggesting that micronutrient has a beneficial effect on stress, psychiatric symptoms, and mood.. Furthermore, high doses of B vitamins may be effective in improving mood states. However the optimal levels of micronutrient intake, optimal doses, and active ingredients are still an open questions to be addressed in future studies on "*Diet and Depression*".

Pregnancy and Depression. Capra et al., (2013) reported that according to the Barker hypothesis, the period of pregnancy and the intrauterine environment are crucial to the tendency to develop diseases like hypertension, diabetes, coronary heart disease, metabolic disorders, pulmonary, renal and mental illnesses including depression. The external environment affects the characteristics that resemble intrauterine conditions. If the extra-uterine environment differs greatly from the intra-uterine one, the fetus is more prone to develop disease. Maternal diseases like depression and anxiety, epilepsy, asthma, anemia and metabolic disorders, like diabetes, can determine alterations in growth and fetal development. Similarly, the maternal lifestyle, particularly diet, exercise, and smoking during pregnancy, have an important role in determining the risk to develop diseases that manifest during childhood and particularly in adulthood. Finally, there are sources of environmental pollutants in which the child lives, which can contribute to an increased probability to the development of several diseases which could be avoided. In addition, sleep disorders during pregnancy influence the risk of insulin resistance and glucose intolerance.

Gylcemic Load and Depression. Depression is a common disorder in elderly, especially in those institutionalized. Nutrition could play an important role in the onset and/or progression of depression, since the intake of carbohydrates with a high glycemic index (GI) or diets with a high glycemic load (GL) may increase the insulin-induced brain serotonin secretion. Aparicio et al., (2013) analyzed the association between dietary GI and GL and the odds of depression in institutionalized elderly people without antidepressant treatment. This study included 140 elderly people (65-90 years of age) whose diets were recorded using a precise weighing method over seven consecutive days. Energy and nutrient intakes were recorded and the GI and GL calculated. The participants' capacity was assessed using the Geriatric Depression Scale (GDS). Subjects were grouped into non-depressed (GDS ≤ 5) and depressed (GDS > 5). Since GDS scores and gender were associated, the data were grouped considering this association. The dietary GL was higher in the non-depressed compared with the depressed group. However, a similar GI was observed between non-depressed and depressed groups. Participants with a dietary GL placed in the second and third tertiles had a 67.4 % and 65.3 %, respectively, less odds of suffering depression than those in the first tertile. GDS scores and dietary GL were inversely related; therefore, an increase in one unit in the dietary GL scale decreased the GDS score by 0.058 units, suggesting that glycemic load is associated with a lower odd of depression.

Overall Effects of Diet. Miyake et al., (2013) examined the relationship between consumption of meat, fish, and specific types of fatty acids and the prevalence of depression during pregnancy. Study subjects were 1745 pregnant women. Depressive symptoms were considered as present when subjects had a Center for Epidemiologic Studies Depression Scale score of 16 or higher. Information on dietary factors was collected using a self-administered diet history questionnaire. The prevalence of depressive symptoms during pregnancy was 19.3%. Higher intake levels of fish, EPA, and DHA were associated with a lower prevalence of depressive symptoms during pregnancy. Higher intake of fat and saturated fatty acids were related to a higher prevalence of depressive symptoms during pregnancy. There were no associations between intake of monounsaturated fatty acids, n-3 PUFAs, α-linolenic acid, n-6 PUFAs, linoleic acid, arachidonic acid, or cholesterol and the ratio of n-3 to n-6 PUFA intake and depressive symptoms during pregnancy. Intake of fish, EPA, and DHA may be inversely associated with depressive symptoms while intake of fat and saturated fatty acids may be positively related to depressive symptoms during pregnancy. Chocano-Bedova et al., (2013) examined whether long-term dietary patterns derived from a food-frequency questionnaire (FFQ) predict the development of depression in middle-aged and older women. These researchers conducted a study in 50,605 participants (age range: 50-77 y) without depression in the Nurses' Health Study at baseline (1996) who were followed until 2008. Long-term diet was assessed by using FFQs. Prudent (*high in vegetables*) and Western (*high in meats*) patterns were identified by using a principal component analysis. Two definitions were used for clinical depression as follows: a strict definition that required both a clinical diagnosis and the use of antidepressants (3002 incident cases) and a broad definition that further included women who reported either a clinical diagnosis or antidepressant use (7413 incident cases). After adjustment for age, BMI, and other potential confounders, no association was noticed between the diet patterns and depression risk under the strict definition. Under the broad definition, women with the highest scores for the Western pattern had 15% higher risk of depression than did women with the lowest scores, but after additional adjustment for psychological scores at baseline, results were insignificant. This study did not support a clear association between dietary patterns from factor analysis and depression risk. Bupropion is mostly used as an antidepressant and smoking cessation therapy. Chevassus et al., (2013) compared the pharmacodynamic properties of Bupropion and the Amphetamine-like Methylphenidate after sustained administration. These authrs used twelve male volunteers who completed the randomized, double-blind, placebo controlled, cross-over study. Bupropion and Methylphenidate were administered for initial half-dose 6-day periods (150 and 10 mg respectively) followed by full-dose 8-day periods (300 and 20 mg respectively). Outcomes were subjective feelings, cognitive performances, autonomic and physiological parameters. Bupropion, like Methylphenidate, decreased asthenia-fatigue, despite an impairment of sleep onset. Both drugs increased resting diastolic BP, body temperature and decreased body weight. No significant change was observed on cognitive functions, appetite and energy consumption. Although it did not share all the properties of stimulant drugs, the profile of Bupropion presented a number of similarities with that of Methylphenidate.

Tryptophan Depletion and Depression. The serotonergic system and HPA axis are involved in the regulation of emotions. Specifically, spontaneous and/or environmentally mediated modulations of the functionality of these systems early in development may favor the onset of depressive- and anxiety-related phenotypes. While the independent contribution of each of these systems to the emergence of abnormal phenotypes has been described in clinical and experimental studies, only rarely has their interaction been investigated. The investigators addressed the effects of reduced serotonin and environmental stress during the early stages of postnatal life on emotional regulations in mice. They administered, to CD1 mouse dams, during their first week of lactation, a tryptophan deficient diet (T) and corticosterone through drinking water (C; 80μg/ml). Four groups of dams (animal facility rearing, AFR; T treated, T; C treated, C; T and C treated, TC) and their male offspring were used in the study. Maternal care was scored throughout treatment and adult offspring were tested for: anhedonia (progressive ratio schedule); anxiety-related behavior (approach-avoidance conflict paradigm); BDNF, dopamine and serotonin concentrations in selected brain areas. T, C and TC treatments reduced active maternal care compared to AFR. Adult TC offspring showed increased anxiety- and anhedonia-related behaviors, reduced striatal and increased hypothalamic BDNF and reduced dopamine and serotonin in the prefrontal cortex and their turnover in the hippocampus, suggesting that neonatal variations in the functionality of the serotonergic system and of HPA axis may contribute to induce emotional disturbances in adulthood.

Melatonin and Metabolic Syndrome. Srinivasan et al., (2013) reported that metabolic syndrome (MetS) is characterized by obesity, insulin resistance, hypertension, dyslipidemia, diabetes mellitus, and depression. The pathophysiological mechanisms involved in MetS are complex and involve dysregulation of many biochemical and physiological regulatory mechanisms. Elevated low density lipoproteins like VLDL, and LDL with reduction of HDL seen in patients with MetS contributing to atherogenic dyslipedemia. Melatonin is effective in improving MetS through its anti-hyperlipidemic action. Melatonin reduced both adiposity, and body weight in animal studies and also attenuated weight gain and obesity-induced metabolic alterations and this effect of Melatonin was attributed to its anti-oxidative effects. Melatonin inhibits insulin release by acting through both MT1 and MT2 receptors on the pancreatic β-cells. Melatonin also increased insulin sensitivity and glucose tolerance in animals fed with either high fat and/or sucrose diet. Melatonin exerted most of its beneficial actions by acting through MT1 and MT2 receptors present in various tissues of the body and some of the metabolic actions of Melatonin were blocked by Melatonin antagonist, Luzindole. In addition, Ramelteon, the newly available Melatonin agonist will have promising role in the control of MetS. Drug related to antidepressant Fluoxetine is used for the treatment of MetS. Anti-oxidants like S-adenosyl-methionine, Vitamin E, and Vitamin C have been found beneficial in treating MetS. Melatonin being a powerful Antioxidant will have a promising role in treating patients with MetS. Melatonin and serotonin urinary metabolites can be estimated to measure total antioxidant capacity. The consumption of cereals containing the higher dose in tryptophan increases sleep efficiency, actual sleep time, immobile time, and decreased total nocturnal activity, sleep fragmentation index, and sleep latency. Urinary 6-sulfatoxymelatonin, 5-hydroxyindoleacetic acid levels, and urinary total antioxidant capacity also increase following tryptophan-enriched cereal ingestion as well as alleviating anxiety and depression. Hence cereals enriched with tryptophan may be useful as a chrononutrition agents for regulating the sleep/wake cycle and mood. Agomelatine is a novel antidepressant acting as an MT1/MT2 Melatonin receptor agonist/5-HT2C serotonin receptor antagonist. Because of its pharmacological profile, this drug resolves the abnormalities of circadian rhythms associated with mood disorders and sleep/wake cycle as shown in Figure 11.

Carbohydrate Solution and Depression. Yildiz et al., (2013) investigated the effects of oral carbohydrate solution (CHO) on perioperative discomfort, biochemistry, hemodynamics, and patient satisfaction in surgery patients under general anesthesia. Sixty cases in ASA I-II group who were planned to have operation under general anesthesia were included in the study. The cases were divided into two groups having 30 subjects in each. The patients were given CHO in the evening prior to the surgery and 2-3 hr before the anesthesia while routine fasting was applied in the control group. 2-3 hr before the surgery; malaise, thirst, hunger, and weakness; just before the surgery malaise, thirst, hunger, and fatigue; 2 hr after the operation thirst, hunger, weakness, and concentration difficulty; 24 hr after the operation malaise and weakness were lower in the study group. Fasting blood glucose level was higher in the control group at the 90th min of the operation. Gastric volumes were higher in the control group whereas gastric pH values were higher in the study group. The level of anxiety and depression risk rate were lower in the study group indicating that CHO reduces perioperative discomfort and improves perioperative wellbeing when compared to overnight fasting.

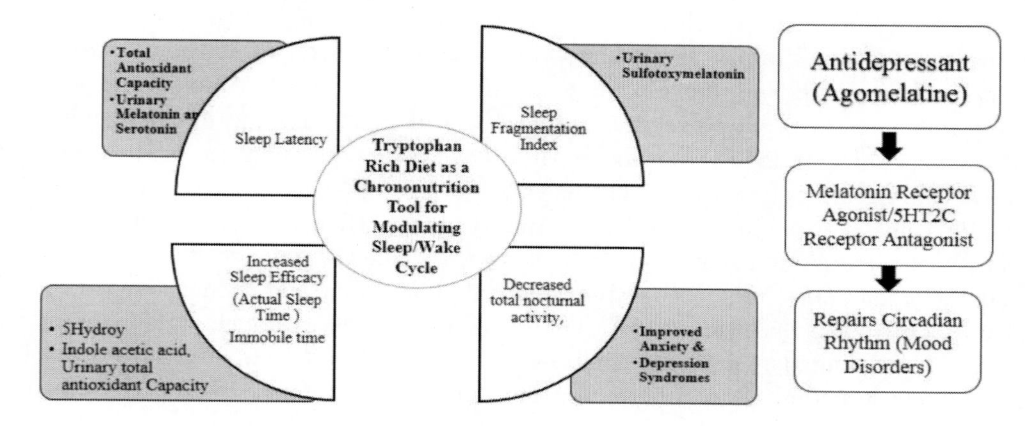

Figure 11. A diagram illustrating that urine can be collected to analyze melatonin and serotonin urinary metabolites to measure total antioxidant capacity. The consumption of cereals containing the higher dose in tryptophan increases sleep efficiency, actual sleep time, immobile time, and decreased total nocturnal activity, sleep fragmentation index, and sleep latency. Urinary 6-sulfatoxymelatonin, 5-hydroxyindoleacetic acid levels, and urinary total antioxidant capacity also increase following tryptophan-enriched cereal ingestion as well as alleviating anxiety and depression. Cereals enriched with tryptophan may be useful as a chrononutrition vehicles for alterations in the sleep/wake cycle. Agomelatine is a novel antidepressant acting as an MT1/MT2 melatonin receptor agonist/5-HT2C serotonin receptor antagonist. Because of its pharmacological profile, this drug alleviates the abnormalities of circadian rhythms associated with mood disorders, and abnormalities of the sleep/wake cycle.

Exercise and Depression. It has been suggested that the antidepressant effect of exercise is attributed to an increase in brain 5-HT; however, the precise mechanism underlying the antidepressant action via exercise is uncertain. In contrast, the effect of 5-HT on antidepressant activity has not been clarified because the therapeutic response to antidepressant drugs has a time window in spite of the acute increase of brain 5-HT upon administration of these drugs. Lee et al. (2013) investigated the contribution of brain 5-HT to the antidepressant effect of exercise. Mice were fed a tryptophan-deficient diet and stressed using chronic unpredictable stress (CUS) for 4 weeks with or without the performance of either moderate or intense exercise on a treadmill for 3 days per week. The onset of depression-like behavior was attributable not to chronic reduction of 5-HT but to chronic stress. Regular exercise prevented depression-like behavior with an improvement of adult hippocampal cell proliferation and survival without recovery of 5-HT. The mice that exercised showed increased hippocampal noradrenaline. Regular exercise prevented the impairment of not long-term memory but short-term memory in a 5-HT-reduced state suggesting that: chronic reduction of brain 5-HT may not contribute to the onset of depression, whereas regular exercise prevents the onset of chronic stress-induced depression-like behavior independent of brain 5-HT and dependent on brain NE. In addition regular exercise prevents chronic tryptophan reduction-induced impairment of not long-term but short-term memory.

Aging and Physical Exercise. Aging is an inevitable process that is associated with loss of functional capacities in the cardiovascular, the skeletal muscle mass, the osteoarticular and the neuro-immune-endocrine systems. Changes appear due to interactions between genetic factors and lifestyle, such as diet and sedentary behavior. Deslandes (2013) provided evidence concerning the importance of physical exercise to reduce the deleterious effects of aging to improve functional performance, prevention of diseases and increased longevity. Moreover, physical exercise improves the cognitive function and the mood. Aerobic and strength training collaborate with the prevention and treatment of mental diseases in older adults, like MDD, dementia, and PD. Prolonged exercise and heavy training are associated with depressed immune function which can increase the risk of infections. To maintain robust immunity, athletes should eat a well-balanced diet sufficient to meet their energy, carbohydrate, protein, and micronutrient requirements. Dietary deficiencies of protein and specific micronutrients have been associated with immune dysfunction and an adequate intake of iron, zinc, and vitamins A, D, E, B_6 and B_{12} is extremely important in the maintenance of immune function. Consuming carbohydrate during prolonged strenuous exercise attenuates rises in stress hormones and limits exercise-induced immune depression. Similar effects can be seen with regular intake of high-dose antioxidant vitamin supplements, though excessive antioxidant intake may impair exercise training adaptations. Hence individual amino acids, colostrum, Echinacea, and zinc are unlikely to boost immunity or reduce infection risk in athletes. The ingestion of carbohydrate during exercise and daily consumption of probiotic and plant polyphenol (e.g. quercetin)-containing supplements or foodstuffs (e.g. non-alcoholic beer) provide success. This approach is most effective for individuals who are highly prone to illness (Gleeson 2013).

Yoga and Depression. Yoga might be beneficial for a number of populations including elderly women and those with chronic health conditions. Yoga has been prescribed in conjunction with other medical treatments in the management of psychosomatic diseases, including cancer, asthma, colitis, and peptic ulcer. It improves strength and flexibility, and may help control BP, lipids, respiration, heart rate, and metabolic rate to improve overall exercise capacity. Ross et al., (2013) conducted a cross-sectional design with anonymous online surveys. 4307 randomly selected individuals from 15 US Iyengar yoga studios (n=18,160), representing 41 states; 1087 individuals responded, with 1045 (24.3%) surveys completed. Participants agreed yoga improved: energy (84.5%), happiness (86.5%), social relationships (67%), sleep (68.5%), and weight (57.3%), and beliefs did not differ according to race or gender. The more they practiced yoga, the higher their odds of believing yoga improved their health, indicating that individuals who practice yoga are not free of health concerns, but most believe their health improved because of yoga. Dhananjai et al., (2013) evaluated the effects of Yogic Practice on anxiety/depression associated with obesity. A total of 272 subjects were divided into two groups: 1) group of 205 subjects (with yogic practice) and 2) a control group of 67 subjects (with aerobic exercise). Assessment of anxiety and depression were done by Hamilton Rating Scale. This study supported yoga as an effective approach with no diet restriction to improve anxiety, depression, and obesity and suggested that incorporating yoga in the treatment protocol of patients suffering from anxiety and depression may prove beneficial.

References

Ahmed, K.E. (2013) The psychology of tooth wear, *Spec Care Dentist.* 33, 28-34.

Allen, K.L; Mori, T.A; Beilin, L; Byrne, S.M; Hickling, S; Oddy, W.H. (2013) Dietary intake in population-based adolescents: support for a relationship between eating disorder symptoms, low fatty acid intake and depressive symptoms., *J Hum Nutr Diet.* 26, 459-469.

Alosco, M.L; Spitznagel, M.B; Raz, N; Cohen, R; Sweet, L.H; Colbert, L.H; Josephson, R; van Dulmen, M; Hughes, J; Rosneck, J; Gunstad, J. (2013) Dietary habits moderate the association between heart failure and cognitive impairment. *J Nutr Gerontol Geriatr.* 32, 106-121.

Aparicio, A; Robles, F; López-Sobaler, A.M, Ortega, R.M. (2013) Dietary glycaemic load and odds of depression in a group of institutionalized elderly people without antidepressant treatment., *Eur J Nutr.* 52, 1059-1066.

Arzoz-Fàbregas, M; Ibarz-Servio, L; Fernández-Castro, J; Valiente-Malmagro, M; Roca-Antonio , J; Edo-Izquierdo, S; Buisan-Rueda, O. (2013) Chronic stress and calcium oxalate stone disease: influence on blood cortisol and urine composition., *Urology,.* 82, 1246-1252.

Badrasawi, M.M; Shahar, S; Abd Manaf , Z; Haron, H. (2013) Effect of Talbinah food consumption on depressive symptoms among elderly individuals in long term care facilities, randomized clinical trial., *Clin Interv Aging.* 8, 279-285.

Beydoun, M.A; Fanelli Kuczmarski, M.T; Beydoun, H.A; Hibbeln, J.R; Evans, M.K; Zonderman, A.B. (2013) ω-3 fatty acid intakes are inversely related to elevated depressive symptoms among United States women,. *J Nutr.* 143, 1743-1752.

Bhattacharyya, M; Marston, L; Walters, K; D'Costa, G; King, M. et al. (2013) Psychological distress, gender and dietary factors in South Asians: a cross-sectional survey., *Public Health Nutrition* 1–9.

Bhatti, S.K; O'Keefe, J.H; Lavie, C.J. (2013) Coffee and tea: perks for health and longevity?., *Curr Opin Clin Nutr Metab Care.* 16, 688-697.

Bichi, E; Hervás, G; Toral, P.G; Loor, J.J; Frutos, P. (2013) Milk fat depression induced by dietary marine algae in dairy ewes: persistency of milk fatty acid composition and animal performance responses., *J Dairy Sci.* 96, 524-532.

Boerman, J.P; Preseault, C.L; Kraft, J; et al. (2014) Short communication: Effect of antioxidant supplementation on milk production, milk fat synthesis, and milk fatty acids in dairy cows when fed a diet designed to cause milk fat depression. [Journal Article]., *J Dairy Sci* 97,:1077-1081.

Bonomi, A.E; Melissa, L; Anderson, M.L; Julianna Nemeth, J; Bartle-Haring, S; Buettner, C; and Schipper, D. (2013) Dating violence victimization across the teen years: Abuse frequency, number of abusive partners, and age at first occurrence. B.M.C Public Health. 12,637.

Boutayeb, A; Boutayeb, S. (2005) The burden of non communicable diseases in developing countries., *Int J Equity Health* 4, 2.

Bravo, R; Matito, S; Cubero, J; Paredes, S.D; Franco, L; Rivero, M; Rodríguez, A.B; Barriga, C. (2013) Tryptophan-enriched cereal intake improves nocturnal sleep, melatonin, serotonin, and total antioxidant capacity levels and mood in elderly humans., *Age (Dordr).* 35, 1277-1285.

Capra, L; Tezza, G; Mazzei, F; Boner, A.L. (2013) The origins of health and disease: the influence of maternal diseases and lifestyle during gestation.,. *Ital J Pediatr.* 39, 7.

Chedraui, P; Prez-Lopez, R. (2013) Nutrition and health during mid life : searching form soultions and meeting challenges for the aging population. *Climatric* 16 (suppl),85-95.

Chen, H.F; Su, H.M. (2013) Exposure to a maternal n-3 fatty acid-deficient diet during brain development provokes excessive hypothalamic-pituitary-adrenal axis responses to stress and behavioral indices of depression and anxiety in male rat offspring later in life., *J Nutr Biochem.* 24, 70-80.

Chocano-Bedoya, P.O; O'Reilly, E.J; Lucas, M; Mirzaei, F; Okereke, O.I; Fung, T.T; Hu, F.B; Ascherio, A. (2013) Prospective study on long-term dietary patterns and incident depression in middle-aged and older women., *Am J Clin Nutr.* 98, 813-820.

Choi S.H; Gang, G.O; Sawyer, J.F; Johnson, B.J; Kim, K.H; Choi, C.W; Smith, S.B. (2013) Fatty acid biosynthesis and lipogenic enzyme activities in subcutaneous adipose tissue of feedlot steers fed supplementary palm oil or soybean oil., *J of Animal Sci* 91, 2091-2098.

Costigan, S.A; Barnett,L; Plotnikoff , R.C; Lubans, D.R. (2013) The health indicators associated with screen-based sedentary behavior among adolescent girls: a systematic review. *J Adolesc Health.* 52, 382-392.

Crichton, G.E; Bryan, J; Hodgson, J.M; Murphy, K.J. (2013) Mediterranean diet adherence and self-reported psychological functioning in an Australian sample., *Appetite.* 70, 53-59.

da Silva Germano, P.C; de Lima e Silva, D; Soares Gde, S; dos Santos, Â.A; Guedes, R.C. (2013) Hypercaloric high-lipid diet and brain development: effects on cortical spreading depression in adult rats. Nutr Neurosci. 16, 275-281.

Dakshinamurti, K, Paulose, C.S; Viswanathan M, Siow Y.L; Sharma S.K; Bolster, B. (1990) Neurobiology of Pyridoxine., *Annals of the New York Academy of Sciences.* 585, 128-144.

Deslandes, A. (2013) The biological clock keeps ticking, but exercise may turn it back., *Arq Neuropsiquiatr.* 71, 113-118.

Dhananjai, S; Sadashiv, Tiwari S, Dutt, K, Kumar, R. (2013) Reducing psychological distress and obesity through Yoga practice., *Int J Yoga.* 6(1).66-70.

Dolinsky, D.H; Armstrong, S.C; Kinra, S. (2013) The clinical treatment of childhood obesity. Indian J Pediatr. 80 Suppl 1, S48-54.

Drieling, R.L; Goldman Rosas, L; Ma, J; Stafford, R.S. (2014) Community resource utilization, psychosocial health, and sociodemographic factors associated with diet and physical activity among low-income obese Latino immigrants. J Acad Nutr Diet. 114, 257-265.

Dulcich, M.S; Hartman, R.E. (2013) Pomegranate supplementation improves affective and motor behavior in mice after radiation exposure. *Evid Based Complement Alternat Med.* 2013, 940830.

Eckart, S; Hörtnagl, H; Kronenberg, G; Gertz, K; Hörster, H; Endres, M; Hellweg, R. (2013) Reduced nerve growth factor levels in stress-related brain regions of folate-deficient mice., *Neuroscience.* 245,129-135.

Eminoglu,T.F; Soysal, S.A; Tumer, L; Okur, I; Hasanoglu, A. (2013) Quality of life in children treated with restrictive diet for inherited metabolic disease., *Pediatr Int.* 55, 428-433.

Fairweather-Tait S., Wawer A., Gillings R., Jennings A., Myint P. K. (2013).Iron status in the elderly. *Mech. Ageing Dev.*

Fairweather-Tait, S.J; Guile, G.R; Valdes, A.M; Wawer ,A.A; Hurst, R; Skinner, J; Macgregor, A.J. (2013) The contribution of diet and genotype to iron status in women: a classical twin study. *PLoS One*. 8, e83047.

Ferreira, C; Pinto-Gouveia, J; Duarte, C. (2013) Physical appearance as a measure of social ranking: the role of a new scale to understand the relationship between weight and dieting., *Clin Psychol Psychother*. 20, 55-66.

Fock, K.M; Khoo, J. (2013) Diet and exercise in management of obesity and overweight. *Journal of Gastroenterology and Hepatology* 28 (Suppl. 4), 59–63.

García-de la Cruz, L; Galvan-Goiz, Y; Caballero-Caballero, S; Zamudio, S; Alfaro, A; Navarrete, A. (2013) Hypericum silenoides Juss. and Hypericum philonotis Cham. & Schlecht. extracts: in-vivo hypolipidaemic and weight-reducing effects in obese rats., *J Pharm Pharmacol*. 65, 591-603.

Gilbert, K; Arseneault-Bréard, J; Flores Monaco, F; Beaudoin, A; Bah, T.M; Tompkins, T.A; Godbout, R; Rousseau, G. (2013) Attenuation of post-myocardial infarction depression in rats by n-3 fatty acids or probiotics starting after the onset of reperfusion., *Br J Nutr.* 109, 50-56.

Giriko, C.A.; Andreoli, C.A.; Mennitti, L.V.; Hosoume, L.F.; Souto, T.d.S.; Silva, A.V.d.; Mendes-da-Silva, C. (2013) Delayed physical and neurobehavioral development and increased aggressive and depression-like behaviors in the rat offspring of dams fed a high-fat diet. *International Journal of Developmental Neuroscience*, 31,731-739.

Glade, M.J. (2013) Vitamin D: health panacea or false prophet?. *Nutrition.* 29, 37-41.

Gleeson, M. (2013) Nutritional support to maintain proper immune status during intense training. *Nestle Nutr Inst Workshop* Ser. 75, 85-97.

Gonnissen, H.K; Hulshof, T; Westerterp-Plantenga. M.S. (2013) Chronobiology, endocrinology, and energy- and food-reward homeostasis., *Obes Rev*. 14, 405-416.

Grosso, C;, Valentão, P; Ferreres, F; Andrade, P.B. (2013) The use of flavonoids in central nervous system disorders., *Curr Med Chem*. 20, 4694-719.

Groves, N.J; Kesby, J.P; Eyles, D.W; McGrath, J.J; Mackay-Sim, A; Burne, T.H. (2013) Adult vitamin D deficiency leads to behavioural and brain neurochemical alterations in C57BL/6J and BALB/c mice., *Behav Brain Res*. 241, 120-131.

Guedes, R.C; Rocha-de-Melo, A.P; de Lima, K.R; de Albuquerque, Jda. M; Francisco, Eda S. (2013) Early malnutrition attenuates the impairing action of naloxone on spreading depression in young rats., *Nutr Neurosci*. 16, 142-146.

Haghighatdoost, F; and Azadbakht, L. (2013) Dietary Treatment Options for Depression among Diabetic Patient, Focusing on Macronutrients. *Journal of Diabetes Research.* Volume 2013 (2013), Article ID 421832, 10 pages.

Halmi, K.A. (2013) Perplexities of treatment resistance in eating disorders., *BMC Psychiatry.* 13, 292.

Halpern, C.H; Tekriwal, A; Santollo, J; Keating, J.G; Wolf, J.A; Daniels, D; Bale, T.L. (2013) Amelioration of binge eating by nucleus accumbens shell deep brain stimulation in mice involves D2 receptor modulation., *J Neurosci.* 33, 7122-7129.

Heal, D.J; Gosden, J; Smith, S.L. (2013) A review of late-stage CNS drug candidates for the treatment of obesity., *Int J Obes (Lond).* 37, 107-117.

Higginbottom, G.M; Morgan, M; O'Mahony, J; Chiu, Y; Kocay, D; Alexandre, M; Forgeron, J, Young, M. (2013) Immigrant women's experiences of postpartum depression in Canada: a protocol for systematic review using a narrative synthesis. Syst Rev. 2, 65.

Hoare, E; Skouteris, H; Fuller-Tyszkiewicz, M; Millar, L; Allender, S. (2014) Associations between obesogenic risk factors and depression among adolescents: a systematic review. *Obes Rev.* 15, 40-51.

Hodge, C.D. (2013) Good Mood Bad Mood: Help and Hope for Depression and Bipolar Disorder. Book (Paper back)

Hötger, K; Hammon, H.M; Weber, C; Görs, S; Tröscher, A; Bruckmaier, R.M; Metges, C.C.(2013) Supplementation of conjugated linoleic acid in dairy cows reduces endogenous glucose production during early lactation. *J Dairy Sci.* 96, 2258-2270.

Hryhorczuk, C; Sharma, S; Fulton, S.E. (2013) Metabolic disturbances connecting obesity and depression. *Front Neurosci.* 7, 177.

Ibrahim, K.S; El-Sayed, E.M. (2013) Proposed remedies for some developmental disorders., *Toxicol Ind Health.* 29, 367-384.

Jacka, F.N; Pasco, J.A; Williams, L.J; Meyer, B.J; Digger, R; Berk, M. (2013) Dietary intake of fish and PUFA, and clinical depressive and anxiety disorders in women. Br J Nutr. 109, 2059-2066.

Jacka, FN, Ystrom, E; Brantsaeter, A.L; Karevold, E; Roth, C; Haugen, M; Meltzer, H.M; Schjolberg, S; Berk, M. (2013) Maternal and early postnatal nutrition and mental health of offspring by age 5 years: a prospective cohort study. J Am Acad Child Adolesc Psychiatry. 52, 1038-1047.

Javelot, H; Messaoudi, M; Jacquelin, C; Bisson, J.F; Rozan, P; Nejdi, A; Lazarus, C; Cassel, J.C; Strazielle, C; Lalonde, R. (2014) Behavioral and neurochemical effects of dietary methyl donor deficiency combined with unpredictable chronic mild stress in rats., *Behav Brain Res.* 261, 8-16.

Jeong, E.M, Monasky, M.M; Gu, L; Taglieri, D.M; Patel, B.G; Liu, H; Wang, Q; Greener, I; Dudley, S.C Jr; Solaro, R.J. (2013) Tetrahydrobiopterin improves diastolic dysfunction by reversing changes in myofilament properties., *J Mol Cell Cardiol.* 56, 44-54.

Katsiardanis, K, Diamantaras, A.A; Dessypris, N; Michelakos, T; Anastasiou, A; Katsiardani, K.P; Kanavidis, P; Papadopoulos, F.C; Stefanadis, C; Panagiotakos, D.B; Petridou, E.T. (2013) Cognitive impairment and dietary habits among elders: the Velestino Study., *J Med Food.* 16, 343-350.

Khodamoradi, Sh; , Fatahnia, F; Taherpour, K; Pirani, V; Rashidi, L; Azarfar, A. (2013) Effect of monensin and vitamin E on milk production and composition of lactating dairy cows., *J Anim Physiol Anim Nutr (Berl).* 97, 666-674.

Kiecolt-Glaser, J.K; Epel, E.S; Belury, M.A; Andridge, R; Lin, J; Glaser, R; Malarkey, W.B; Hwang, B.S; Blackburn, E. (2013) Omega-3 fatty acids, oxidative stress, and leukocyte telomere length: A randomized controlled trial. *Brain Behav Immun.* 28, 16-24.

Knibb, R.C; Semper, H. (2013) Impact of suspected food allergy on emotional distress and family life of parents prior to allergy diagnosis., *Pediatr Allergy Immunol.* 24, 798-803.

Kramer, R; Wolf , S; Petri, T; von Soosten, D; Dänicke, S; Weber, E.M; Zimmer, R; Rehage, J; Jahreis, G. (2013) A commonly used rumen-protected conjugated linoleic acid supplement marginally affects fatty acid distribution of body tissues and gene expression of mammary gland in heifers during early lactation., *Lipids Health Dis.* 12, 96.

Lai, J.S; Hiles, S; Bisquera, A; Hure, A.J; McEvoy, M; Attia, J. (2014) A systematic review and meta-analysis of dietary patterns and depression in community-dwelling adults. *Am J Clin Nutr.* 99, 181-197.

Lambrecht, J.T; Greuter, C; Surber, C. (2013) Antidepressants relevant to oral and maxillofacial surgical practice. *Ann Maxillofac Surg.* 3, 160-166.

Lee, H; Ohno, M; Ohta, S; Mikami, T. (2013) Regular moderate or intense exercise prevents depression-like behavior without change of hippocampal tryptophan content in chronically tryptophan-deficient and stressed mice., *PLoS One.* 8, e66996.

Long, S.J; Benton, D. (2013) Effects of vitamin and mineral supplementation on stress, mild psychiatric symptoms, and mood in nonclinical samples: a meta-analysis., *Psychosom Med.* 75, 144-153.

Lopresti, A.L; Hood, S.D; and Drummond, P.D. (2013) A review of lifestyle factors that contribute to important pathways associated with major depression: Diet, sleep and exercise. *Journal of Affective Disorders*, 148,12-27.

Lucas, M; Chocano-Bedoya; P; Shulze, M.B; Mirzaei, F; O'Reilly, E.J; Okereke, O.I; Hu, F.B; Willett, W.C; Ascherio, A. (2014) Inflammatory dietary pattern and risk of depression among women. *Brain Behav Immun.* 36, 46-53.

Lustig, RH. (2010) Fructose: metabolic, hedonic, and societal parallels with ethanol., *J Am Diet Assoc.* 110, 1307-1321.

Mairesse, J; Silletti, V; Laloux, C; Zuena, A.R; Giovine, A; Consolazione, M; van Camp, G; Malagodi, M; Gaetani, S; Cianci, S; Catalani, A; Mennuni, G; Mazzetta, A; van Reeth, O; Gabriel, C; Mocaër, E; Nicoletti, F; Morley-Fletcher, S; Maccari, S. (2013) Chronic agomelatine treatment corrects the abnormalities in the circadian rhythm of motor activity and sleep/wake cycle induced by prenatal restraint stress in adult rats., *Int J Neuropsychopharmacol.* 16, 323-338.

Martínez-Lapiscina E.H; Clavero, P; Toledo, E; Estruch, R; Salas-Salvadó, J; San Julián, B; Sanchez-Tainta, A; Ros, E; Valls-Pedret, C; Martinez-Gonzalez, M.Á. Mediterranean diet improves cognition: the PREDIMED-NAVARRA randomised trial. *J Neurol Neurosurg Psychiatry.* 84, 1318-1325.

McMartin, S.E; Jacka, F.N; Colman, I. (2013) The association between fruit and vegetable consumption and mental health disorders: evidence from five waves of a national survey of Canadians. *Prev Med.* 56, 225-230.

Mediterranean Diet, Stroke, Cognitive Impairment, and Depression: A Meta-Analysis. *Ann. Neurol* 74, 580-591.

Miller, BJ, Murray, L; Beckmann, M.M; Kent, T; Macfarlane, B. (2013) Dietary supplements for preventing postnatal depression. *Cochrane Database Syst Rev.* 2013 Oct 24;10:CD009104.

Miyake, Y; Tanaka, K; Okubo, H; Sasaki, S; Arakawa, M. (2013) Fish and fat intake and prevalence of depressive symptoms during pregnancy in Japan: baseline data from the Kyushu Okinawa Maternal and Child Health Study., *J Psychiatr Res.* 47, 572-578.

Miyaki, K; Yixuan Song, Y; and Shimbo, T. Socioeconomic Status is Significantly Associated with Dietary Salt Intakes and Blood Pressure in Japanese Workers (J-HOPE Study).,*Int J. Environ.Res Public Health* 10, 980-993.

Monro, J.A; Leon, R; Puri, B.K. (2013) The risk of lead contamination in bone broth diets. Med Hypotheses. 80, 389-390.

Moran L,J; Ko, H; Misso, M; Marsh, K; Noakes, M; Talbot, M; Frearson, M; Thondan, M; Stepto, N; Teede, H.J. (2013) Dietary composition in the treatment of polycystic ovary syndrome: a systematic review to inform evidence-based guidelines. *J Acad Nutr Diet.* 113, 520-545.

Morgan, A.J; Reavley, N.J; Jorm, A. F. (2014) Beliefs about mental disorder treatment and prognosis: comparison of health professionals with the Australian public,. *Aust N Z J Psychiatry.* 48, 442-451.

Navarro, ZS; Pérez Llamas, PF. [Importance of sucrose in cognitive functions: knowledge and behavior. *Nutr Hosp.* 4, 106-111.

Niu, K; Guo, H; Kakizaki, M; Cui, Y; Ohmori-Matsuda, K; Guan, L; Hozawa, A; Kuriyama, S; Tsuboya, T; Ohrui, T; Furukawa, K; Arai, H; Tsuji, I; Nagatomi, R. (2013) A tomato-rich diet is related to depressive symptoms among an elderly population aged 70 years and over: a population-based, cross-sectional analysis. *J Affect Disord.* 144, 165-170.

Orr, S.K; Trépanier, M.O; Bazinet, R.P. (2013) n-3 Polyunsaturated fatty acids in animal models with neuroinflammation. *Prostaglandins Leukot Essent Fatty Acids.* 88, 97-103.

Ota, K.T; Duman, R.S. (2013) Environmental and pharmacological modulations of cellular plasticity: role in the pathophysiology and treatment of depression. *Neurobiol Dis.* 57, 28-37.

Ota, K.T, Duman, R.S. (2013) Environmental and pharmacological modulations of cellular plasticity: role in the pathophysiology and treatment of depression., Neurobiol Dis. 57, 28-37.

Peltzer, K; and Phaswana-Mafuya, N (2013) conducted a national population-based study with a sample of 3,840 individuals aged 50 years or above in South Africa. *Glob Health Action.* 6,1-9.

Persons, J.E; Robinson, J.G; Ammann, E.M; Coryell, W.H; Espeland, M.A; Harris, W.S; Manson, J.E; Fiedorowicz, J.G. (2014) Omega-3 fatty acid biomarkers and subsequent depressive symptoms., *Int J Geriatr Psychiatry.* 29, 747-757.

Persons, J.E; Robinson, J.G; Ammann, E.M; Coryell, W.H; Espeland, M.A; Harris, W.S; Manson, J.E; Fiedorowicz, J.G. (2014) Omega-3 fatty acid biomarkers and subsequent depressive symptoms., *Int J Geriatr Psychiatry.* 29, 747-57.

Pipatpiboon, N; Pintana, H; Pratchayasakul, W; Chattipakorn, N; Chattipakorn, S.C. (2013) DPP4-inhibitor improves neuronal insulin receptor function, brain mitochondrial function and cognitive function in rats with insulin resistance induced by high-fat diet consumption,. *Eur J Neurosci.* 37, 839-849.

Psaltopoulou, T; Sergentanis, T.N; Panagiotakos, D.B; Sergentanis, I.N; Kosti, R; Scarmeas, N. (2013)

Quirk, S.E; Williams, L.J; O,Neil, A; Pasco, J.A; Jacka, F.N; Housden, S; Berk, M; Brenan, S.L. (2013) The association between diet quality, dietary patterns and depression in adults: a systematic review. *BMC Psychiatry* 13,175.

Ramage-Morin, P.L, Garriguet, D. (2013) Nutritional risk among older Canadians.,. *Health Rep.* 24, 3-13.

Rico, D.E; Harvatine, K.J. (2013) Induction of and recovery from milk fat depression occurs progressively in dairy cows switched between diets that differ in fiber and oil concentration., *J Dairy Sci.* 96, 6621-6630.

Rienks, J; Dobson, A.J; and G D Mishra, G.D. (2013) Mediterranean dietary pattern and prevalence and incidence of depressive symptoms in mid-aged women: results from a large community-based prospective study, *European Journal of Clinical Nutrition* 67, 75-82.

Rintamäki, R; Kaplas, N; Männistö, S; Montonen, J; Knekt, P; Lönnqvist, J; Partonen, T. (2014) Difference in diet between a general population national representative sample and individuals with alcohol use disorders, but not individuals with depressive or anxiety disorders., *Nord J Psychiatry.* 68, 391-400.

Rosenberg, D; Lin, E; Peterson, D; Ludman, E; Von Korff, M; Katon, W. (2014) Integrated medical care management and behavioral risk factor reduction for multicondition patients: behavioral outcomes of the TEAMcare trial. *Gen Hosp Psychiatry.* 36, 129-134.

Ross, A; Friedmann, E; Bevans, M; Thomas, S. (2013) National survey of yoga practitioners: mental and physical health benefits. Complement., *Ther Med.* 21, 313-323.

Rutkowska, M; Trocha, M; Szandruk, M; Słupski, W; Rymaszewska, J.(2013) Effects of supplementation with fish oil and n-3 PUFAs enriched egg yolk phospholipids on anhedonic-like response and body weight in the rat chronic mild stress model of depression., *Pharmazie.* 68, 685-688.

Sánchez-Villegas, A; Galbete, C; Martinez-González, M.A; Martinez, J.A; Razquin, C; Salas-Salvadó, J; Estruch, R; Buil-Cosiales, P; Martí, A. (2011) The effect of the Mediterranean diet on plasma brain-derived neurotrophic factor (BDNF) levels: the PREDIMED-NAVARRA randomized trial., *Nutr Neurosci* 14, 195-201.

Sanhueza, C; Ryan, L; Foxcroft, D.R. (2013) Diet and the risk of unipolar depression in adults: systematic review of cohort studies. *Journal of Human Nutrition & Dietetics.* 26, 56-70.

Sharma S; Rais A, Nel W, Sandhu R; Ebadi, M. (2013) Clinical significance of metallothioneins in cell therapy and nanomedicine., *Int J. Nanomed.* 8, 1477-1488.

Sharma, S.K; Dakshinamurti, K. (1992) Determination of vitamin B6 vitamers and pyridoxic acid in biological samples., *J Chromatogr.* 578, 45-51.

Sharma, S; and Ebadi, M. (2014) Antioxidants as Potential Therapeutics in Neurodegeneration. *System Biology of Free Radicals and Antioxidants.* Springer-Verlag pp. 2191-2273. Chapter: 97.

Sharma, S; Ebadi, M. (2014) Significance of metallothioneins in aging brain., *Neurochem Int.* 65:40-48.

Sharma, S; Fulton, S. (2013) Diet-induced obesity promotes depressive-like behaviour that is associated with neural adaptations in brain reward circuitry. *Int J Obes (Lond).* 37, 382-389.

Sharma, S; Moon, C.S; Khogali, A; Haidous, A; Chabenne, A; Ojo, C; Jelebinkov, M; Kurdi, Y; Ebadi, M. (2013) Biomarkers in Parkinson's disease (recent update). Neurochem Int. 63, 201-229.

Srinivasan, V; Ohta, Y; Espino, J; Pariente, J.A; Rodriguez, A.B; Mohamed, M; Zakaria, R. (2013) Metabolic syndrome, its pathophysiology and the role of melatonin., *Recent Pat Endocr Metab Immune Drug Discov.* 7, 11-25.

Stahel, P; Purdie, N.G; Cant, J.P. (2013) Use of dietary feather meal to induce histidine deficiency or imbalance in dairy cows and effects on milk composition., *J Dairy Sci.* 97, 439-445.

Sullivan, S; Stein, R; Jonnalagadda, S; Mullady, D; Edmundowicz, S. (2013) Aspiration therapy leads to weight loss in obese subjects: a pilot study., *Gastroenterology.* 145,1245-1252.

Toyoda, A; Iio, W. (2013) Antidepressant-like effect of chronic taurine administration and its hippocampal signal transduction in rats. *Adv Exp Med Biol.* 775, 29-43.

Van Hees, N.J.M; der Does, W.V; Giltay, E.J. (2013) Coeliac disease, diet adherence and depressive symptoms. Journal of Psychosomatic Research. 74, 155-160.

Vekovischeva, O.Y; Peuhkuri, K; Bäckström, P; Sihvola, N; Pilvi, T; Korpela, R. (2013) The effects of native whey and α-lactalbumin on the social and individual behaviour of C57BL/6J mice., *Br J Nutr.* 110, 1336-1346.

Vyas, D; Moallem, U; Teter, B.B; Fardin-Kia, A.R; Erdman, R.A. (2013) Milk fat responses to butterfat infusion during conjugated linoleic acid-induced milk fat depression in lactating dairy cows., *J Dairy Sci.* 96, 2387-2399.

Wise, R.A. (2013) Dual Roles of Dopamine in Food and Drug Seeking: The Drive-Reward Paradox. Biol Psychiatry 73, 819-826.

Wojciak, R.W. (2014) Effect of short-term food restriction on iron metabolism, relative well-being and depression symptoms in healthy women., *Eat Weight Disord.* 19, 321-327.

Xu, S.L; Zhu, K.T; Bi, C.W; Choi, R.C; Miernisha, A; Yan, A.L; Maiwulanjiang, M; Men, S.W; Dong, T.T; Tsim, K.W. (2013) Flavinoids induce the expression of synaptic proteins, synaptotagmin, and postsynaptic density protein-95 in cultured rat cortical neuron., Planta Med. 79, 1710-1714.

Yildiz, H; Gunal, S.E; Yilmaz, G; Yucel, S. (2013) Oral carbohydrate supplementation reduces preoperative discomfort in laparoscopic cholecystectomy. *J Invest Surg.* 26, 89-95.

Yu, Y; Wu, Y; Patch, C; Wu, Z; Szabo, A; Li, D; Huang, X.F. (2013) DHA prevents altered 5-HT1A, 5-HT2A, CB1 and GABAA receptor binding densities in the brain of male rats fed a high-saturated-fat diet. *J Nutr Biochem.* 24, 1349-1358.

Ziv, L; Muto, A; Schoonheim, P.J; Meijsing, S.H; Strasser, D; Ingraham, H.A; Schaaf, M.J; Yamamoto, K.R; Baier, H. (2013) An affective disorder in zebrafish with mutation of the glucocorticoid receptor. *Mol Psychiatry.* 18, 681-691.

Chapter 8

Antidepressant Diets

Abstract

In this chapter recent knowledge about various risk factors in depression and its alleviation by intake of antidepressant diets is discussed. Patients with obesity, premenstrual syndrome, inflammatory bowel disease, and zinc deficiency suffer severely from depression. In addition to diet and conventional antidepressant therapy, curcumin, and electroconvulsive therapy can be used in certain major depressive disorders. The emerging knowledge along these therapeutic regimens is highlighted in this chapter.

Keywords: Risk factors, Zinc deficiency, Electroconvulsive Therapy, Major depression

Obesity is a causative factor in morbidity, disability and premature death. Obesity imposes health, financial and social burdens globally unless effective interventions are implemented. For many obese individuals, diet and behavioral modification need to be supplemented by pharmacotherapy. Heal et al., (2013) described the therapeutic approaches to tackle obesity. These investigators discussed drugs for the treatment of obesity and also future directions. Preclinical research revealed understanding of the complex nature of the hypothalamic regulation of food intake and has generated new molecular targets for the development of drug candidates for the treatment of obesity. Some approaches, for example, fixed-dose drug combinations deliver levels of efficacy that are not achievable with the anti-obesity drug therapies. The regulatory and marketing landscape for development, registration and commercialization of novel centrally acting drugs for the treatment of obesity and related metabolic disorders has changed substantially in recent years. More emphasis is placed on tolerability and safety, as well as efficacy. The serotonergic system and the HPA axis are involved in the regulation of emotions. Specifically, spontaneous and/or environmentally mediated modulations of these systems early in development may favor the onset of depressive- and anxiety-related phenotypes. While the contribution of each of these systems to the abnormal phenotypes has been described in clinical and experimental studies, there is limited information regarding their interactions. Zoratto et al., (2013) studied the effects of reduced serotonin and environmental stress during early stages of postnatal life on emotional regulations in mice. They administered, to CD1 mouse dams, during their first week of lactation, a tryptophan deficient diet (T) and corticosterone in the drinking water (C; 80 μg/ml). Four groups of dams (animal facility rearing, AFR; T treated, T; C treated, C; T and C treated, TC) and their male offspring were used in the study. Maternal care was scored throughout treatment and adult offspring were tested for: anhedonia (progressive ratio schedule); anxiety-related behavior (approach-avoidance conflict paradigm); BDNF, dopamine and serotonin in selected brain areas. T, C and TC treatments reduced active maternal care compared to AFR. Adult TC offspring showed increased anxiety-and anhedonia-related behaviors, reduced striatal and increased hypothalamic BDNF and reduced dopamine and serotonin in the prefrontal cortex and their turnover in the hippocampus suggesting that neonatal variations in the serotonergic system and of HPA axis may contribute to induce emotional disturbances in obesity.

Type-2 Diabetes and Depression. Recently Liu et al., 2013) reported that MDD and type II diabetes mellitus (T2DM) are co-morbid, and there may be a bi-directional connection between the two. These investigators described a mouse model of a depression-like and insulin-resistant (DIR) state induced by high-fat diet (HFD) and corticosterone (CORT). 5-Aminoimidazole-4-carboxamide-1-β-d- ribofuranoside (AICAR), a pharmacological activator of AMP-activated protein kinase (AMPK), was used to improve insulin resistance (IR). Their results demonstrated a potential for AICAR as an antidepressant with action on the DIR mice. In contrast to the traditional antidepressants, AICAR avoided reducing insulin actions of skeletal muscle in long-term HFD. Exercise also produced antidepressant effects. To investigate the association between depressive symptoms and diet quality, physical activity, and body composition, Yu et al., (2013) recruited 4511 men and women aged 35-69 years from 2009 through 2010 in Nova Scotia, Canada. These investigators assessed depressive symptoms by using the Patient Health Questionnaire. Anthropometric indices and body composition. Antidepressant use, habitual diet intake, physical activity, and potential confounders were collected. Depressive symptoms were positively associated with obesity indices after controlling for potential confounders. Compared with non-depressed individuals, those with mild and MDD had increased odd ratios (ORs) for both obesity and abdominal obesity. Depressed individuals were less likely to have a high quality diet or engage in high levels of physical activity compared with their non-depressed controls.

Mezuk et al., (21013) examined the association between undiagnosed prediabetes and Type 2 diabetes with depression and antidepressant medication use. Data come from the National Health and Nutrition Examination Study (2005 and 2007), a population-based cross-sectional survey. Analysis was limited to adults aged 30 and older (n = 3,183, Mean age = 52.1 year). Depression syndrome was measured by the Patient Health Questionnaire-9. Participants were categorized using fasting glucose levels as normoglycemic (glucose <100 mg/dL), undiagnosed prediabetes (glucose 100-125.9), prediabetes (glucose 100-125.9 plus clinician diagnosis), undiagnosed Type 2 diabetes (glucose >126), and Type 2 diabetes (glucose >126 plus clinician diagnosis or use of antidiabetic medications). Health behaviors included smoking, poor diet, excessive alcohol use, and obesity. Health promotion behaviors included efforts to change diet, lose weight, and increase physical activity. Clinically identified diabetes was associated with 4.3-fold greater odds of depression, but undiagnosed diabetes was not significantly associated with depression. This relationship was more pronounced for prediabetes. Clinically identified diabetes was associated with 1.8-fold greater odds of antidepressant use, but undiagnosed diabetes was not associated with antidepressant use. Health behaviors were not related to depression syndrome. The relationship between diabetes status and depression and antidepressant use depends on whether the diabetes has been clinically identified. Findings were consistent with the hypothesis that the relationship between diabetes and depression may be attributable to factors related to disease management.

Premenstrual Dysphoric Disorder. Premenstrual dysphoric disorder (PMDD) afflicts ~7% of reproductive-age women resulting in impaired relationships, diminished overall quality of life, and disability-adjusted life years lost on par with other major psychiatric disorders. It is known that response to pharmacological treatment is inadequate in ~50% of women with PMDD. Brownley et al., (2013) evaluated the effects of short-term chromium supplementation-on menstrual cycle-related mood and physical symptoms. Five women were studied under single-blind conditions (2 of them were referred specifically for treatment-resistant menstrual-related symptoms); 6 women completed a double-blind crossover study of chromium plus placebo versus chromium plus Sertraline. Treatments were administered from mid-cycle to onset of menses in 1-month intervals. Symptom ratings were obtained by using daily symptom checklists, and by clinical assessment, using the Hamilton Psychiatric Rating Scale for Depression (HAM-D) and the Clinical Global Impressions (CGI) scale. Chromium treatment was associated with reduced mood symptoms and improved overall health satisfaction. In some cases, chromium was associated with marked clinical improvement; in others, chromium in combination with an antidepressant resulted in better improvement than either chromium alone or an antidepressant alone suggesting that chromium may be useful for women suffering from menstrual cycle-related symptoms.

Lucas et al., (2013) identified a dietary pattern that was related to plasma levels of inflammatory markers (C-reactive protein, IL-6, TNF-α receptor 2), and analyzed the relationship of this pattern and depression risk among participants in the Nurses' Health Study. A total of 43,685 women (aged 50-77) without depression at baseline (1996) were included and followed up until 2008. Diet information was obtained from food frequency questionnaires completed between 1984 through 2002 and computed as cumulative average of dietary intakes with a 2-year latency. These investigators used a strict definition of depression that required both self-reported physician-diagnosed depression and use of antidepressants, and a broader definition that included women who reported either clinical diagnosis or antidepressant use. During the 12-year follow-up, they documented 2594 incident cases of depression using the stricter definition and 6446 using the broader definition. After adjustment for BMI and other potential confounders, relative risks comparing extreme quinties of the inflammatory dietary pattern were 1.41 for the broader definition of depression suggesting that inflammatory dietary pattern is associated with a higher depression risk and that chronic inflammation may underlie the association between diet and depression. Various biomarkers of systemic inflammation (C-reactive protein (CRP), IL-1β, IL-6, IL-8, IL-10, IL-12, plasminogen activator inhibitor-1 (PAI-1), serum amyloid A, TNF-α, and vascular adhesion molecule-1) IL-8. Inflammation. C-reactive protein (CRP), IL-6, tumor necrosis factor-α, eotaxin, interferon γ-induced protein-10, monocyte chemotactic protein-1 (MCP-1), and macrophage inflammatory protein 1-β have been estimated in CSF samples from PD patients. Increased inflammatory biomarkers in CSF are associated with severe symptoms of depression, anxiety, fatigue, and cognition in the PD group. After controlling for PD duration, age, gender, somatic illness and dementia diagnosis, high CRP was associated with symptoms of depression and fatigue, and high MCP-1 was associated with severe depression suggesting that non-motor features of PD such as depression, fatigue, and cognitive impairment are associated with higher CSF inflammatory biomarkers such as TNFα. In addition, Gong-Tone Music improved immunological function in depression as presented in Figure 12.

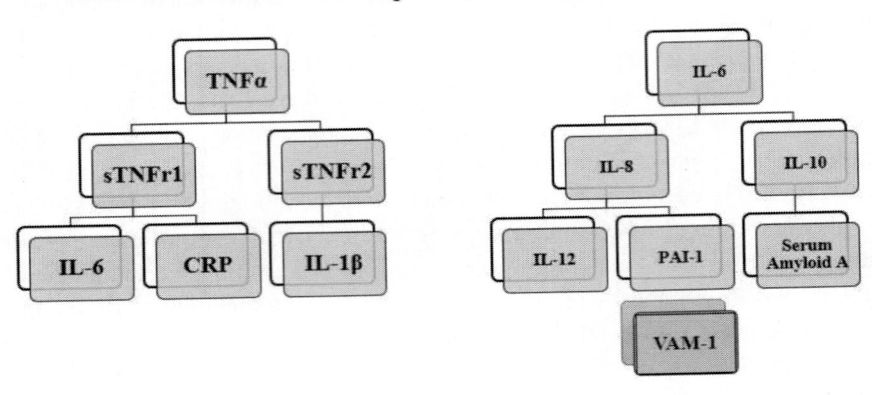

Figure 12. A diagram illustrating biomarkers of systemic inflammation (C-reactive protein (CRP), IL-1β, IL-6, IL-8, IL-10, IL-12, plasminogen activator inhibitor-1 (PAI-1), serum amyloid A, TNF-α, and vascular adhesion molecule-1) IL-8, inflammation. C-Reactive protein (CRP), IL-6, tumor necrosis factor-α, eotaxin, interferon γ-induced protein-10, monocyte chemotactic protein-1 (MCP-1), and macrophage inflammatory protein 1-β were estimated in CSF samples from PD patients. Increased inflammatory biomarkers in CSF are associated with severe symptoms of depression, anxiety, fatigue, and cognition in the PD group. After controlling for PD duration, age, gender, somatic illness and dementia diagnosis, high CRP is associated with symptoms of depression and fatigue, and high MCP-1 is associated with severe depression suggesting that non-motor features of PD such as depression, fatigue, and cognitive impairment are associated with higher CSF inflammatory biomarkers such as TNFα. Gong-Tone Music improves imunological function in depression.

Serotonergic medications can mitigate the negative affective biases in disorders such as depression or anxiety, but the neural mechanism by which this occurs is largely unknown. In line with recent advances demonstrating that negative affective biases may be driven by specific medial prefrontal-amygdala circuitry, Robinson et al., (2013) investigated whether serotonin manipulation can alter affective processing within dorsal medial prefrontal-amygdala circuit: the putative human homologue of the rodent prelimbic-amygdala circuit or 'aversive amplification' circuit. In a double-blind, placebo-controlled crossover pharmaco-fMRI design, subjects performed a forced-choice face identification task with word distractors in an fMRI scanner over two separate sessions. On one session subjects received dietary depletion of the serotonin precursor tryptophan while on the other session they received a balanced placebo control diet. Dorsal medial prefrontal responding was elevated in response to fearful relative to happy faces under depletion but not placebo. This was accompanied by a corresponding increase in positive dorsal medial prefrontal-amygdala functional connectivity suggesting that serotonin depletion engages a prefrontal-amygdala circuit during the processing of fearful relative to happy face stimuli. This same 'aversive amplification' circuit is also engaged during anxiety induced by shock anticipation. As such, serotonergic projections may inhibit engagement of the 'aversive amplification' circuit and dysfunction in this projection may contribute to the negative affective bias in mood and anxiety disorders providing explanation for the role of serotonin and serotonergic medications in the neurocircuitry of negative affective bias. Apter and Steingart (2013) reported that psychiatric medications have many implications on weight and growth. Stimulant medications may produce appetite loss and thus affect growth. Second-generation antipsychotics widely used for psychosis and many other indications may cause weight gain and subsequent metabolic disease. Weight loss such as that seen in anorexia nervosa may severely interfere with the efficacy of antidepressants.

Electroconvulsive Therapy. (ECT) is an important treatment option for MDDs, acute mania, mood disorders with psychotic features, and catatonia. Several hypotheses have been proposed as electroconvulsive therapy's mechanism of action. Hoirisch-Clapauch et al., (2014) hypothesized many converging pathways facilitated by increased synthesis and release of TPA. Human and animal experiments revealed that TPA participates in many mechanisms of action of ECT or its animal variant, electroconvulsive stimulus, including improved N-methyl-D-aspartate receptor-mediated signaling, activation of both brain-derived neurotrophic factor (BDNF) and vascular endothelial growth factor (VEGF), increased bioavailability of zinc, purinergic release, and increased mobility of dendritic spines. As a result, TPA promotes neurogenesis in limbic structures, modulates synaptic transmission and plasticity, improves cognitive function, and mediates antidepressant effects. ECT influences TPA metabolism. For example, it increases the expression of glutamate decarboxylase 65 isoform in γ-aminobutyric acid-releasing neurons, which enhances the release of TPA, and the expression of p11, a protein involved in plasminogen and TPA assembling. Interventions aiming at increasing TPA levels or its bioavailability - such as daily aerobic exercises together with a carbohydrate-restricted diet, or normalization of homocysteine levels - be evaluated in assessing response and remission duration in patients who undergo ECT.

References

Aparicio, A; Robles, F; López-Sobaler, A.M; Ortega, R.M. (2013) Dietary glycaemic load and odds of depression in a group of institutionalized elderly people withoutantidepressant treatment., *Eur J Nutr.* 52, 1059-1066.

Apter, A; Steingart, L. (2013) Interaction between weight and medications in psychological illnesses of children. *World Rev Nutr Diet.* 106, 174-180.

Atrahimovich, D; Vaya, J; Khatib, S. (2013) The effects and mechanism of flavonoid-rePON1 interactions. Structure-activity relationship study., *Bioorg Med Chem.* 21, 3348-3355.

Basic, D; Schjolden, J; Krogdahl, A; von Krogh, K; Hillestad, M; Winberg, S; Mayer, I; Skjerve, E; Höglund, E. (2013) Changes in regional brain monoaminergic activity and temporary down-regulation in stress response from dietary supplementation with l-tryptophan in Atlantic cod (Gadus morhua)., *Br J Nutr.* 109, 2166-2174.

Bello, N.T; Walters, A.L; Verpeut, J.L; Cunha, P.P. (2013) High-fat diet-induced alterations in the feeding suppression of low-dose nisoxetine, a selective norepinephrine reuptake inhibitor., *J Obes.* 2013, 457047.

Betancourt, J; Ríos, J.L; Pagán, I; Fabián, C; González, A.M; Cruz, S.Y; González, M.J; Rivera, W.T; Palacios, C. (2013) Non-medical use of prescription drugs and its association with socio-demographic characteristics, dietary pattern, and perceived academic load and stress in college students in Puerto Rico. *P R Health Sci J.* 32, 89-94.

Brownley, K.A; Girdler, S.S; Stout, A.L; McLeod, M.N. (2013) Chromium supplementation for menstrual cycle-related mood symptoms., *J Diet Suppl.* 10, 345-356.

Butt, M.S; Pasha, I; Sultan, M.T; Randhawa, M.A; Saeed, F; Ahmed, W. (2013) Black pepper and health claims: a comprehensive treatise., *Crit Rev Food Sci Nutr.* 53, 875-886.

Chevassus, H; Farret, A; Gagnol, J.P; Ponçon, C.A; Costa, F; Roux, C; Galtier, F; Petit, P. (2013) Psychological and physiological effects of bupropion compared to methylphenidate after prolonged administration in healthy volunteers., *Eur J Clin Pharmacol.* 69, 779-787.

Chocano-Bedoya, P.O; O'Reilly, E.J; Lucas, M; Mirzaei, F; Okereke, O.I; Fung, T.T; Hu, F.B; Ascherio, A. (2013) Prospective study on long-term dietary patterns and incident depression in middle-aged and older women., *Am J Clin Nutr.* 98, 813-820.

Clapper, J.R; Athanacio, J; Wittmer, C; Griffin, P.S; D'Souza, L; Parkes, D.G; Roth, J.D. (2013) Effects of amylin and bupropion/naltrexone on food intake and body weight are interactive in rodent models. *Eur J Pharmacol.* 698, 292-298.

Ford, A.C; Moayyedi, P. (2013) Dyspepsia., *Curr Opin Gastroenterol.* 29, 662-668.

García-de la Cruz, L; Galvan-Goiz, Y; Caballero-Caballero, S; Zamudio, S; Alfaro, A; Navarrete, A. (2013) Hypericum silenoides Juss. and Hypericum philonotis Cham. & Schlecht. extracts: in-vivo hypolipidaemic and weight-reducing effects in obese rats., *J Pharm Pharmacol.* 65, 591-603.

Gracida, X; Eckmann, C.R. (2013) Fertility and germline stem cell maintenance under different diets requires nhr-114/HNF4 in C. elegans., *Curr Biol.* 23, 607-613.

Hainerová IA, Lebl J. Treatment options for children with monogenic forms of obesity. *World Rev Nutr Diet.* 2013;106: 105-112.

Heal, D.J; Gosden, J; Smith, S.L. (2013) A review of late-stage CNS drug candidates for the treatment of obesity. *Int J Obes (Lond).* 37, 107-117.

Hoirisch-Clapauch, S, Mezzasalma, M.A; Nardi, A.E. (2013) Pivotal role of tissue plasminogen activator in the mechanism of action of electroconvulsive therapy., *J Psychopharmacol.* 2013 Oct 9.

Howland, R.H. (2013) Therapies for obesity and medication-associated weight gain., *J Psychosoc Nurs Ment Health Serv.* 51, 13-16.

Imayama, I; Alfano, C.M; Mason, C; Wang, C; Duggan, C; Campbell, K.L; Kong, A; Foster-Schubert, K.E; Blackburn, G.L; Wang, C.Y; McTiernan, A. (2013) Weight and metabolic effects of dietary weight loss and exercise interventions in post-menopausal antidepressant medication users and non-users: a randomized controlled trial., *Prev Med.* 57, 525-532.

Kalinowska, M; Hawrylak-Nowak, B; Szymańska, M. (2013) The influence of two lithium forms on the growth, L-ascorbic acid content and lithium accumulation in lettuce plants., *Biol Trace Elem Res.* 152, 251-257.

Kaplan, G. (2013) What is new in adolescent psychiatry? Literature review and clinical implications., *Adolesc Med State Art Rev.* 24, 29-42.

Kumar, J; Chuang, J.C; Na, E.S; Kuperman, A; Gillman, A.G; Mukherjee, S; Zigman, J.M; McClung, C.A; Lutter, M. (2013) Differential effects of chronic social stress and fluoxetine on meal patterns in mice. *Appetite.* 64, 81-88.

Lee, H; Ohno, M; Ohta, S; Mikami, T. (2013) Regular moderate or intense exercise prevents depression-like behavior without change of hippocampal tryptophan content in chronically tryptophan-deficient and stressed mice. *PLoS One*. 8, :e66996.

Lehto, S.M; Ruusunen, A; Tolmunen, T; Voutilainen, S; Tuomainen, T.P; Kauhanen, J. (2013) Dietary zinc intake and the risk of depression in middle-aged men: a 20-year prospective follow-up study., *J Affect Disord*. 150, 682-585.

Liu, W; Zhai, X; Li, H; Ji, L. (2013) Depression-like behaviors in mice subjected to co-treatment of high-fat diet and corticosterone are ameliorated by AICAR and exercise., *J Affect Disord*.

Lucas, M; Chocano-Bedoya, P; Shulze, M.B; Mirzaei, F; O'Reilly, E.J; Okereke, O.I; Hu, F.B; Willett, W.C; Ascherio, A. (2014) Inflammatory dietary pattern and risk of depression among women. *Brain Behav Immun*. 36, 46-53.

Mezuk, B; Johnson-Lawrence, V; Lee, H; Rafferty, J.A; Abdou, C.M; Uzogara, E.E; Jackson, J.S. (2013) Is ignorance bliss? Depression, antidepressants, and the diagnosis of prediabetes and type 2 diabetes., *Health Psychol*. 32, 254-263.

Młyniec, K; Budziszewska, B; Reczyński, W; Doboszewska, U; Pilc, A; Nowak, G. (2013) Zinc deficiency alters responsiveness to antidepressant drugs in mice., *Pharmacol Rep*. 65, 579-592.

Oberholzer, H.M; Van Der Schoor, C; Pretorius, E. (2013) The effect of sibutramine on platelet morphology of Spraque-Dawley rats fed a high energy diet., *Microsc Res Tech*. 76, 653-657.

Ota, K.T; Duman, R.S. (2013) Environmental and pharmacological modulations of cellular plasticity: role in the pathophysiology and treatment of depression., *Neurobiol Dis*. 57, 28-37.

Pałucha-Poniewiera, A; Brański, P; Wierońska, J.M; Stachowicz, K; Sławińska, A; Pilc, A. (2013) The antidepressant-like action of mGlu5 receptor antagonist, MTEP, in the tail suspension test in mice is serotonin dependent., *Psychopharmacology (Berl)*. 2013 Aug 20.

Perveen, T; Hashmi, B.M; Haider, S; Tabassum, S; Saleem, S; Siddiqui, M.A. (2013) Role of monoaminergic system in the etiology of olive oil induced antidepressant and anxiolytic effects in rats., *ISRN Pharmacol*. 10, 615685.

Robinson, O.J; Overstreet, C; Allen, P.S; Letkiewicz, A; Vytal, K; Pine, D.S; Grillon, C. (2013) The role of serotonin in the neurocircuitry of negative affective bias: serotonergic modulation of the dorsal medial prefrontal-amygdala 'aversive amplification' circuit., *Neuroimage*. 78, 217-223.

Siebenhofer, A; Jeitler, K; Horvath, K; Berghold, A; Siering, U; Semlitsch, T. (2013) Long-term effects of weight-reducing drugs in hypertensive patients., *Cochrane Database Syst Rev*. 2013 Mar 28;3:CD007654.

Sihvola, N; Korpela, R; Henelius, A; Holm, A; Huotilainen, M; Müller, K; Poussa, T; Pettersson, K; Turpeinen, A; Peuhkuri, K. (2013) Breakfast high in whey protein or carbohydrates improves coping with workload in healthy subjects., *Br J Nutr*. 110, 1712-1721.

Skarupski, K.A; Tangney, C.C; Li, H; Evans, D.A; Morris, M.C. (2013) Mediterranean diet and depressive symptoms among older adults over time., *J Nutr Health Aging*. 17, 441-445.

Srinivasan, V; Ohta, Y; Espino, J; Pariente, J.A; Rodriguez, A.B; Mohamed, M; Zakaria, R. (2013) Metabolic syndrome, its pathophysiology and the role of melatonin., *Recent Pat Endocr Metab Immune Drug Discov.* 7, 11-25.

Terakata, M; Fukuwatari, T; Kadota, E; Sano, M; Kanai, M; Nakamura, T; Funakoshi, H; Shibata, K. (2013) The niacin required for optimum growth can be synthesized from L-tryptophan in growing mice lacking tryptophan-2,3-dioxygenase., *J Nutr.* 143, 1046-1051.

Toyoda, A; Iio, W. (2013) Antidepressant-like effect of chronic taurine administration and its hippocampal signal transduction in rats. *Adv Exp Med Biol.* 775, 29-43.

Trigueros, L; Peña, S; Ugidos, A.V; Sayas-Barberá, E; Pérez-Álvarez, J.A; Sendra, E. (2013) Food ingredients as anti-obesity agents: a review., *Crit Rev Food Sci Nutr.* 53, 929-942.

Vekovischeva, O.Y; Peuhkuri, K; Bäckström, P; Sihvola, N; Pilvi, T; Korpela, R. (2013) The effects of native whey and α-lactalbumin on the social and individual behavior of C57BL/6J mice., *Br J Nutr.* 110, 1336-1346.

Witkin, J.M; Li, X. (2013) Curcumin, an active constiuent of the ancient medicinal herb Curcuma longa L.: some uses and the establishment and biological basis of medical efficacy., *CNS Neurol Disord Drug Targets.* 12, 487-497.

Yu, Z.M; Parker, L; Dummer, T.J. (2013) Depressive symptoms, diet quality, physical activity, and body composition among populations in Nova Scotia, Canada: Report from the Atlantic Partnership for Tomorrow's Health., *Prev Med.* 61,106-113.

Zoratto, F; Fiore, M; Ali, S.F; Laviola, G; Macrì, S. (2013) Neonatal tryptophan depletion and corticosterone supplementation modify emotional responses in adult male mice., *Psychoneuroendocrinology.* 38, 24-39.

Chapter 9

Diets to Prevent Primary Depression

Abstract

The prevention of mental disorders is crucial due to significant health, social and economic burden. Among them, unipolar major depression is the global leading cause of loss of productivity as a result of disability and it is projected to also be the leading cause of disability-adjusted life years lost in 2030. Relatively little etiological research has been conducted to assess which are the dietary or lifestyle determinants of depression. Only limited studies have analyzed the relationship between dietary patterns, such as the Mediterranean diet, and prevention of depression. To confirm these findings, further studies with improved methodology, and randomized prevention trials, with interventions based on changes in the diatary pattern, including participants at high risk of mental disorders are needed. Dietary factors are likely to play a significant role. Although the role of diet in the prevention of other noncommunicable diseases, such as cardiovascular disease (CVD) has been investigated for the last 50 years, the relationship between diet and depression is a new field that has only emerged very recently. This chapter describes various chronic diseases and their direct association with depression and its alleviation for the better clinical prognosis.

Keywords: Diet, Cardiovascular Disease, Depression, metabolic syndrome, and obesity

There are studies suggesting that depression seems to share common mechanisms with the metabolic syndrome (MetS), obesity, and CVD. Several major cardiovascular risk factors (including obesity and MetS) are prevalent among patients who are depressed. Metabolic and inflammatory processes, such as reduced insulin sensitivity, elevations in plasma homocysteine levels, increased production of proinflammatory cytokines, and endothelial dysfunction may be responsible for the link between depression and cardiometabolic disorders.

Proinflammatory cytokines interfere with neurotransmitters metabolism and decrease the availability of some precursors such as tryptophan. Moreover, low-grade inflammatory status and endothelial dysfunction inhibit the expression of BDNF because it is the endothelial cells that synthesize and secrete BDNF. An emerging concept in neuroscience is that perturbations in the health of the cerebral endothelium (including loss of the neuroprotection by BDNF) may mediate progressive neuronal dysfunction. Several meta-analyses have established that BDNF levels are reduced in patients with depression, and that antidepressant medication seems to up-regulate their levels.

Role of Diet. To date, most of the evidence relating diet to depression is similar to that demonstrating the role that diet plays on MetS or CVD as both diseases seem to share several common physiopathological mechanisms. This analogy is supported by the beneficial effects reported for lipids with anti-inflammatory properties, such as omega-3 fatty acids or olive oil. Conversely, the intake of trans fatty acids or the consumption of foods rich in this kind of fat, like fast food or commercial bakery products, have been reported as contributors to higher depression risk.

The mediators of adverse effects of trans fatty acids on CVD include increases in plasma concentrations of low density lipoprotein-cholesterol, reductions in high density lipoprotein-cholesterol, proinflammatory changes, and endothelial dysfunction. Because depression is also associated with a low-grade inflammatory status, endothelial dysfunction and worse lipid profiles, the adverse biological modifications caused by trans fatty acids could also be responsible for detrimental effects on depression. However, it is important to study the overall dietary pattern rather than isolated nutrients. In this context, it is reasonable to think that dietary patterns that foster cardiometabolic health could also be inversely related to depressive disorders. Similarly, those dietary patterns involved in cardiometabolic risk could also exert a detrimental effect on depression.

Life Style Choices & Depression

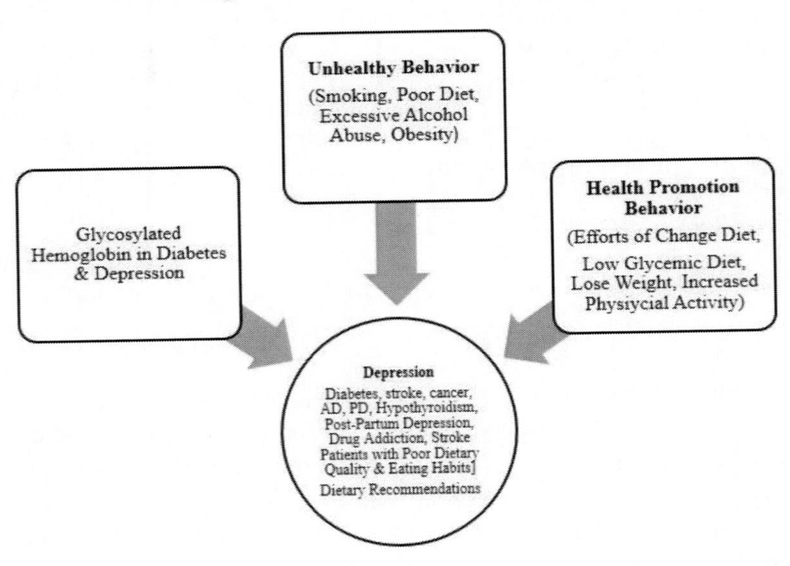

Figure 13. A diagram illustrating life style choices and the risk of depression. Unhealthy behavior is associated with smoking, poor diet, excessive alcohol abuse, and obesity. Health promotion behavior includes efforts to changes dietary pattern (Mediterranean diet), diet with low glycemic index, increased physical activity. The severity of depression in diabetes can be assessed by estimating the glycosylated hemoglobin. Patients suffering from chronic diabetes, stroke, cancer AD, PD, hypothyroidism, drug addiction with poor dietary quality and eating habits need to be provided with specific dietary recommendations.

A few epidemiological studies have negatively related healthy dietary patterns, including the Mediterranean Diet, or directly related the Western dietary pattern to the risk of developing depression. Significant differences in plasma BDNF levels have been observed for patients with depression who were assigned to the Mediterranean diet compared with those assigned to a control diet.

Nevertheless, these evidences are sparse and not definitive, because some of these studies were not well-controlled against diverse sources of bias. The risk of depression is associated with life style choices such as unhealthy behavior is associated with smoking, poor diet, excessive alcohol abuse, and obesity. Health promotion behavior includes efforts to change dietary pattern (Mediterranean diet), diet with low glycemic index, increased physical activity. The severity of depression in diabetes can be assessed by estimating the glycosylated hemoglobin. Patients suffering from chronic diabetes, stroke, cancer AD, PD, hypothyroidism, drug addiction with poor dietary quality and eating habits need to be provided with specific dietary recommendations as illustrated in Figure 13.

In postpartum women depressive symptoms are associated with body image; diet and physical activity; substance abuse including smoking and alcohol intake, body mass index (BMI), not exclusively breastfeeding, ethnicity, education level, and parity. Low-income postpartum women have poor nutritional status. Furthermore, reduced intake of sea food during post-partum period can significantly impact self care. Hence low omega-3 index in pregnancy is a possible risk factor for postpartum depression as Figure 14 illustrates.

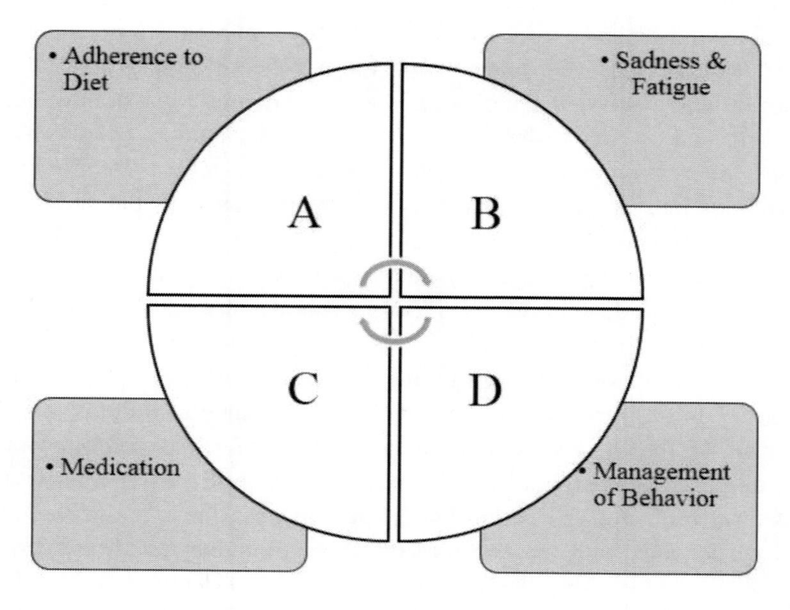

Figure 14. A diagram illustrating depressive symptoms; body image; diet and physical activity; substance abuse including smoking and alcohol intake, body mass index (BMI), not exclusively breastfeeding, ethnicity, education level, and parity. Low-income postpartum women with poor nutritional status. Furthermore, reduced intake of sea food during post-partum period can significantly impact self care. Low omega-3 index in pregnancy is a possible risk factor for postpartum depression.

Epidemiological Evidence. Some of the associations between diet and depression have been found in studies with large sample sizes. These studies use questionnaires to collect information on the outcome (depression) and/or the exposure (diet). Food frequency questionnaires are used, but they have some potential for misclassification bias. The use of adequately-validated questionnaires is encouraged to minimize misclassification biases. Depression assessment is usually based on depressive symptoms scales. Quite often this information is self-reported and the choice of a cut-off point to define depression is generally arbitrary. This cut-off point depends on the sample characteristics and limits the ability to conduct comparisons between studies carried out in different populations. Thus, the use of medical diagnoses of depression ascertained via clinical assessments or the use of a validated self-reported medical diagnosis of depression could be appropriate approach to reduce misclassification problems in epidemiological studies. Most of the evidence suggesting a link between nutrition and depression comes from studies with a cross-sectional design. This design usually precludes the possibility to infer a truly causal relationship. In these studies exposure is ascertained simultaneously with disease and, therefore, results could be interpreted as a consequence of reverse causation bias, that is, depression may lead to poorer dietary habits. Only a few longitudinal studies have analyzed the role of diet on depression risk. One of these epidemiological studies is the Seguimiento Universidad de Navarra (SUN) Project, a dynamic prospective cohort of university graduates, with a median follow-up of 6 years including >10,000 participants in longitudinal assessments. Several diet components were associated with depression risk in this cohort. Whereas trans fatty acids or fast food and commercial bakery products were associated with higher depression risk, omega-3 fatty acids and olive oil intake showed inverse associations. This project reported that adherence to the Mediterranean dietary pattern was associated with reduced depression risk. Almost immediately after, investigators from the Whitehall II longitudinal study (another prospective cohort in the UK) reported a detrimental role for a Western dietary pattern. Recently, the divergent roles of healthy or Western dietary patterns on depression risk have been confirmed in a longitudinal analysis of Australian adolescents. Other studies conducted on adults in Australia (*Geelong Osteoporosis Study*) and Norway (*Hordaland Health Study*) reported similar associations between dietary patterns and depression risk, but they were based on cross-sectional assessments. Thus, these findings need to be confirmed in future prospective assessments. Finally, the effect of dietary patterns on depression could be explained by the co-occurrence of other lifestyle-related factors such as physical activity alcohol intake, smoking or the use of illicit drugs; by sociodemographic factors such as social networks, marital status or socioeconomic level; or by medical conditions such as the presence of CVD. Thus, one of the most important aspects in observational epidemiology is to obtain an adequate control of these possible confounders. Most of these confounders are usually collected in well-designed epidemiological studies and controlled using multivariable models. Restriction is an even better procedure that is used on occasion. This procedure consists of excluding all participants with the presence of the confounding condition (that is, cases of prevalent CVD) before assessing the role of diet on incident depression. Nevertheless, when the lack of or inadequate control for some of these potential confounders and the presence of residual confounding exist, the interpretation of the findings obtained from observational studies need caution.

Prevention or treatment. Whereas the above-mentioned studies have analyzed the role of diet in the primary prevention of depression, clinical trials have been designed to assess the impact of nutritional interventions on the clinical course of depression. However, most available trials are based on small samples and have been carried out in a controlled clinical setting with a short follow-up period. Moreover, with the exception of a recent clinical trial, none of these trials has analyzed the effect of an overall dietary pattern. Instead they have assessed isolated nutrients, mainly omega-3 fatty acids or B vitamins.

Interaction between diet and genetic factors. To date, there are no studies that ascertain the possible interaction between diet and genetic factors on depression risk. Nevertheless, effect modification of genetic factors by diet on several diseases related to depression, such as obesity or CVD, has been reported. This new line of nutrigenetics research based on the hypothesis that visceral obesity or MetS share some etiological mechanisms, including diet and genes, with unipolar depressive disorder should be developed in future. This would help to better understand the role of diet on the risk and prognosis of major depression.

Craving and Self-Injury. People have engaged in self-injury-defined as direct and deliberate bodily harm in the absence of suicidal intent-for thousands of years; however, systematic research on this behavior has been lacking. Recent theoretical and empirical work on self-injury has advanced the understanding of this perplexing behavior. Self-injury is most prevalent among adolescents and young adults, typically involves cutting or carving the skin, and has a consistent presentation cross-nationally. Behavioral, physiological, and self-report data suggest that the behavior serves both an intrapersonal function (i.e., decreases aversive affective/cognitive states or increases desired states) and an interpersonal function (i.e., increases social support or removes undesired social demands). There is no evidence-based psychological or pharmacological treatment for self-injury. Nock (2010) presented an integrated theoretical model of the development and maintenance of self-injury that synthesizes prior findings and proposed several testable hypotheses for future research.

Clinical Management of Cravings. Alcoholism is a progressive neurological disorder that represents one of the leading preventable causes of morbidity and mortality in the USA. Individuals with alcohol dependence may exhibit differences in their sensitivity to intoxication, the age at which they begin heavy drinking or the presentation of comorbid psychiatric illness. The heterogeneous nature of the disorder has complicated efforts to predict treatment outcomes, indicating a need for improved diagnostic and therapeutic approaches. Pharmaceutical development has focused on treating the symptoms of alcohol withdrawal, reducing consumption of and craving for alcohol, preventing relapse and treating associated psychiatric problems. Current therapies may be optimized by combining psychosocial and pharmacologic approaches to treat alcoholic patients with the most appropriate regimen to achieve the desired therapeutic outcome. The neurobiological mechanisms of dependence on alcohol in brief and review major medications approved for the treatment of alcoholism with regard to recent clinical evidence for the therapeutic efficacy of each agent has been explored by Clapp (2012). Investigations on the use of drugs with other indications (e.g., *antidepressants and anticonvulsants*) to target alcohol-dependent subtypes were also discussed. Treatment strategies are based on pharmacological interventions to reduce craving and relapse in alcohol-dependent patients. First a historical overview about relapse prevention strategies was provided and the development of Disulfiram, Naltrexone, Acamprosate, and Nalmefene with their neurobiological modes of action. Then the concept of convergent genomic analysis has been introduced for the discovery of new molecular treatment targets. Finally, convincing evidence for the use of N-methyl-D-aspartate (NMDA) receptor channel blockers as substitution drugs has been provided. Important conclusions of this review are: (i) learning from other addictive substances is very helpful-e.g., substitution therapies as applied to opiate addiction for decades could also be translated to alcoholics, (ii) the glutamate theory of alcohol addiction provides a convincing framework for the use of NMDA receptor antagonists for alcohol-dependent patients, (iii) a combination of behavioral and pharmacological therapies may be the optimal approach for future treatment strategies-one promising example concerns the pharmacological disruption of reconsolidation processes of alcohol cue memories, (iv) given that many neurotransmitter systems are affected by chronic alcohol consumption, numerous druggable targets have been identified; consequently, a "cocktail" of different compounds will improve the treatment options, (v) in psychopharmacology, such as drug will yield new medications, and finally, (vi) the whole organism has to be taken into consideration to provide personalized treatment.

There is no other field in psychiatric research that has yielded so many novel, druggable targets and innovative treatment strategies than for alcohol addiction. However, it will still be several years before the majority of the "treatment-seeking population" will benefit from those developments (Spanagel., 2013). Alcohol addiction is a chronically relapsing disorder characterized by compulsive alcohol seeking and use. Alcohol craving and long-lasting vulnerability to relapse present a great challenge for the successful treatment of alcohol addiction. Therefore, relapse prevention has emerged as a critically important area of research, with the need for effective and valid animal models of relapse. This chapter provides an overview of the animal models of craving and relapse presently available and employed in alcoholism research. These models include conditioned reinstatement, stress-induced reinstatement, ethanol priming-induced reinstatement, conditioned place preference, Pavlovian spontaneous recovery, the alcohol deprivation effect, and seeking-taking chained schedules. Thus, a wide array of animal models is available that permit investigation of behaviors directed at obtaining access to alcohol, as well as neurobehavioral mechanisms and genetic factors that regulate these behaviors. These models also facilitate identifying pharmacological treatment targets and as tools for evaluating the efficacy of potential medications for the prevention of alcohol craving and relapse (Martin-Fardon and Weiss 2013). While stress significantly impacts alcoholism risk, there is also evidence that increasing levels of alcohol use affect peripheral and central stress and reward pathways thereby setting up a reciprocal relationship among the effects of alcohol consumption of the development, course of recovery from alcoholism. Efforts in assessing the integrity of stress pathways in alcoholism by examining whether altered responses of the stress pathways play a role in relapse risk have been highlighted. Using validated human laboratory procedures to model two of the most common situations that contribute to relapse risk, these researchers reviewed how such models in the laboratory can predict subsequent alcohol relapse. Empirical findings from laboratory and brain imaging studies reviewed to show that specific stress-related dysregulation accompanies the alcohol craving state in alcohol-dependent individuals, and such dysregulation along with increases in alcohol seeking are predictive of increased alcohol relapse risk. Finally, the implications of these findings for the development of novel treatment interventions that target stress processes and alcohol craving to improve alcoholism relapse outcomes have been discussed (Sinha, 2013).

Designer drugs are currently marketed as substitutes for stimulant drugs as cocaine, amphetamine, MDMA. Unlike compounds listed as narcotics, these new substances are synthesized to avoid anti-drug laws. Among them, Mephedrone (4-methylmethcatinone) that belongs to cathinone family, has been recently introduced in France. Users report positive euphoric and entactogenic effects. They also describe negative effects such as increased dependence and larger craving for tobacco and alcohol. The adverse effects include psychoactive, digestive, cardiovascular effects. Some fatality cases have been reported and attributed to mephedrone in association with other substances. Mephedrone has been listed as narcotic in several European countries and recently in France (Debruyne et al., 2010). Varenicline is a partial agonist of the α(4)β(2) nicotinic acetylcholine receptor approved by the FDA for the treatment of nicotine dependence. While the clinical efficacy of Varenicline for smoking cessation is well-supported, its biobehavioral mechanisms of action remain poorly understood. This randomized, crossover, placebo-controlled, human laboratory study combined guided imagery stress exposure with in vivo presentation of cigarette cues to test the effects of Varenicline on stress-induced and cue-induced craving for cigarettes. A total of 40 (13 females) daily smokers (>/=10 cigarettes per day) completed a guided imagery exposure (stress and neutral) followed by the presentation of cigarette cues at the target dose of Varenicline (1mg twice per day) and on matched placebo. Multilevel regression models revealed a main effect of Varenicline such that it reduced cigarette craving across the experimental paradigm, compared to placebo. Varenicline attenuated cue induced craving following neutral imagery but not when cues were preceded by stress induction (i.e., stress+cues). These results elucidate the biobehavioral effects of Varenicline for nicotine dependence and suggest that Varenicline-induced amelioration of cigarette craving is unique to tonic and cue-induced craving following neutral imagery but does not extend to the combination of stress plus cues (Giuliano et al., 2013).

Clinical Management of Cravings. Early editions of the American Psychiatric Association's Diagnostic and Statistical Manual of Mental Disorders (DSM) described addiction as a physical dependency to a substance that resulted in withdrawal symptoms in its absence. Recent editions, including DSM-IV, have been focsed toward a diagnostic instrument that classifies such conditions as dependency, rather than addiction. The American Society of Addiction Medicine recommends treatment for people with chemical dependency based on patient placement criteria (currently listed in PPC-2), which attempt to match levels of care according to clinical assessments in six areas, including: Acute intoxication and/or withdrawal potential; Biomedical conditions or complications; Emotional/behavioral conditions or complications; Treatment acceptance/resistance; Relapse potential; Recovery environment. Some medical systems, including those of at least 15 states of the United States, refer to an Addiction Severity Index to assess the severity of problems related to substance use. The index assesses problems in six areas: medical, employment/support, alcohol and other drug use, legal, family/social, and psychiatric. While addiction or dependency is related to seemingly uncontrollable urges, and may have roots in genetic predisposition, treatment of dependency is always classified as behavioral medicine. Early treatment of acute withdrawal often includes medical detoxification, which can include doses of anxiolytics to reduce symptoms of withdrawal. In chronic opiate addiction, a surrogate drug such as Methadone is sometimes offered as a form of opiate replacement therapy. But treatment approaches universally focus on the individual's ultimate choice to pursue an alternate course of action. Therapists often classify patients with chemical dependencies as either interested or not interested in changing. Treatments usually involve planning for specific ways to avoid the addictive stimulus, and therapeutic interventions intended to help a client learn healthier ways to find satisfaction. Doctors have attempted to tailor intervention approaches to specific influences that effect addictive behavior, using therapeutic interviews in an effort to discover factors that led a person to embrace unhealthy, addictive sources of pleasure or relief from pain. Baclofen is an anti-spastic drug that acts as an agonist of GABA-B receptors. It also seems to decrease the appetence for alcohol (anti-craving effect), although this effect has not been certified by Authorities for drug approval in France (AMM). However, Baclofen receives a great deal of demand by patients hoping to reduce their alcohol consumption. Nonetheless, the lack of AMM and the high doses of baclofen supposed to exert an anti-craving effect often discourage practitioners from prescribing this drug. Therefore, it is preferable for a drug like Baclofen to be prescribed under specific regulations. As such, certain criteria similar to those required in clinical trials are necessary to protect patients as well as the prescribing doctors. The criteria that are proposed are: the use of drugs without AMM approval as a last resort (all other treatments must have failed), the collegiate decision for the drug prescription, knowledge of the potency of the drug as well as record keeping of patients and proper supervision. The departments of addiction, pharmacology and pharmacovigilance of the University Hospital of Lille, France present a medical process named "multidisciplinary consultations for resort treatments of addictions" (CAMTEA). This process is designed to meet all the above mentioned criteria and to allow the use of Baclofen as an anti-craving drug. If this proves to be successful with Baclofen, it is possible to extend the use of CAMTEA to other drugs without AMM approval in addictologic pathologies (Debruyne et al., 2010). Treatment strategies that are based on pharmacological interventions to reduce craving and relapse in alcohol-dependent patients have been described. The development of Disulfiram, Naltrexone, Acamprosate, and Nalmefene and their neurobiological modes of action has been discussed. Then the concept of convergent genomic analysis, has been introduced for the discovery of new molecular treatment targets. Finally, these authors provided convincing evidence for the use of NMDA receptor channel blockers as substitution drugs. Learning from other addictive substances is very helpful-e.g., substitution therapies as applied to opiate addiction for decades could also be translated to alcoholics, (ii) the glutamate theory of alcohol addiction provides a convincing framework for the use of NMDA receptor antagonists as substitution drugs for alcohol-dependent patients, (iii) a combination of behavioral and pharmacological therapies may be the optimal approach for future treatment strategies-one promising example concerns the pharmacological disruption of reconsolidation processes of alcohol cue memories, (iv) given that many neurotransmitter systems are affected by chronic alcohol consumption, numerous targets have been identified; consequently, a "cocktail" of different compounds will further improve the treatment situation, (v) in silico psychopharmacology, such as drug repurposing will yield new medications, and finally, (vi) the whole organism has to be taken into consideration to provide the best therapy for our patients. There is no other field in psychiatric research that has, in recent years, yielded so many novel, drug targets and innovative treatment strategies than for alcohol addiction. However, it will still be several years before the majority of the "treatment-seeking population" will benefit from those developments (Gass et al., 2012). Baclofen has shown promise in treating substance abuse disorders and also reduced binge frequency in an open-label trial. This placebo-controlled, double-blind, crossover study further assessed the effects of Baclofen on binge eating. Twelve individuals who self-reported binge eating completed the study. Data were collected during a run-in period (no drug or placebo), placebo phase (48 days), and Baclofen phase (titrated up to 60 mg daily or the maximum tolerated dose, 48 days). All the participants were exposed to all conditions.

Participants completed a binge diary daily, and the Binge Eating Scale (BES), Food Craving Inventory-II (FCI-II), and Hospital Anxiety and Depression Scale (HADS) at regular intervals throughout the study. Baclofen significantly reduced binge frequency relative to placebo and run-in confirming results from the previous open-label trial. Baclofen also produced slight increases in depression symptomatology as assessed by the HADS. Binge severity (BES scores) and craving (FCI-II scores) were reduced during placebo and Baclofen phases. Both measures exhibited significant placebo effects. Tiredness, fatigue, and upset stomach were the most common side-effects. These results indicate that Baclofen may be a useful treatment for binge eating in some patients (Xu et al., 2012).

Food Craving & Sleep Quality. The purpose of this study was to evaluate the effects of acute, oral Modafinil (200 mg) exposure on daytime sleepiness in Methamphetamine (Meth)-dependent individuals. Eighteen Meth-dependent subjects were enrolled in a 7-d inpatient study and were administered placebo or Modafinil on day 6 and the counter-condition on day 7 (randomized) of the protocol. Subjects completed several subjective daily assessments (*such as the Epworth Sleepiness Scale Pittsburgh Sleep Quality Index, Beck Depression Inventory and visual analogue scale)* throughout the protocol as well as objective assessments on days 5-7, when the Multiple Sleep Latency Test was performed. The results of this study suggested that short-term abstinence from Meth is associated with increased daytime sleepiness and that a single dose of 200 mg Modafinil reduces daytime somnolence. In addition, a positive correlation was found between the likelihood of taking a nap and craving and desire for Meth, as well as the likelihood of using Meth and whether Meth would make the participant feel better (Clausius et al., 2012).

Acceptance and Commitment Therapy. (ACT) provides a theoretical rationale for "acceptance" of thoughts and feelings, and proscribes suppression, a more intuitive and commonly used coping strategy. Suppression has negative consequences not applicable to acceptance, including depletion in self-control and ironic post suppression rebound effects. However, it remains unknown whether these strategies differentially affect frequency of drug-related thoughts, craving intensity, drug use behavior, or other relevant outcomes. Adult smokers received a brief laboratory-based coping intervention (acceptance or suppression) or were not given coping instructions (control group) and then were exposed to smoking cues. The suppression group was successful at suppressing thoughts of smoking, as they reported fewer thoughts of smoking than the other two groups. Also, both coping strategies were associated with benefits with respect to craving and affect. However, there were no group differences in depletion, and rebound effects did not occur when coping was discontinued. Following the laboratory session, all participants attempted to quit or at least reduce their smoking for 3 days; the acceptance and suppression groups resumed use of their strategy. At 3-day follow-up, the acceptance and suppression groups reported greater self-efficacy for avoiding smoking when experiencing craving compared to the control group. However, there were no group differences in the number of cigarettes smoked during the 3 days. This study provided support for the value of acceptance-based coping, but it also suggested that more research is needed to differentiate its benefits compared to suppression (Kavanagh et al., 2013). Self-expanding experiences like falling in love or engaging in novel, exciting and interesting activities activate the same brain reward mechanism (mesolimbic dopamine pathway) that reinforces drug use and abuse, including tobacco smoking suggesting the possibility that reward from smoking is substitutable by self-expansion (through competition with the same neural system), potentially aiding cessation efforts. Using a model of self-expansion in the context of romantic love, the fMRI experiment examined whether, among nicotine-deprived smokers, relationship self-expansion is associated with deactivation of cigarette cue-reactivity regions. Among participants who were experiencing moderate levels of craving, cigarett cue-reactivity regions (e.g., cuneus and posterior cingulate cortex) showed less activation during self-expansion conditions compared with control conditions. These results provided evidence that rewards from one domain (self-expansion) can act as a substitute for reward from another domain (nicotine) to attenuate cigarette cue reactivity. Varenicline is believed to work by reducing craving responses to smoking cues and by reducing general levels of craving; however, these hypotheses have never been evaluated with craving assessed in the natural environments of treatment-seeking smokers. Ecological momentary assessment procedures were used to assess the impact of Varenicline on cue-specific and general craving in treatment-seeking smokers prior to quitting. For 5 weeks prior to quitting, 60 smokers carried personal digital assistants that assessed their response to smoking or neutral cues. During week 1 (baseline), participants did not receive medication; during weeks 2-4 (drug manipulation), participants were randomized to receive varenicline or placebo; during week 5 (standard therapy), all participants received Varenicline. Craving was assessed before each cue; cue-specific craving and attention to cue were assessed after each cue. During all phases, smoking cues elicited greater craving than neutral cues; the magnitude of this effect declined after the first week. General craving declined across each phase of the study. Relative to the placebo condition, Varenicline was associated with a greater decline in craving over the drug manipulation phase. Varenicline did not attenuate cue-specific craving during any phase of the study. Smoking cues delivered in the natural environment elicited strong craving responses in treatment-seeking smokers, but cue-specific craving was not affected by Varenicline administered prior to the quit attempt suggesting that the clinical efficacy of Varenicline is not mediated by changes in cue-specific craving during the pre-quit period of treatment-seeking smokers (Sweitzer et al., 2013). This study evaluated the factor structure of the Brief Questionnaire of Smoking Urges (QSU-Brief) within a sample of Black light smokers (1-10 cigarettes per day). The QSU-Brief was administered to 540 (mean age = 46.5; 66.1% women) urban Black light smokers upon entering a smoking cessation clinical trial. An exploratory factor analysis (EFA) was conducted to evaluate the factor structure of this 10-item measure. An EFA indicated that as in other samples, the construct of craving in a Black sample is defined by 2 factors; 1 factor emphasizing the positive reinforcement of smoking and the other factor emphasizing the negative reinforcement properties of smoking. These findings replicated a 2-factor structure of craving seen in smokers from other racial/ethnic groups, demonstrating the clinical utility of the QSU-Brief in measuring craving in Black light smokers (Martin-Fardon and Weiss 2013). Noninvasive brain stimulation of the dorsolateral prefrontal cortex with repetitive transcranial magnetic stimulation and transcranial direct current stimulation can modify decision-making behaviors in healthy subjects. The same type of noninvasive brain stimulation can suppress drug craving in substance user patients, who display impaired decision-making behaviors. The implications of these studies for the cognitive neurosciences and their translational applications to the treatment of addictions were discussed and proposed a neurocognitive model that can account for findings and suggested a promising therapeutic role of brain stimulation in the treatment of substance abuse and addictive behavior disorders (Rolland et al., 2010).

Alcohol and tobacco dependence are highly comorbid disorders, with preclinical evidence suggesting a role for nicotinic acetylcholine receptors (nAChRs) in alcohol consumption. Varenicline, a partial nicotinic agonist with high affinity for the α4β2 nAChR receptor, reduced ethanol intake in rodents. It was tested whether Varenicline would reduce alcohol consumption and alcohol craving in humans. This double-blind, placebo-controlled investigation examined the effect of Varenicline (2 mg/day vs. placebo) on alcohol self-administration using an established laboratory paradigm in non-alcohol-dependent heavy drinkers (n = 20) who were daily smokers. Following 7 days of medication pretreatment, participants were first administered a priming dose of alcohol (.3 g/kg) and subjective, and physiologic responses were assessed. A 2-hour alcohol self-administration period followed during which participants could choose to consume up to 8 additional drinks (each .15 g/kg). Varenicline significantly reduced the number of drinks consumed compared to placebo and increased the likelihood of abstaining from any drinking during the self-administration period. Following the priming drink, Varenicline attenuated alcohol craving and reduced subjective reinforcing alcohol effects (high, like, rush, feel good, intoxicated). Adverse events associated with Varenicline were minimal and, when combined with alcohol, produced no significant effects on physiologic reactivity, mood, or nausea, suggesting that Varenicline reduced alcohol self-administration and was well tolerated, alone and in combination with alcohol in heavy-drinking smokers. Hence Varenicline should be investigated as a potential treatment for alcohol use disorders (Fecteau et al., 2010).

Future Research Directions. Large randomized prevention trials with interventions based on changes in the overall food pattern and participants at high risk of mental disorders could provide the most definitive answer to confirm or refute experimentally the findings reported by observational studies. Though ideal, these trials might not seem feasible. However, similar trials have been conducted in cardiovascular fields, as it has been the case for the Dietary Approaches to Stop Hypertension (DASH) diet or the Prevención con Dieta Mediterránea (PREDIMED) trial. Similar trials can be designed for the prevention of depression. Although a few prospective cohort studies have analyzed the role of dietary patterns on depression risk, their contributions are still scarce. Further observational studies with improved methodology (*including repeated measurements of diet, better validation of measuring instruments, longer follow-up periods, larger sample sizes and adequate control of confounders*) as well as large randomized primary prevention trials with interventions based on changes in the overall food pattern and including participants at high risk of mental disorders are necessary to confirm the findings.

References

Clapp, P. (2012) Current progress in pharmacologic treatment strategies for alcohol dependence., *Expert Rev Clin Pharmacol.* 2012 Jul;5(4):427-435.

Clausius, R.L; Krebill, R; Mayo, M.S; Bronars, C; Martin, L; Ahluwalia, J.S; Cox, L.S. (2012) Acute modafinil exposure reduces daytime sleepiness in abstinent methamphetamine-dependent volunteers,. *Nicotine Tob Res.* 14, 1110-1114.

Debruyne, D; Courne, M.A; Le Boisselier, R; Djezzar, S; Gerardin, M; Boucher, A; Karila, L; Coquerel, A; Mallaret, M. (2010) [A system of prescriptions without drug approval: example of baclofen]., *Therapie.* 65, 519-524.

Fecteau, S; Fregni, F; Boggio, P.S; Camprodon, J.A; Pascual-Leone, A. (2010) Varenicline reduces alcohol self-administration in heavy-drinking smokers., *Subst Use Misuse*.45, 1766-1786.

Gass, J. C; Wray, J.M; Hawk, L.W; Mahoney, M.C; Tiffany, S.T. (2012) New pharmacological treatment strategies for relapse prevention., *Psychopharmacology (Berl)*.223, 107-116.

Giuliano, C; Robbins, T.W; Wille, D.R; Bullmore, E.T; Everitt, B.J. (2013) The effects of varenicline on stress-induced and cue-induced craving for cigarettes., *Psychopharmacology (Berl)*. Jan 9.

Giuliano, C; Robbins, T.W; Wille, D.R; Bullmore, E.T; Everitt, B.J. (2013) Attenuation of cocaine and heroin seeking by mu-opioid receptor antagonism., *Psychopharmacology (Berl)*.

Martin-Fardon, R; and Weiss, F. (2013) Evaluation of the brief questionnaire of smoking urges in Black light smokers., *Curr Top Behav Neurosci*. 13, 403-432.

Nock, MK. (2010) Self-injury., *Annu Rev Clin Psychol*. 6, 339-63

Rolland, B; Deheul, S; Danel, T; Bordet, R; Cottencin, O. (2010) Un dispositif de prescriptions hors-AMM : exemple du baclofene., *Therapie. Neuromodulation of decision-making in the addictive brain*.65, 511-518.

Sinha, R. (2013) Mephedrone: a designer drug of recent use in France]., *Curr Top Behav Neurosci*.13,379-402.

Spanagel, R; Vengeliene, V. (2013) New pharmacological treatment strategies for relapse prevention., *Curr Top Behav Neurosci*. 13, 583-609.

Sweitzer, M.M; Denlinger, R.L; Donny, E.C. (2013) Impact of varenicline on cue-specific craving assessed in the natural environment among treatment-seeking smokers., *Nicotine Tob Res*.15, 36-43.

Xu, X; Wang, J; Aron, A; Lei, W; Westmaas, .JL; Weng, X. (2012) Baclofen reduces binge eating in a double-blind, placebo-controlled, crossover study., *PLoS One*. 7, e42235

Chapter 10

Clinical Symptoms and Treatment of Depression

Abstract

In certain major depressive disorders (MDDs) a combinatorial treatment including special diet, psychotherapy, pharmacotherapy, and even electroconvulsive therapy (ECT) may alleviate deleterious symptoms of MDD, avoids progressive morbidity and early mortality and improves quality of life. Clinically, depression is characterized by hopelessness, negative thoughts, loss of apettite, impaired sleep, and loss of motivation. The most common symptoms of depression if these remain persistent are: sleep disturbance, anhedonia (loss of interest in pleasure seeking events), guilt, thoughts of worthlessness, fatigue, impaired concentraton, apettite, weight changes, psychomotor disturbances, and suicidal ideation. Five out of these nine symptoms should be present to confirm the diagnosis of depression. There are several ways to clinially manage depression for example: physiological (moderate exercise), psychological (counseling), pharmacological (specific serotonin reuptake inhibitors: SSRIs Fluoxetine, Paroxetine), phototherapy (sunlight or photolamp), and by dietary manipulation (by prescribing tryptophan, vitamin B_6, niacin, folate, iron, vitamin B_{12}, vitamin D, magnesium, and zinc-supplemted diet). Although pharmacological treatment to manage depression is effective, it is costly and has lot of adverse effects. In general, various antidepressants have low margin of safety and reduced therapeutic index. Weight loss, anorexia, diabetes, cardiovascular diseases can occur in patients on antidepressants. In addition, antidepressants can induce osteoporosis particularly in post-menopausal women. Hence alternative therapeutic strategies including specific dietary interventions are currently being encouraged and discovered. The most common approach about which very little information is available is the disease specific dietary manipulation in depression. Although several dietary constituents are essential for the health and wellbeing; tryptophan-rich Mediterranean diet proved highly effective in the clinical management of depression. This chapter is written with a primary intention to emphasize that when various dietary interventions as described in this book become unsuccessful and the patient suffering from MDD is difficult to manage with diet alone and needs hospital admission. In this situation a psychiatrist who is expert in the clinical management of depression may prescribe a selective antidepressant drug therapy with or without specific dietary interventions. These antidepressant drugs may have synergistic, antagonistic, and/or no interaction with the specific diet chosen for a particular patient with depressive symptoms.

Keywords: Anhedonia, Pyridoxine, Niacin, Specific serotonin Reuptake Inhibitors (SSRIs), Mediterranean Diet

Depression is the most common psychiatric disorder and has significant burden of treatment costs, effect on families and care providers, loss of workplace productivity, and is ranked fourth in global disease burden by the WHO. It may become a chronic disorder with disability, particularly in inadequately treated patients. More than 80% of patients with depression are managed and treated in primary care units, with those seen in secondary care being skewed towards more severe disease (Timonen and Liukkonen, 2008).

Although depression is one of the most common illnesses, it is often overlooked. A significant suspicion is essential in clinical evaluation. Very few patients present with a straightforward complaint of depression. The majority is seen for other complaints and may never mention depressed mood unless questioned for the symptoms. Vague somatic complaints or complaints that do not fit any clear clinical criteria should prompt consideration of the diagnosis of depression. Depression can be evaluated by investigating the symptoms such as changes in sleeping patterns, appetite, and energy levels. A positive response should elicit further questioning. The primary objective is to identify the common symptoms of depression.

Depression refers to both negative affect (*low mood*) and/or absence of positive affect (*loss of interest and pleasure*) and is accompanied by emotional, cognitive, physical, and behavioral symptoms. Depression is one of a group of disorders known as the affective mood disorders, and the internalizing disorders – other examples include: *(i) Affective mood disorder (ii) Depression (iii)* Anxiety *(iv)* Bipolar Disorder. The symptoms of these conditions are quite similar as there is considerable overlap. The actual combination of symptoms determines the diagnosis. This can occur as a single episode, or as ongoing condition with bauts of *'relapse' and 'remission'*. Depressed patients have a poor quality of life, as well as increased morbidity and mortality. Although the exact etiopathogenesis remains unknown; (i) genetic susceptibility (ii) life factors –i.e. social situation – e.g. single mothers (iii) alcohol/drug dependence (iv) abuse (sexual or not) – particularly in childhood (v) unemployed (vi) previous psychiatric history of chronic disease (vii) lack of a confiding relationship, (viii) urban population. More than 10% of post-partum women suffer from depression.

Epidemiology of Depression. Annually, 6% of adults have an episode of depression, and >15% experience depression during their lifetime (Depression*; NICE CKS, February 2010*). Most depressive states are at the mild-to-moderate level of the spectrum and generally seen in primary care units. Chronic illness increases the risk of depression. Recently specific guidelines have been issued regarding depression in adults with a chronic physical health problem. About 10-16% of men, and 20-24% of women have typical symptoms of depression. 2-4% of men and 7-8% of women can have actual depression. It is the common diagnosis – and accounts for about 12% of new illnesses, which accounts for 45% of psychiatric diagnoses. The prevalence of MD is between 5% *and 10%, and two to three times as many subjects have depressive symptoms but do not meet the* criteria for MD (Katon and

Schulberg, 1992). It is the third most common reason for a consultation in primary care units. Weissman et al., (1996) provided cross-national epidemiologic data on MD as well as bipolar disorder, and detailed statistics on prevalence, onset, comorbidity, gender, age, and other demographic feature. Murray et al., (1997) described the *Global Burden of Disease Study*, which provides a standardized review of mortality, disability, and risk factors for 107 disorders. Among psychiatric disorders, burden and disability related to depression have been reviewed. Furthermore, Nolen-Hoeksema (2001) provided an overview of gender differences in depression, including epidemiological data and explanations for gender differences in prevalence. The *Diagnostic and Statistical Manual of Mental Disorders* (DSM-IV) provides an overview of epidemiological statistics and features associated with depression, as well as diagnostic criteria. It is considered the gold standard by which psychiatric disorders are diagnosed in the US (*American Psychiatric Association; 2000*). About two thirds of adults experience severe depressed mood to influence their activities (Stewart et al., 2004). Boland et al., (2009) provided outcome of depression, including relapse and remission rates, definitions of relapse and recovery, and factors related to the disorder. Kessler and Wang (2009) provided an overview of the epidemiology of depression, including prevalence rates, clinical severity, subtypes, comorbidity, and adverse prognosis of depression. These authors also reviewed epidemiological data from national sample on MDD and associated factors, including gender differences (Kessler et al., 2003).

Risk factors. Depression is more common in people from the *African-Caribbean, Asian, refugees and asylum seeker communities.* Women have a higher prevalence, incidence, and morbidity associated with depressive disorders compared with men. The gender difference is controversial and may be attributed to differences in likelihood of reporting symptoms and help seeking/illness behavior, but there may also be differences in biological, psychological and sociocultural vulnerabilities (Piccinelli and Wilkinson, 2000). There is an increased incidence of depression during pregnancy and in the postnatal period and past history of depression, physical illnesses causing disability or pain, other mental health problems include dementia.

Classification of Depression. National Institute for Health and Clinical Excellence (NICE) guidance uses the Diagnostic and Statistical Manual Fourth Edition (DSM-IV) classification (Depression in adults*; NICE Clinical Guideline' October 2009*). To diagnose MD, this requires at least one of the core symptoms: (a) Persistent sadness or low mood nearly every day, or (b) Loss of interests or pleasure in most activities and few of the following symptoms: (a) *Fatigue or loss of energy (b) Worthlessness, excessive or inappropriate guilt (c)* suicidal *thoughts, actual suicide attempts, recurrent thoughts of death, (d) reduced ability to think/concentrate or increased indecision (e) psychomotor agitation or retardation (f)* insomnia/hypersomnia (h) changes *in appetite and/or weight loss.* These symptoms should be present for at least two weeks and must have caused distress and impairment. These symptoms should not be due to a physical/organic factor (e.g., *substance abuse*) or *illness* (*although illness and depression may coexist*). Severity is based on the extent of symptoms and their functional impact: (a) **subthreshold depressive symptoms** - <five symptoms. **Mild depression -** few, if any, symptoms in excess of the five required to make the diagnosis with symptoms resulting in minor functional impairment. (b) **Moderate depression** - symptoms or functional impairment are between 'mild' and 'severe'. (c) **Severe depression** - most symptoms present and interfere with normal function. It can occur with or without psychotic symptoms. Normal sadness exists along with depression: differentiation is

based on the severity, persistence, the degree of functional impairment, and disability associated with the low mood.

Differential Diagnosis of Depression. The differentials for low mood are (a) *Hypothyroidism and (b) Bipolar disorder.* To differentially diagnose a patient with depression; lab tests are needed such as: FBC,U+E's, Hemotinics – folate and vitamin B_{12}; LFT's– for alcohol / drugs / cancer; CXR – to investigate for chronic infection (e.g. TB), ECG – can provide evidence of metabolic disturbances, mental state and a complete history. There are three major symptoms incluing: (a) *Low mood* (b) *Anhedonia* (*reduced pleasure from normal activities*), and (c) *Low energy levels*. Usually depression is present when two or more of these symptoms exist for more than two weeks. Minor symptoms can be either cognitive or functional. Cognitive symptoms include: *Feelings of guilt, uselessness, worthlessness; and suicide ideation.* If the patient says having suicidal thoughts or have acted upon any of these thoughts – e.g. have they 'stock up' on paracetomol and poor concentration, these should be taken seriously.

Molecular Mechanism of Depression: (a) The Monoamine theory. Although it has its own limitations, monoamine theory is generally accepted. It states that depression results from reduced activity of monoamine transmitters, and that mania results from overactivity of monoamine transmitters. The primary neurotransmitter involved is 5-HT although it is thought that NE is also involved. (a) Most serotonergic neurons arise in the Raphe area of the midbrain, and project to the limbic system and cerebral cortex. (b) Most adrenergic neurons are found in the locus cereleus and lateral tegmental areas of the brainstem. There is link between Raphe and locus cereleus areas. Evidence for the theory comes from the fact that: *There is reduced levels of 5-HT in the brains of depressed people*. There is increased number of 5-HT-ergic receptors in the brains of suicidal patients. The theory is also supported by the medications used to treat depression, although there are some discripancies. Both NE and 5-HT treatments are equally effective, although some patients respond better to some types of drugs than others. When patients take medications the level of the NT in the brain is altered very quickly, but the clinical effect takes weeks to appear, suggesting that there are secondary adaptive changes which are responsible for depression, and not just the actual level of neurotransmitter in the brain. These changes may involve the downregulation of receptors. There are also probably altered signalling pathways in response to 5-HT in depressed patients–G-protein coupling may not function properly. ***(b) Hypothalamic Involvement.*** Hypothalamic neurons receive 5-HTergic input, which alters their output (*5-HT is inhibitory on these neurons*). They release corticotropic releasing hormone (CRH)), which controls ACTH, and eventually, steroid levels. In depressed patients, cortisol levels are often high, because the hypothalamic neurons are not suppressed as much as normal, and just as in Cushing's, these patients fail to be suppressed by the Dexamethasone suppression test. CRH itself in higher concentrations causes some of the symptoms of depression – such as *anxiety, loss of appetite, reduced activity* etc. and CRH levels are also elevated in depression. **(c) *Neuroplasticity and Hypotrophy.*** Generally, there is loss of neurons in the hippocampus and prefrontal cortex in the depressed patients. Also, many of the therapies used to treat depression and ultimately 5-HT itself promote hippocampal neurogenesis. Electroconvulsive therapy *(ECT)*) also promotes hippocampal neurogenesis. Many of the studies have been conducted in animals, and thus it is only a hypothesis. ***(d) Major Depression*** Depression - Major; Unipolar depression; Major Depressive Disorder (MDD). Depression may be described as feeling sad, blue, unhappy, miserable, or down in the dumps. Although most of us feel this way at one time or another for short periods (Fava and Cassano, 2008), true clinical depression is an illness. It is a mood disorder in which *feelings of sadness, loss, anger, or frustration* interfere with daily life for weeks or longer. We do not know the exact causes of depression. It is believed that neurochemical changes in the brain are responsible, it may be due to impaired genes, or it may be triggered by stressful events. More likely, it is a combination of both. *Certain types of depression run in families.* Other types occur, even if there is no family history. Anyone including children and teens can develop depression. Depression may be caused by: (a) Alcohol or drug abuse (b) certain medical conditions, including hypothyrodism, chronic pain and cancer (iii) certain medicines, such as steroids (iv) sleeping problems (v) stressful life events, such as death or illness of near and dear relative, divorce, childhood abuse or neglect, loneliness (*common in the elderly*), relationship breakup. Depression can change or distort the way one sees himself, his/her life, and those around. With depression, one often sees everything in a negative way. Symptoms of depression may include: *agitation, restlessness, and irritability, anger; becoming withdrawn or isolated; fatigue and lack of energy; feeling hopeless and helpless, worthless, guilty, self-hate; loss of interest or pleasure in activities; sudden change in appetite, often with weight gain or loss; thoughts of death or suicide, dificulty concentrating; insomnia or hypersomnia.* It is difficult to identify depression among adolescents. Problems with school, behavior, or alcohol or drug use can all be signs. If depression is severe, one may have hallucinations and delusions (*false beliefs*).

This condition is called depression with psychotic features. The health care provider may ask about medical history and symptoms. These answers can help doctor diagnose depression and determine how severe it may be. Blood and urine tests are done to rule out other conditions that have symptoms similar to depression. Treatment of depression includes pharmacotherapy, psychotherapy or both. If some one is thinking about suicide or significantly depressed and cannot function, this patient may need to be treated in a hospital. After a patient has been on treatment, if symptoms are getting worse, a doctor should be consulted. Treatment plan may need to be changed under these circumstances.

Common Clinical Symptoms of Depression: These symptoms can be categorized as (SIGECAPS) *Give Energy Capsules S: sleep disturbance; I: loss of interest/pleasure; G: guilt feelings or thoughts of worthlessness; E: energy changes/fatigue, A: concentration /attention impairment; A: appetite/weight changes; P: psychomotor disturbance; S: suicidal thoughts and depressed mood.* These are the nine for depression. Five of these nine must be present to meet the basic criteria of diagnosis. All patients with depression should be evaluated for suicidal risk.

Questions should begin with the assessment of thoughts of hurting self. If the response is positive, the patient should be questioned whether they have a specific plan and intent and emergency admission must be required. Some assessment of the degree of risk for suicide can be attempted by evaluating the lethality of the plan and the chance of rescue. Many suicide attempts are made with the hope of the rescue, which can be useful in assessing how receptive the patient may be to therapy. However plans can have a fatal outcome and any suicide risk must be given immediate attention. Some patients take action once their energy level has increased in response to therapy.

Medical and Family History. Patients with a history of depressive episode have an increased risk of having a subsequent episode. The family medical history may be positive for depression, substance abuse, and/or suicidal attempts. Chronic medical problems are often associated with depressive symptoms.

Medications. Various medications can induce depressive symptoms. For example; R*eserpine, β-Blockers, α-Methyldopa, Levodopa, and Estrogens*. Alcohol abuse, prescription drugs, or illegal substances can be either a risk factor for depression or the result of attempts at self-medication.

Social History. Discussion of the emotional and mental stressors can provide clues to the patient's state of mind. Investigating the family and/or social support structures is important in determining the patient's prognosis. Lack of support can increase the risk of suicide and may undermine effective therapy of depression. The patient should be questioned for the use of alcohol or other mood and/or mind-modifying substances. In some cases the patient may have been self-medicating prior to diagnosis and such substances may increase the risk of suicide. If the use is continued after treatment begins, the chances for successful treatment may be compromised.

Physical Examination. There could be several causes of depression such as medications (Reserpine, β-Blockers, α-Methyl DOPA, Levo DOPA, and Estrogen), drugs of abuse (*Alcohol, Sedative-Hypnotics, Cocaine*), toxic-metabolites (hyperthyroidism, hypothyroidism, Cushing's syndrome, hypercalcemia, hyponatremia, diabetes mellitus), neurological disorders (stroke, subdural hematoma. Multiple sclerosis, brain tumors especially frontal, PD, Huntington's disease, uncontrolled epilepsy, syphilis, dementias), nutritional disorders (vitamin B_{12} deficiency (pellagra), other (viral infection, carcinoma) to name a few. Hence a comprehsive history and physical examination is required to rule out organic causes of depression. Adults diagnosed with depression and with negative findings on physical examination do not need further testing. A complete blood count, metabolic panel and thyroid function tests may be required to rule out anemia and thyroid disease and to assess the nutritional status.

We need to consider following while evaluating for depression such as CBC (*to rule out anemia*), electrolytes (*to rule out electrolyte abnormalities*), creatine/BUN (*to assess renal function*), LFTs (*to rule out hepatitis and drug effects*), TFTs (*to rule out thyroid disease*), EKG (*as a baseline if pharmacotherapy with a TCA is being considered*), EEG (*to rule out seizure disorder*). Generally depressive symptoms and severity are evaluated with screening questionnaires. These screening tools are: *(a) Becks's Depression Inventory (BDI), (b) Zung Self-Rating Depression Scale (c) Hamilton Depression Scale (Ham-D).* For a diagnosis of MDD, five of the nine (SIGECAPS) must be present for at least two weeks and one of those five must be loss of interest or pleasure or depressed mood. *(Source: Son, Sung E. and Jeffery T. Kirchner. Depression in Children and Adolescents. American Family Physician. November 15, 2000. Vol 62, no 10. Pp 2303).*

There are primarily eight clinical symptoms of depression. They are represented as SIGECAPS: S: sleep disturbance; I: loss of interest/pleasure; G: guilt feelings or thoughts of worthlessness; E: energy changes/fatigue, A: concentration/attention impairment; A: appetite/weight changes; P: psychomotor disturbance; S: suicidal thoughts and depressed mood. (*Give Energy Capsules*). As discussed above, for a diagnosis of major depression five of the nine (*SIGECAPS)* must be present for at least two weeks and one of those five must be loss of interest or pleasure or depressed mood as presented in Figure 15.

Clinical Symptoms of Depression SIGECAPS

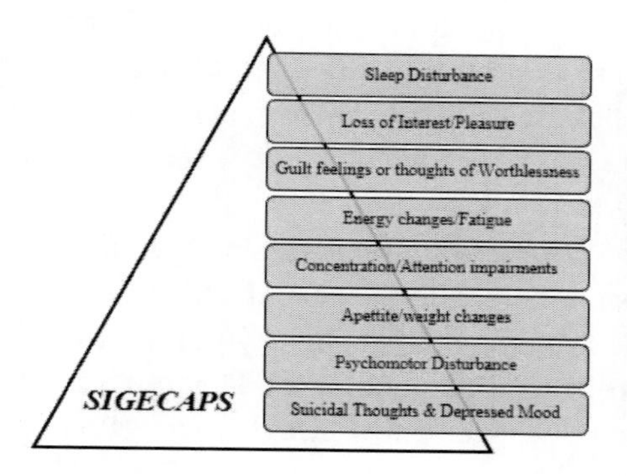

Figure 15. A diagram illustrating primarily eight major clinical symptoms of depression. They are represented as SIGECAPS: S: sleep disturbance; I: loss of interest/pleasure; G: guilt feelings or thoughts of worthlessness; E: energy changes/fatigue, A: concentration/attention impairment; A: appetite/weight changes; P: psychomotor disturbance; S: suicidal thoughts and depressed mood. (Give Energy Capsules). For a diagnosis of major depression five of the nine (SIGECAPS) must be present for at least two weeks and one of those five must be loss of interest or pleasure or depressed mood.

Screening Tools For Depression

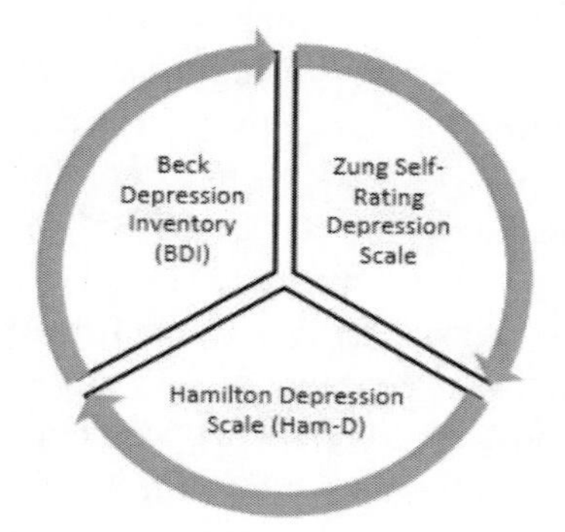

Figure 16. A diagram illustrating screening tools: (a) Beck's Depression Inventory (BDI) ; (b) Zung Self-Rating Depression Scale; and (c) Hamilton Depression Scale (Ham-D) that are generally employed to evaluate the symptomes and their severity with screening questionnaires. The diagnosis of severity not only depends on the symptoms, but also on the impact on normal functioning. (a) Mild depression – 1 core symptom, and 3 other symptoms for at least 2 weeks. Reduced ability to perform at work, reduced willingness to socialize. (b) Moderate Depression - 1 core symptom and 4-7 other symptoms (major or minor), for at least 2 weeks severe depression - 1 core symptoms and 7+ other symptoms (major or minor), for at least 2 weeks. There may also be: (a) psychotic symptoms (b) hallucinations (c) delusions. The diagnosis of severity also depends on the impact on normal functioning.

Various screening tools: *(a) Beck's Depression Inventory (BDI); (b) Zung Self-Rating Depression Scale; and (c) Hamilton Depression Scale (Ham-D)* are generally employed to evaluate the symptomes and their severity with screening questionnaires as shown in Figure 16. The diagnosis of severity not only depends on the symptoms, but also on the impact on normal functioning. (a) Mild depression – one core symptom, and three other symptoms for at least two weeks, reduced ability to perform at work, reduced willingness to socialize. (b) Moderate Depression - one core symptom and four-seven other symptoms (major or minor), for at least two weeks severe depression - one core symptoms and seven+ other symptoms (major or minor), for at least two weeks. There may also be: (a) psychotic symptoms (b) hallucinations (c) and delusions. The diagnosis of severity also depends on the impact on normal functioning as illustrated in Figure 17.

Clinical Assessment of Depression*:** Becks's Depression Inventory-Short Form **(b)** The Harvard National Depression Screening Scale (HANDS) **(c)** The Inventory to Diagnose Depression (IDD) (d) The Mood and Feelings Questionnaire (MFQ) **(e)** PHQ-9 Patient Questionnaire **(f)** The Primary Care Evaluation of Mental Disorders (PRIME-MD) [Source:*** Monograph - Diagnosis and Management of Depression; Monograph #2 2000; Michele R. Webb; AAFP; McCulloch J, Ramesar S, Peterson H. Psychotherapy in primary care: The BATHE technique. Am Fam Physician. 1998;57(9):2131-4. http://lib-sh.lsumc.edu/fammed/intern/antidepr.html**;** Lieberman J, Stuart M, Robinson S. Enhance the Patient Visit with Counseling and Listening Skills. Fam Pract Manag (United States), Nov/Dec 1996. 3(10)**;** PDR Monthly Prescribing Guide. June 2002. Vol 1, no 6. pp 256-262, 268-275.**;** Nease, Don. Anxiety and Depression. In: Sloane, P, et al., eds. Essentials of Family Medicine. 4th ed. Lippincott Williams & Wilkins. 2002. pp 345-355.. URL: http://www.nlm.nih.gov/medlineplus/ency/article/000945.htm **(Modified from D.L. Powell, MD**)

Functional Symptoms of Depression. **(a)** Sleep disturbance: Difficulty getting to asleep (b) Waking up several times during the night. **Early Waking** - *This is important if the patient regularly wakes up two hours before 'normal'* **Weight loss** - *This will be because the patient is eating less, either because he/she takes no pleasure in eating and/or feels nauseous.* In some patients weight gain can also occur. Patients may 'comfort eat'. It is important to ask if the weight loss/gain is intentional. Weight change of >5% is significant. **Loss of libido. Psychomotor retardation** – the patient can be very 'slow' both in their thoughts and actions, to a degree that is noticeable by others. **Agitated and fidgety** – this can be both in their thoughts and physically. Patients may keep going over and over the same thoughts, or they may e.g. stand up and sit down constantly. Patient may complain of **memory problems**, but it is probably not their memory that is the issue. If you test them on memory things you may notice they do not concentrate when the information is given, thus the information is not processed, and so they are unable to recall it – however it is the **information processing** and not the memory recall that is at fault. Other clinical characteristics include: **Diurnal variation of symptoms**. Generally, symptoms are worse early in the morning and late at night than at other times during the day. **Hallucinations and delusions**–may be present, and are generally congruent to the current mood. **Schneider's positive symptoms** can occur in severe depression. Some patients may experience **melancholia**–when the patient feels unable to experience any emotions at all (*emotional numbness*).

Clinical Investigation. Investigations are used to exclude organic causes for depression; they are not mandatory and should be used according to clinical judgement. (a) Blood tests may include blood glucose, U&Es, LFTs, thyroid function tests, calcium levels, FBC and inflammatory and other rccently deveoped biomarkers as disussed in Volume-2 of this Book. (b) Other tests may include magnesium levels, HIV or syphilis serology, or drug screening. (c) Imaging (MRI or CT brain scanning) may be recommended where presentation or examination is atypical or where there are suspicious of an intracranial lesion (*headache or personality change*). A specialist's advice may be saught in such cases of depression.

Clinical Diagnosis. The diagnosis of severity not only depends on the symptoms, but also on the impact on normal functioning. (a) Mild depression – 1 core symptom, and 3 other symptoms for at least 2 weeks, reduced ability to perform at work, reduced willingness to socialize. (b) Moderate Depression - 1 core symptom and 4-7 other symptoms (major or minor), for at least 2 weeks severe depression - 1 core symptoms and 7+ other symptoms (major or minor), for at least 2 weeks. There may also be: (a) psychotic symptoms (b) hallucinations (c) delusions. The diagnosis of severity also depends on the impact on normal functioning. Typical symptoms of clinical depression according to WHO guidelines. It is characterized by hopelessness, negative thoughts, loss of apettite, impaired sleep, and loss of motivation. The most common symptoms of depression if these remain persistent are: sleep disturbance, anhedonia (loss of interest in pleasure seeking events), guilt, thoughts of worthlessness, fatigue, impaired concentraton, apettite, weight changes, psychomotor disturbances, and suicidal ideation. Five out of these nine symptoms should be present to confirm the diagnosis of depression as illustrated in Figure 17.

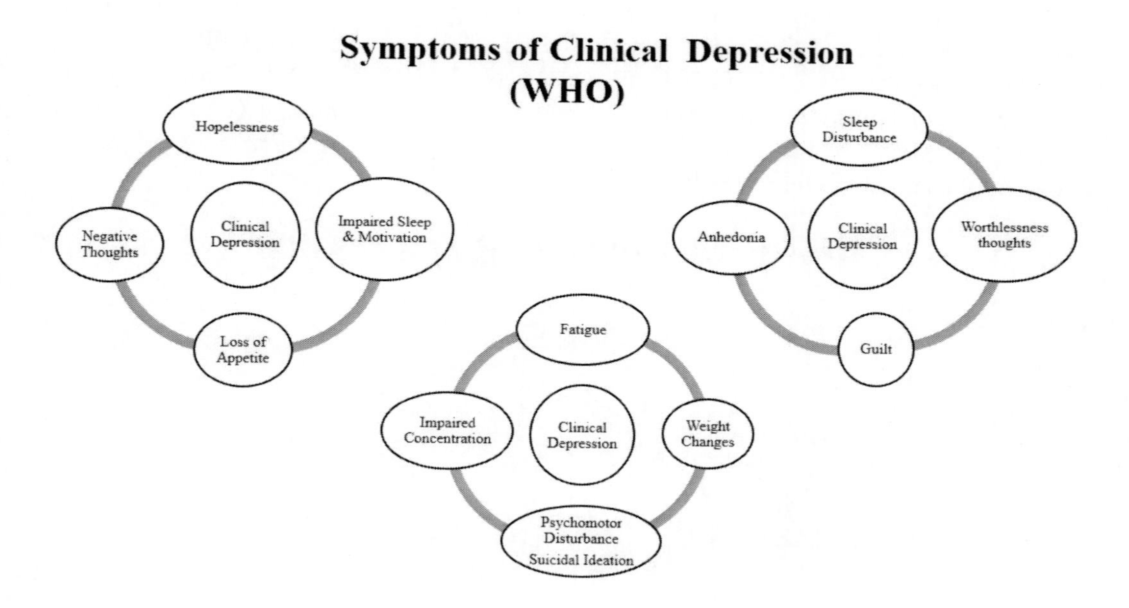

Figure 17. A diagram illustrating typical symptoms of clinical depression according to WHO guidelines. It is characterized by hopelessness, negative thoughts, loss of apettite, impaired sleep, and loss of motivation. The most common symptoms of depression if these remain persistent are: sleep disturbance, anhedonia (loss of interest in pleasure seeking events), guilt, thoughts of worthlessness, fatigue, impaired concentraton, apettite, weight changes, psychomotor disturbances, and suicidal ideation. Five out of these nine symptoms should be present to confirm the diagnosis of depression.

Screening Mothods. In general, screening tools are used to assess if a patient is suffering from depression, as well as to track the course of the condition over time. Two examples of screening tools are: Hospital Anxiety and Depression score (HADS) (external link) – despite its name is still used in general practice. (b) Patient Health Questionnaire (PHQ-9) – (*external link*) (c) ICD-10 depression Inventory (MDI) (*external link*). Other variations may be used. Patients may complete these questionnaires on paper or on the computer. The second method is more widely used, as you easily and quickly compare progress over time. These methods provide a rough idea to the severity of the depression, as well as to assess risk. The following questions may be asked while taking the history: (a) Have you felt 'low' or miserable recently? (b) Have you lost your emotions? (c) Does it happen everyday? (d) Does anything seem to have brought it on? (e) Have you lost interest in things you usually enjoy? - *Do you still see your friends often?* (f) Does your current mood/experience interfere with your normal life? (Sleep, Weight loss), feelings of guilt, feelings of worthlessness). Mental State: Appearance and behavior – poor self care, lack of eye contact, does not 'engage' in conversation, little movement, or lots of fidgeting – monotone, hesitant, and low speech.

Various approaches are employed to evaluate depression such as CBC (*to rule out anemia*), Electrolytes (*to rule out electrolyte abnormalities*), Creatine/BUN (*to assess renal function*), LFTs (*to rule out hepatitis and drug effects*), TFTs (*to rule out thyroid disease*), EKG (*as a baseline if pharmacotherapy with a TCA is being considered*), EEG (*to rule out seizures*). Investigations are performed to exclude organic causes for depression; they are not mandatory and should be used according to clinical judgement. (a) Blood tests may include blood glucose, U&Es, LFTs, thyroid function tests, calcium levels, FBC and inflammatory biomarkers. (b) Other tests may include magnesium levels, HIV or syphilis serology, or drug screening. (c) Imaging (MRI or CT brain scanning) where presentation or examination is atypical or where there are suspicious of an intracranial lesion (*headache or personality change*) as illustrated in Figure 18.

Clinical Evaluation of Depression

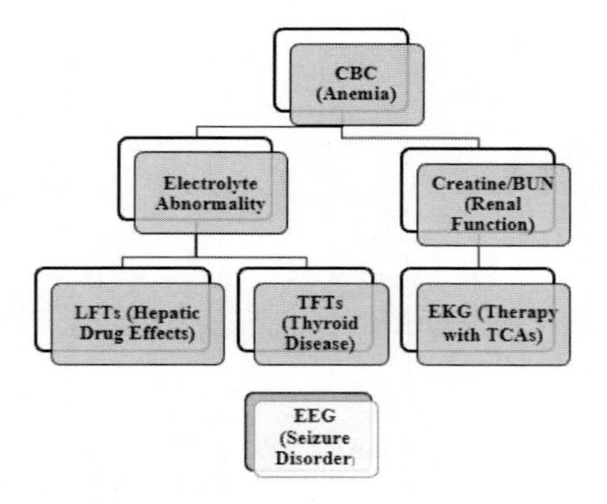

Figure 18. A diagram illustrating different approaches to evaluate depression such as CBC (*to rule out anemia*), Electrolytes (*to rule out electrolyte abnormalities*), Creatine/BUN (*to assess renal function*), LFTs (*to rule out hepatitis and drug effects*), TFTs (*to rule out thyroid disease*), EKG (*as a baseline if pharmacotherapy with a tricyclic antidepressant is being considered*), EEG (*to rule out seizure disorder*). Investigations are used to exclude organic causes for depression; they are not mandatory and should be used according to clinical judgement. (a) Blood tests may include blood glucose, U&Es, LFTs, thyroid function tests, calcium levels, FBC and inflammatory markers. (b) Other tests may include magnesium levels, HIV or syphilis serology, or drug screening. (c) Imaging (MRI or CT brain scanning) may be recommended where presentation or examination is atypical or where there are suspicious of an intracranial lesion (*headache or personality change*).

In addition, homeostatic assessment of insulin resistance (HOMA) is done because chronic diabetes is the primary cause of depression; Spielberger State- Trait anxiety inventory, FMDw, and Hamilton Anxiety Scale, and Beck Depression Inventory are generally used for the neurobehavioral assessment as Figure 19 illustrates.

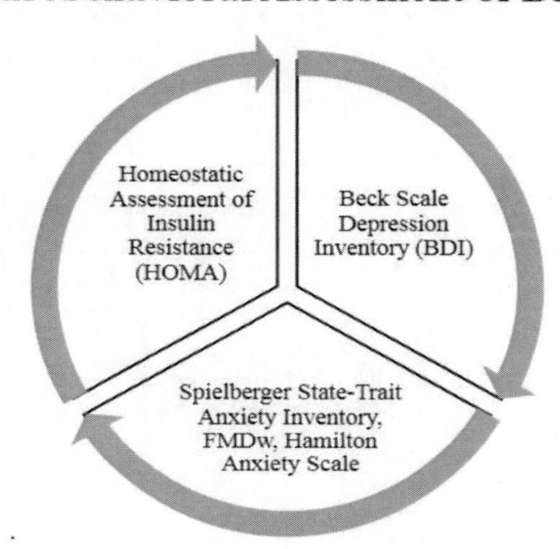

Figure 19 A diagram illustrating homeostatic assessment of insulin resistance (HOMA) [as chronic diabetes is the primary cause of depression]; Spielberger State- Trait anxiety inventory, FMDw, and Hamilton Anxiety Scale, and Beck Depression Inventory are generally used for the neurobehavioral assessment.

***DEAD SWAMP** –A*sk all these questions: D – depressions; E – energy levels; A – anhedonia; D – death – thoughts about death and self harm – i.e. Risk! ; S – sleep pattern; W – worthlessness, guilt, A – appetite, M – mentation – decreased ability to think and concentrate, P – psychomotor agitation and retardation. Post natal depression, post natal blues – occurs 3-4 days after birth. Post natal depression – occurs about 1 year after baby. Post natal psychosis – can occur at any time, and involves delusions/hallucinations. ECT works particularly well for these patients. (DEAD SWAMP): D – depressions; E – energy levels; A – anhedonia; D – death – thoughts about death and self harm – i.e. Risk! ; S – sleep pattern; W – worthlessness, guilt, A – appetite, M – mentation – decreased ability to think and concentrate, P – psychomotor agitation and retardation. Postnatal depression, postnatal blues – occurs 3-4 days after birth. Post natal depression – occurs about 1 year after baby. Post natal psychosis – can occur at any time, and involves delusions/hallucinations. ECT works particularly well for these patients as illustrated in Figure 20.

Screening for Depression. Depression is common but is often undetected - only about half of individuals with MDD are identified by their general physicians. However, a diagnosis of depression in primary care has a sensitivity of about 50% and specificity of 81%, with the risk of misidentification outweighing the risk of missed cases. In other words, ruling out those without depression but may need to consider more cautiously cases where depression might be present. Somatisation is the most important cause of missed diagnosis but about two thirds of depressed patients with somatic symptoms, making it critical always to consider emotional health in a differential (Timonen and Liukkonen, 2008).

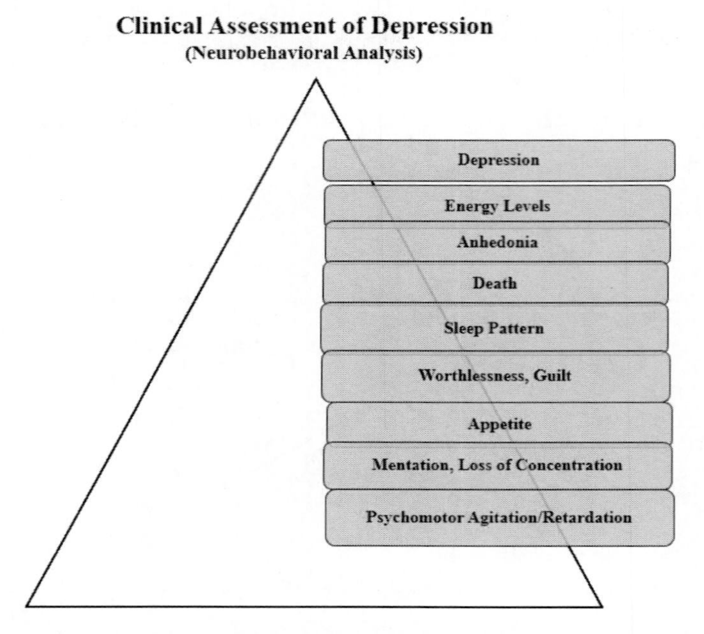

Figure 20. A diagram illustrating (DEAD SWAMP): D – depressions; E – energy levels; A – anhedonia; D – death – thoughts about death and self harm – i.e. Risk! ; S – sleep pattern; W – worthlessness, guilt, A – appetite, M – mentation – decreased ability to think and concentrate, P – psychomotor agitation and retardation. Post natal depression, post natal blues – occurs 3-4 days after birth. Post natal depression – occurs about 1 year after baby. Post natal psychosis – can occur at any time, and involves delusions/hallucinations. ECT works particularly well for these patients.

Many patients have a pre-existing physical illness which can also divert attention away from their mental state. In the elderly, depression can present as pseudodementia, with abnormalities of memory and behavior that are typical of true dementia. By using a two question approach: During the past month, have you: Felt low, depressed or hopeless? Had little interest or pleasure in doing things? Where there is a positive answer to either question, further evaluation should be initiated. However negative response does not exclude depression. Kaplan (2013) provided a review of seminal psychiatric research and its clinical relevance to ADHD, autism, bipolar disorder, tic disorders, and MDDs, which focuses on conditions commonly encountered by adolescent medicine physicians such as:

Self Assessment. Self-report symptom scales are widely used and include: a) *The Patient Health Questionnaire (PHQ-9) (b) The Hospital Anxiety and Depression (HAD) Scale (Hospital Anxiety and Depression (HAD) Scale, NHS Specialist Libraries). (c) The Beck Depression Inventory.* While these can be helpful in staging depression, one should not *rely on a symptom count alone* to make a diagnosis of depression. An individual considered to have depression should be completely assessed, including: (a) Full history and examination, including mental state examination, enquiring about suicidal ideas, delusions, and hallucinations. Consider organic causes of depression such as hypothyroidism or drug side-effect. Establish the duration of the episode. (b) Review of related functional, interpersonal and social difficulties. Involve family members or carers, with the patient's consent, to obtain third-party history if appropriate. Is there evidence of self-neglect, psychosis or severe agitation? Consider cultural factors. (c) Past psychiatric history including episodes of depression or mood elevation, response to previous treatment and comorbid mental health conditions. Patient safety and risk to others - suicidal intent should be assessed regularly. Depression may be assessed as mild, moderate, or severe depending on the extent and impact of symptoms and level of functional impairment and/or disability which will determine the line of treatment.

Differential diagnosis of Depression. *(a)* Bipolar affective disorder, (b) schizophrenia (depression may coexist). (c) dementia may present as depression and vice versa. (d) seasonal affective disorder (e) bereavement: depressive symptoms begin within 2-3 weeks of a death (uncomplicated bereavement and major depression share many symptoms but active suicidal thoughts, psychotic symptoms and profound guilt are rare with uncomplicated bereavement), (f) organic cause, e.g., hypothyroidism. Drug adverse effects are rare cause of depression. Medications that may cause depressed mood include: (a) centrally acting antihypertensives (e.g., Methyldopa). (b) lipid-soluble β-blockers (e.g., Propranolol). (c) Benzodiazepines or other CNS depressants. (d) Progesterone contraceptives, especially Medroxyprogesterone injection.

Associated diseases. Dysthymia is a chronic depressive state of more than 2 years' duration, which does not meet full criteria for MD and is not the consequence of a partially resolved MDD. People with dysthymia are likely to experience episodes of depression. Dysthymia increases with age. **(b) Eating disorders**: anorexia nervosa and bulimia nervosa. (a) **Substance misuse** is generally associated with depression. (b) Other psychiatric conditions may coexist with depression (e.g., *generalized anxiety disorder, panic disorder, obsessive-compulsive disorder, personality disorders*). (c) Some medical conditions have known associations with depression: (a) PD (d) **Chronic diseases such as diabetes and cardiac disease**. (c) **Cerebrovascular disease**. (e) **Endocrine disorders such as hyperthyroidism, Cushing's syndrome, Addison's disease and hyperparathyroidism.** (f) **Cancer,** especially pancreatic. (g) **Autoimmune conditions** have depression as a major complaint.

Treatment of Depression. The major *goals of antidepressant therapy are to (a) relief of acute symptoms, (b) prevention of relapse (c) return patient to normal functioning level (c) decrease risk of suicide.* The treatment of depression depends on the severity of the symptoms as described above.

Management Decision Aids. Doctors and patients can use decision aids together to help choose the best course of action. Compare the options for depression. Conventional primary care management of depression has been concentrated on the use of antidepressants. There is now evidence supporting the efficacy of non-pharmaceutical management of depression, Scottish Intercollegiate Guidelines Network – SIGN; January 2010; Cuijpers et al., 2009). But these are inadequate. The Government has targeted additional money to develop new local services, known as *'Improving Access to Psychological Therapies'* (IAPT) (Department of Health*; Improving Access to Psychological Therapies implementation plan, February 2008*). A brief summary of the stepped management proposed by NICE guidance (Depression in adults*; NICE Clinical Guideline; October 2009*).

Treatment of Mild-to-Moderate Depression. ***(a)*** Consider watchful waiting, assessing again normally within 2 weeks. (b) Offer one or more low-intensity psychosocial interventions, guided by patient preference: (c) Guided self-help based on cognitive behavioural therapy (CBT) principles - book prescription schemes, or internet resources. (a) Computerized CBT (Depression and anxiety - computerized cognitive behavioural therapy (CCBT); NICE Technology Appraisal (2006). (b) Relaxation therapy - more effective than no, or minimal, treatment (Jorm et al., 2008), (c) Brief psychological interventions (6-8 sessions) including problem-solving therapy, brief CBT and counselling. Antidepressants should not be recommended for the initial treatment of mild depression, because the risk-benefit ratio is low. However, their use may be considered: (a) If mild depression persists after other interventions including diet and exercise, or is associated with psychosocial and medical problems. (b) In mild depression complicating the care of physical health problems. (c) When a patient with a history of moderate or severe depression presents with mild depression. (d) With subthreshold depressive symptoms exist for at least two years or persisting even after other interventions.

Treatment of Moderate-to-Severe Depression. (a) Offer antidepressant medication *combined with* high-intensity psychological treatment (CBT or interpersonal therapy (IPT)). (For an individual with a chronic health problem and moderate depression, this should be high-intensity psychological treatment *alone* in the first instance (Depression with a chronic physical health problem, *NICE Clinical Guideline (October 2009)*; *American Psychiatric Association. Practice guideline for the treatment of patients with MDD, third edition. October 2010.* ***(b)*** Make an urgent psychiatric referral if the patient has active suicidal ideas or plans, is putting themself or others at immediate risk of harm, is psychotic, severely agitated or is self-neglecting. The use of the Mental Health Act may be necessary in some instances. (c) Electroconvulsive treatment (**ECT**) may be used to gain fast and short-term improvement of severe symptoms when all other treatment options have failed, or when the situation is thought to be life-threatening (The clinical effectiveness and cost effectiveness of ECT for depressive illness, schizophrenia, catatonia and mania). The advice about exercise as a treatment is conflicting. In addition to the above treatments, regular exercise as a possible treatment. A Cochrane review published in 2012 supports this advice that exercise seems to improve depressive symptoms (Rimer et al., 2012). However, the Cochrane review summerizes "*caution is required in interpreting these results*". In contrast, a research trial published in 2012 found that the addition of an exercise programme to the usual care for depression did not improve the outcome of depression or reduce the use of antidepressants compared with usual care alone (Chalde et al., 2012; Daley and Jolly., 2012).

Duration of Treatment. (a) For patients who have benefited from the use of an antidepressant, they should be continued for at least 6 months after remission to reduce the risk of relapse. ***(b)*** Patients who have had two or more depressive episodes in the recent past, and who have experienced significant functional impairment during the episodes, should be advised to continue antidepressants for 2 years. A longer duration of treatment may be required for some patients. (c) Patients who are considered to be at substantial risk of relapse or who have residual symptoms, should be considered for referral for either individual CBT or mindfulness-based cognitive therapy. When stopping antidepressants: (a) reduce doses gradually over a 4-week period; some people may require longer periods, while Fluoxetine can be stopped over a shorter period. (b) For mild discontinuation/withdrawal symptoms, reassure the patient and monitor symptoms. For severe symptoms, consider reintroducing the original antidepressant at the effective dose (or another antidepressant with a longer half-life from the same class) and reduce gradually while monitoring symptoms.

Psychotherapy. First line of therapy for depression is psychotherapy, not pharmacotherapy. Counseling is essential in all age groups but access is limited. Some counseling can be done in routine office visits. One method of addressing patient concerns is the BATHE technique. This is by no means a substitute for professional counseling but it may be helpful when other options are limited. BATHE is an easy and quick procedure of allowing patients to express their concerns and empathy. The physican is not expected to be able to solve all of the patient's problems. It takes 5-10 minutes to complete the questions and ancedotal evidence shows that patients' satisfaction with their physician is increased. **B: Bother/Background**: *What is bothering you the most now*? This question is meant to elicit any history of current problems. Some will use an alternate form like "*Tell me what is happening now*?" This may result in a seeming avalance of problems. Do not let this overwhelm. Listen patiently for 3-5 minutes and then ask the next question. Asking the patient to identify the most troubling aspect of numerous problems/stressors can be therapeutic of itself for the patient. **A**: **Affact:** *How is that affecting you*? This question I aimed at clarifying the patient's emotional state. An alternative form would be "*How do you feel about that*? For some patients this may be first time they consciously admit that they are affected. **T: Trouble**: *What is it about this that trouble you the most*? With this question we hope to further focus and clarify the patient's reaction to stressors and identify major area of concern. **H: handle;** *How are you handling that*? This question carries an implicit belief that the patient is handling the situation in some manner. This assists in establishing a working rapport with the patient and may allow brief discussion of alternative coping strategies or resources. E: **Empathy**: express/understanding of the patient's concern: The common statement could be "*I can see how that would make you angry or "that might be very frustrating*" The genuine concern can be as therapeutic as offering a detailed plan of care. **Talk therapy** is counseling to talk about your feelings and thoughts, and help you learn how to deal with them. Types of talk therapy include: (i) Cognitive behavioral therapy teaches how to fight off negative thoughts. The patient will learn how to become more aware of symptoms and how to spot things that make depression worse. Patients are also taught problem-solving skills. (ii) Psychotherapy can help understand the issues that may be behind thoughts and feelings. (iii) **At group therapy**, the patient shares with others who have problems like himslef/herself.

For mild depression: Watchful waiting, CBT (not usually practical on the NHS due to long waiting lists), computerized CBT, self-help, exercise, short psychological interventions; Moderate and severe depression: Medication, psychological interventions, consider getting social support; and for Treatment-resistant, atypical/psychotic depression, those at risk: Medication, complex psychological interventions, combined rugs treatment; High risk: All the above, plus consider ECT. Drug treatments: *There are details about mechanisms and side effects of medications in the* Psychiatric medications article_SSRI's – 1st line. E.g. Fluoxetine, Citalopram. Side effects include: (a) Nausea (b) Vomiting (c) Abdominal pain (d) Sexual dysfunction (e) Allow 4-6 weeks for beneficial effects (f) Patient's may describe how low feelings are not as pronounced, but the drugs do not increase' happy' feelings. (f) If one SSRI is not successful, attempt another SSRI, before trying other drugs. If these are unsuccessful you can consider the following types of medication: (a) TCAs (b) MAOI (c) NASSA (d) St John's Wort Medications are effective in 70% of patients – but you need to try them for at least 4-6 weeks. If this is unsuccessful try another drug in the same class, before trying a drug in a different class. There are various drugs that are used for the clinical management of depression. These drugs alleviate the mood and have different pharmacological mechanism of action. (i) TCAs block NE and 5-HT re-uptake at the synaptic teminals; MAOIs increased the NE and 5-HT stores; resperpine increases NE synthesis; a α-Methyltyrosine inhibits NE synthesis and downregulates the mood like Methyl DOPA which inhibits NE synthesis; ECT increases CNS responsiveness to 5-HT and NE; whereas tryptophan increases 5-HT synthesis to to alleviate mood. Methyl-DOPA and α-Methyltyrosine are used to help calm manic patients. These drugs in general cause *(a) increased monoamine levels in the brain (b) reversed impaired intracellular signalling pathways (c) reduced CRF production and (d) inhibit NMDA release.*

Drugs Causing Depression. Using alcohol, recreational drugs, and even prescription medications can cause depression. Long-term or heavy use of alcohol is known to cause severe depression. Stopping alcohol use often clears up depression within a few weeks. Stopping heavy alcohol use should only be done under a doctor's care. Withdrawal from recreational drugs, such as Cocaine, or stimulants, such as Amphetamines, may also trigger depression. Depression is also associated with long-term use of certain antibiotics, including Tetracycline and Sulfonamides. Some prescription medications can change brain chemistry and cause depression. If a patient with depression is taking medication and feeling depressed, he/she should consult the doctor about whether the medicine may be causing the problem. The doctor may make changes in medication to help decrease the side effects. The antidepressant drug treatment should never be stopped without consulting the doctor because it could be dangerous.

Cocktail phenomenon –Anecdotally, doctors report that the antidepressive effect is greatest when you mix the medications together Particularly MAOI's in conjunction with other anti-depressants as they can cause a serotonin syndrome. It is also recommended not to use another anti-depressant within 2 weeks of stopping an MAOI inhibitor.

***Drug Treatment of Depression*:** SSRIs are used as first-line antidepressants in routine care because they are as effective as tricyclic antidepressants and less likely to be discontinued because of side-effects, and are less toxic in overdose. Recent meta-analyses have concluded that SSRIs have benefit in severely depressed patients (Fournier et al., 2010) but evidence for their efficacy in mild-to-moderate depression above placebo effects is much less clear (Kirsch et al., 2008), suggesting that we choose a generic SSRI (e.g., *Citalopram, Fluoxetine, Paroxetine, or Sertraline*) when treating an individual with antidepressants for the first time, with the assumption that they have equivalent efficacy (Gartlehner et al., 2008). However, a recent meta-analysis suggested that there are clinically significant differences in efficacy and acceptability between new-generation antidepressants in favor of *Sertraline and Escitalopram*, although there are cost implications (Cipriani et al., 2009). Where a patient has concurrent physical health problems, *Citalopram or Sertraline* may be preferred as they have less risk of drug interactions (Depression*; NICE CKS, February 2010*).

Where a patient has previously been treated for depression, be guided by past patterns of response/non-response to antidepressants. Treatments such as *Dosulepin, Phenelzine*, combined antidepressants, and *Lithium* augmentation of antidepressants should be initiated only by specialist. St John's wort should not be recommended because of uncertainty about appropriate doses, variation in the nature of preparations, and potential serious interactions with other drugs. Prior to initiating any medication, discuss the patient's fears of addiction or other concerns about medication; over a quarter of patients newly prescribed an antidepressant never obtain their prescription or take more than a single dose (van Geffen et al., 2009). Warn about expected side-effects and discontinuation reactions. Inform patients about the delay in onset of effect, the time course of treatment and the need to take medication as prescribed.

Monitoring of Depressive Patients. See patients who are not considered to be at increased risk of suicide 2 weeks after starting treatment and continue to review regularly as appropriate. (b) Monitor for signs of akathisia, suicidal ideas, and increased anxiety and agitation, particularly in the early stages of treatment with an SSRI. (c) Watch patients who are considered to be at increased risk of suicide or who are younger than 30 years old 1 week after starting treatment. Regularly review (every 2-4 weeks) in the first 3 months or until the risk is no longer significant. Where there is a high risk of suicide, prescribe a limited quantity of antidepressants and consider additional support such as more frequent contacts with primary care staff, or telephone contacts. Where there is partial or no response to medication at 2-4 weeks: (a) Check adherence to and side-effects from the treatment. (b) Consider increasing the dose of the antidepressant. (c) Consider switching to an alternative antidepressant - either another SSRI, Mirtazapine, Moclobemide, Reboxetine, Venlafaxine or a Tricyclic. Check guidance regarding switching and the need for 'wash out times' and careful dosage adjustment. Avoid TCAs or Venlafaxine when there is a risk of overdose.

Antidepressant Drugs. Antidepressants work by bringing back the neurotransitters in the brain to the right levels. This helps relieve symptoms. If the patient has delusions or hallucinations, the doctor may prescribe additional medicines. Tell the doctor about any other medicines being taken. Some medicines can change the way antidepressants work in the body. Allow medicine time to work. It may take a few weeks before you feel better. Keep taking medicine as instructed. Do not stop taking it or change the amount (dosage) you are taking without talking to your doctor. Ask the doctor about possible side effects, and what to do if you have any. If the patient feels medicine is not working, doctor should be consulted. The medicine or its dosage may need to be changed. Do not stop taking medicines suddenly. Children, teens, and young adults should be watched closely for suicidal behavior. This is especially true during the first few months after starting medicines for depression. Women being treated for depression who are pregnant or thinking about becoming pregnant should not stop taking antidepressants without first talking to their physician. Beware of natural remedies such as St. John's wort. This is an herb sold without a prescription. It may help some people with mild depression. But it can change the way other medicines work in the body, including antidepressants. Some of the most commonly prescribed antidepressant drugs are described below:

(i) Selective serotonin reuptake inhibitors (SSRIs): Sertraline (Zoloft)' Fluoxetine (Prozac), Paroxetine (Paxil), Citalopram (Celexa) are indicated for depression. Some SSRIs have indications for conditions that may be comorbid with depression such as anxiety, panic disorder, bulimia nervosa, or obsessive-compulsive disorder. These drugs are commonly used. Possibly the most popular class for treatment of depression with or without anxiety. Maximize benefits by considering possible comorbid conditions. Fluoxetine has a weekly dosing which may improve compliance in some patients. The possible side effects of these drugs may be associated with undesirable behavioral changes (nervousness/anxiety, increased energy, restlessness/akathisia, insomnia, irritability/agitation, silliness/euphoria, disinhibition). Sexual dysfunction may occur and can be extremely distressing to the patient.

(ii) Tricyclic Antidepressants. (TCAs) [Amitriptyline (Elavil)] can also be used for the treatment of depression. However it is rarely used as a single therapy. Highly sedating and often used in patients with sleep disturbance. However, it should be avoided in patients with cardiovascular disorders. Multiple possible side effects and interactions with medications limit usefulness. Overdosage is potentially fatal and should be avoided in patients with significant suicidal risks.

(iii) Aminoketone: Bupropion (Welbutrin, Zyban) This drug is used for Depression and smoking cessation. It should be considered for patients who express a desire to stop smoking. The drug should not be used in patients with a history of seizure disorder, bulimia or anorexia nervosa. Common side effects include insomnia, dry mouth, dizziness, and constipation.

(iv) Triazolopyridine derivative: Trazodone (Desyrel) It is used for the treatment of depression. Sedating property utilized for sleep disturbance or anxiety in some patients. It should be used cautiously in patients with CVDs. It has a risk of priapism, nausea, xerostomia, dizziness, postural hypotension, and constipation.

(v) Piperazino-azepine: Mirtazapine (Remeron) Depression can cause agranulocytosis in patients - watch for symptoms of sore throat. Has some sedative properties and may be useful in patients with anxiety or insomnia.

(v) Serotonin and Norepinephrine reuptake inhibitor: Nefazodone (Serzone) Considered with comorbid anxiety or insomnia. It should be used cautiously in patients with cardiovascular disorders. It has a risk of priapism, nausea, dry mouth, dizziness, postural hypotension, and constipation.

(vi)Venlafaxine: Effexor Depression & Generalized Anxiety Disorder. Considered with comorbid anxiety or insomnia. Monitor BP closely - may cause sustained increases. Risks include sweating, nausea, constipation, anorexia, sexual dysfunction, and dream disturbance.

Follow-up. Patients with severe depression and suicidal risk should be considered for admission while initiating therapy. If admission is not necessary, initial outpatient follow-up would be in 1-2 weeks depending on the severity of the symptoms. It can take several (possibly 8-10) weeks for therapy to have an impact and patients may benefit from follow-up and encouragement while awaiting relief of symptoms. If the patient does not have access to psychotherapy or counseling, follow-up may be even more important to provide support and encouragement. Once symptoms have begun to remit, follow-up can be scheduled at intervals of 2 to 4 months. Consider referral for (a) High risk of suicide; (b) Lack of response to appropriate therapy; (c) Symptoms or signs of psychosis; (d) Symptoms or signs of OCD. (**Source**: Sung, E. Son. Depression in Children and Adolescents. Am Fam Physician. 2000;62(10):2297 – 2308).

Other Therapeutic Options for Depression. Electroconvulsive therapy (ECT) may improve mood in people with severe depression or suicidal thoughts who do not get better with any other treatments. ECT is generally safe. Light therapy may relieve depression symptoms in the winter time. This type of depression is called seasonal affective disorder (SAD) as discussed earlier.

Electroconvulsive therapy (ECT). ECT is mainly used in severe depression. It is mostly reserved for depression that fails to respond to drug intervention. Although controversial, ECT has been proven in several studies to be more effective than antidepressant medications. It is thought that it induces grand mal type seizures, and that these are necessary for anti-depressant effect. It is also thought that seizures that originate in lower brain areas are less effective than seizures that originate in higher brain areas at reducing depression. Using a high electrical current increases the therapeutic effect, but increases the risk of memory loss and confusion. (a) Unilateral treatment to the non-dominant hemisphere also reduces the risk of confusion and memory loss, but has reduced efficacy. Patients who undergo this type of treatment require 2-4 more sessions than other individuals.'Sub-seizure' currents do not have therapeutic benefit. ECT increases the activity of 5-HT cell, and increases the number of post-synaptic 5-HT receptors. It also enhances dopamine activity, and has similar effects on NE to anti-depressant drugs (*particularly reduction in β receptors*). It is particularly effective in illness that has: (a) Psychomotor retardation (b) Early-morning wakening (c) Psychotic features (d) Severe weight loss. It is also used in: (a) Schizophrenia with severe depressive symptoms (b) Schizophrenia with clouding of consciousness (c) Mania; when drug treatments (*both neuroleptics and Lithium*) have been ineffective. ECT It is given under a short acting general anesthetic (Succinyl Choline). Patients are also given a muscle relaxant (Pancuronium, Rocuronium) to reduce the risk of injury and are usually starved from at least midnight the night before. They are also given Atropine (*anticholinergic*) to reduce salivary and bronchial secretions, and to prevent bradycardia. Before the treatment begins, patients are ventilated with 100% O_2. This has been proven to reduce amnesia. Electrodes are placed: (a) Unilateral – one on temporal region, one near vertex (b) Bilateral – on each temporal region. They are moistened to allow good contact with the skin. Almost all patients have bilateral ECT. The usual treatment regimen is 2x per week until improvement is seen which is usually noticed after 6-8 treatments.

Adverse Effects of ECT. ECT is relatively safe, but there is a mortality associated with it (1 in 20,000). However, this is extremely low, roughly equal to that of a minor procedure involving a short-acting general anaesthetic. General physiological effects include; increase in BP, massive increase in cerebral blood flow, altered pulse rate. Hence ECT is contraindicated in patients with previous MI, arryhtmias, aneurysms, cerebral haemorrhage and raised intracranial pressure (ICP). Although rare, serious physical complications can include: MI, Cardiac arrhythmias, PE, Pneumonia, Dislocations and fractures – in cases where the muscle relaxant was not administered correctly or was ineffective, increased BP during treatment can cause: cerebral haemorrhage, bleeding of peptic ulcer.

Psychological Side Effects Mania – Results from 5% of cases of ECT. This is a similar risk to anti-depressants, and occurs in those at risk of bipolar disorder. Confusional state – occurs in almost all patients, but only lasts about half an hour. May be associated with headache. Memory loss – there is usually both retrograde amnesia (*can't remember what happened just prior to treatment*) as well as anterograde amnesia (*unable to lay down new memories for a short time after the procedure*). Some patients may report difficulty recalling previously well-known materal – e.g. telephone numbers, although in objective tests, there is no obvious problems. Factors that increase the risk of memory loss include: Bilateral shock, shock to dominant hemisphere.>12 treatments. >3 treatments per week, with <48 hours between treatments. Not giving O_2 before treatment. Using large current. ECT is useful in the short-term, but does not give an indication as to what treatments might be useful in the longer term. TMS – transcranial magnetic stimulation –does not provide proven benefit in depression, nor does electrical stimulation of the vagus nerve.

Risks of ECT. Managing risk is important in depression. The risk to others is usually low, but risk of self-harm is increased. One needs to specifically ask about thoughts of self harm and suicide. As well as active self-harm, many depressed patients suffer self neglect, secondary to the core symptoms of depression (loss of interest in normal activities). In many cases, this can be managed with carers and home support, but in severe cases, where the patient's physical well-being is at risk, then inpatient care may be necessary.

Prognosis. Prognosis for depression is very good. Most patients make a good recovery. The greatest risk is usually death from suicide before treatment has had time to take effect. Outcome and time scales are variable, but many patients on anti-depressant drugs will be symptom free within just 4-6 weeks. However, treatment should be continued for a minimum of 9 months, otherwise there is an 80% risk of relapse. Despite this, recurrence is common, especially in those with previous depressive episodes in the last 5 years. Clinicians have to make decisions on a personalized basis as to whether or not to continue treatment beyond the 9 month period. Factors that point to a good outcome are: Large loss event precipitating the depression.

Normal pre-morbid personality. The patient may start feeling better a few weeks after starting treatment. If he/she takes medicine, the patient will need to stay on the medicine for several months to feel good and prevent depression from returning. If depression keeps coming back, there is need to stay on medicine for a long period. Chronic depression may make it harder to manage other illnesses such as diabetes or heart disease. Ask the doctor for help in managing these health problems. Alcohol or drug use can make depression worse. Talk to doctor about getting help. If thoughts of suicide or harming or others; call local emergency number (such as 911) right away. Or go to the hospital emergency room. Call the doctor right away if: (a) hear voices not coming from people around you. (b) have frequent crying spells with little or no reason. (c) depression is disrupting work, school, or family life. (d) think that current medicine is not working or is causing side effects. Do not stop or change medicine without talking to doctor. The outlook varies with the severity of the condition: (a) The average length of an episode of depression is 6-8 months and, with mild depression, spontaneous recovery is likely. (b) For major depression: approximately 80% of people who have received psychiatric care for an episode will have at least one more episode in their lifetime, with a median of four episodes. (c) The outcome for those seen in primary care also seems to be poor, with only about a third remaining well over 11 years and about 20% having a chronic course (*Evidence-based guidelines for treating bipolar disorder: revised second edition, British Association for Psychopharmacology; March 2009*). In light of this, some argue for a model of chronic disease management for depression, akin to that for diabetes or asthma (Tylee and Walters 2007). Risk factors for depression recurrence include: ≥3 episodes of major depression (b) High prior frequency of recurrence (c) An episode in the previous 12 months (d) residual symptoms during continuation treatment (d) severe episodes, e.g., 'suicidality', psychotic features (e) long previous episodes (f) relapse after drug discontinuation.

Prevention Do not drink alcohol or use illegal drugs. These substances make depression worse and may lead to thoughts of suicide. Take medicine exactly as the doctor instructed. Learn to recognize the early signs that your depression is getting worse. Continue going to talk therapy sessions. Counseling is just as effective as taking medicine. The following tips may help feel better: (i) Get more exercise, (ii) Maintain good sleep habits, (iii) Do activities that bring pleasure, (iv) Volunteer or get involved in group activities, (v) Talk to someone trustworthy for expresing feelings, (v) Try to be around people who are caring and positive. Learn more about depression by contacting a local mental health clinic. Workplace employee assistance program (EAP) is also a good resource. Online resources and relavent literature survey can also provide good information.

Advice to Patient. Be as thorough and honest as possible when giving medical history. Include any allergies or illnesses you've had or currently have. Also include all of the alcohol, recreational drugs, and prescription or over-the-counter medications, supplements (such as V*itamins*), and herbal remedies that were taken. Medical history may reveal the cause of depression. If depression is associated with another medical illness, doctor may be able to treat the illness and relieve your depression. If depression is associated with medications, doctor may be able to change the medication or dosage to deal with the depression. About 10% to 15% of all depressions may be caused by medications or other medical problems. If substance abuse is the cause of depression, getting help for substance abuse may improve depression, often as soon as stop using drugs or alcohol. It is common for depression to be associated with certain medical conditions. Let doctor know about any conditions that could be linked with depression.

Referral. In addition to the urgent referral when an individual is actively suicidal, referral to secondary care may be necessary where there is: (a) Uncertain diagnosis, including possible bipolar disorder (b) Failed response to two or more interventions (c) Recurrence of depression <1 year from previous episode (c) More persistent suicidal thoughts c) Comorbid substance, physical, or sexual abuse. (d) Severe psychosocial problems. (d) Rapid deterioration cognitive impairment complications: (a) Depression is a major cause of impaired quality of life and reduced productivity. Social difficulties are common (e.g., social stigma, loss of employment, marital break-up). Associated problems, such as anxiety symptoms and substance absuse, may cause further disability. Depression is also associated with increased morbidity and mortality. More than half of all individuals who commit suicide have evidence of major depressive illness. Depressed men are at higher risk of suicide than women, particularly in combination with alcohol misuse and impulsive or aggressive personality traits (Hawton van Heeringen, 2009). Clinical predictors of suicide in people with depression include: (a) A history of attempted suicide (b) High levels of hopelessness (c) High ratings of suicidal tendencies. Depression increases the risk of developing and dying from coronary heart disease (Barth et al., 2009). This volume has attempted to provide some basic guideleines of how depression can develop in an individual and its possible prevention and/or treatment with dietary interventions in addition to psychotherapy and pharmacotherapy; hence it is logical to choose the title "Beyond Diet and Depression". How far beyond, only time will tell.

Source: A.D.A.M., Inc. is the American Accreditation HealthCare Commission (www.urac.org). URAC's accreditation program is an independent audit to verify that A.D.A.M. follows rigorous standards of quality and accountability. A.D.A.M. is among the first to achieve this important distinction for online health information and services. The information provided herein should not be used during any medical emergency or for the diagnosis or treatment of any medical condition. A licensed physician should be consulted for diagnosis and treatment of any and all medical conditions. Call 911 for all medical emergencies. Links to other sites are provided for information only -- they do not constitute endorsements of those other sites. Copyright 1997-2013, A.D.A.M., Inc. *Updated by: Fred K. Berger, MD, Addiction and Forensic Psychiatrist, Scripps Memorial Hospital, La Jolla, California. Also reviewed by A.D.A.M. Health Solutions, Ebix, Inc., Editorial Team: David Zieve, MD, MHA, Bethanne Black, Stephanie Slon, and Nissi Wang.*

Disclaimer

This chapter is for information only and should not be used for the diagnosis or treatment of medical conditions. EMIS has used all reasonable care in compiling the information but make no warranty as to its accuracy. Consult a doctor or other health care professional for diagnosis and treatment of medical conditions. (Source: original author: Dr. Colin Tidy Document ID: 2037)

References

American Psychiatric Association. (2000) *Diagnostic and statistical manual of mental disorders.* 4th ed. Washington, DC: American Psychiatric Association.

American Psychiatric Association. Practice guideline for the treatment of patients with major depressive disorder, third edition. October 2010. Available at http://psychiatryonline.org/content.aspx?bookid=28§ionid=1667485.

Barth, J; Schumacher, M; Herrmann-Lingen, C. (2004) Depression as a risk factor for mortality in patients with coronary heart disease. *Psychosom Med.* 66, 802-813.

Boland, R. J; and M. B. Keller. M.B. (2009) Course and outcome of depression. In *Handbook of depression.* Edited by I. H. Gotlib and C. L. Hammen, 23–43. 2d ed. New York: Guilford.

Chalder, M; Wiles, N.J; Campbell, J. et al., (2012) Facilitated physical activity as a treatment for depressed adults: randomized. *BMJ.* 6, 344:e2758.

Cipriani, A; Furukawa, T.A; Salanti, G. et al., (2009) Comparative efficacy and acceptability of 12 new-generation antidepressants: *Lancet.* 373m 746-758.

Cuijpers, P; van Straten, A; van Schaik, A et al., (2009) Psychological treatment of depression in primary care: a meta-analysis., *Br J Gen Pract.* 59, e51-60.

Daley, A; Jolly, K. (2012) Exercise to treat depression. BMJ. 344, e3181.

Department of Health; Improving Access to Psychological Therapies implementation plan (February 2008).

Depression and anxiety - computerised cognitive behavioural therapy (CCBT); *NICE Technology Appraisal* (2006).

Depression in adults; *NICE Clinical Guideline* (October 2009).

Depression with a chronic physical health problem, NICE Clinical Guideline (October 2009).

Depression; NICE CKS, February 2010.

Evidence-based guidelines for treating bipolar disorder: revised second edition, British Association for Psychopharmacology (March 2009)

Fava, M; Cassano, P. (2008) Mood disorders: Major depressive disorder and dysthymic disorder. In: Stern TA, Rosenbaum JF, Fava M, Biederman J, Rauch SL, eds. *Massachusetts General Hospital Comprehensive Clinical Psychiatry.* 1st ed. Philadelphia, Pa: Elsevier Mosby; Chapter 29.

Fournier, J.C; DeRubeis, R.J; Hollon, S.D, et al., (2010) Antidepressant drug effects and depression severity: a patient-level., *JAMA.* 303, 47-53.

Gartlehner, G; Gaynes, B.N; Hansen, R.A, et al., (2008) Comparative benefits and harms of second-generation antidepressants: background Ann Intern Med. 149, 734-750.

Hawton, K; van Heeringen, K; (2009) Suicide. *Lancet.* 373, 1372-1381.

Hospital Anxiety and Depression (HAD) Scale, GL Assessments; for purchase of questionnaire from copyright owners.

Hospital Anxiety and Depression (HAD) Scale, NHS Specialist Libraries; MS Word document.

Jorm, A.F; Morgan, A.J; Hetrick, S.E. (2008) Relaxation for depression., *Cochrane Database Syst Rev.* 8(4), CD007142.

Information about NICE Technology Appraisal (2006) Computerised cognitive behaviour therapy for depression and anxiety Understanding NICE guidance – information for people with depression and anxiety, their families and carers, and the public. National Institute for Health and Clinical Excellence.

Katon, W; Schulberg, H. (1992) Epidemiology of depression in primary care. Gen Hosp Psychiatry. 14, 237-247.

Kessler, R. C, P; Berglund, O; Demler, et al. (2003) The epidemiology of major depressive disorder: Results from the National Comorbidity Survey Replication (NCS-R)., *Journal of the American Medical Association* 289, 3095–3105.

Kessler, R. C; and Wang. P.S. (2009) Epidemiology of depression. In *Handbook of depression.* Edited by I. H. Gotlib and C. L. Hammen, 5–22. 2d ed. New York: Guilford.

Kirsch, I; Deacon, B.J; Huedo-Medina, T.B. (2008) Initial severity and antidepressant benefits: a meta-analysis of data submitted to the Food and Drug Administration. *PLoS Med.* 5(2), e45.

Mitchell, A.J; Vaze, A; Rao, S. (2009) Clinical diagnosis of depression in primary care: a meta-analysis., *Lancet.* 374, 609-619.

Murray, C. J; and A. D. Lopez. A.D. (1997) Global mortality, disability and the contribution of risk factors: Global burden of disease study. *Lancet* 349,1436–1442.

Nolen-Hoeksema, S.(2001) Gender differences in depression., *Current Directions in Psychological Science* 10, 173–176.

Non-pharmaceutical management of depression, Scottish Intercollegiate Guidelines Network - SIGN (January 2010)

Piccinelli, M; Wilkinson, G. (2000) Gender differences in depression., Critical review. *Br J Psychiatry.* 177, 486-492.

Rimer, J; Dwan, K; Lawlor, D.A. et al., (2012) Exercise for depression., *Cochrane Database Syst Rev.* 11, 7:CD004366.

Stewart, D.E; Gucciardi, E; Grace, S.L. (2004) Depression. BMC Womens Health. 4 Suppl 1:S19.

The clinical effectiveness and cost effectiveness of electroconvulsive therapy (ECT) for depressive illness,schizophrenia, catatonia and mania; NICE (2003)

Timonen, M; Liukkonen, T. (2008) Management of depression in adults., *BMJ.* 336, 435-439.

Tylee, A; Walters, P. (2007) We need a chronic disease management model for depression in primary care., *Br J Gen Pract.* 57, 348-350.

Van Geffen, E.C; Gardarsdottir, H; van Hulten, R. et al., (2009) Initiation of antidepressant therapy: do patients follow the GP's prescription?., *Br J Gen Pract.* 59, 81-87.

Weissman, M. M., R. C; Bland, G. J; Canino, et al. (1996) Cross-national epidemiology of major depression and bipolar disorder. *Journal of the American Medical Association* 276, 293–299.

Index

#

A

B

C

D

E

F

G

I

J

P

Q

T

U

V

W

X

Y

Z